PSYCHOLOGICAL DISTURBANCE IN ADOLESCENCE

WILEY SERIES ON PSYCHOLOGICAL DISORDERS

IRVING B. WEINER, Editor
School of Medicine and Dentistry
The University of Rochester

PSYCHOLOGICAL DISTURBANCE IN ADOLESCENCE

IRVING B. WEINER, Ph.D.

Professor of Psychiatry, Pediatrics, and Psychology
University of Rochester School of Medicine and Dentistry

Wiley-Interscience

A DIVISION OF JOHN WILEY & SONS

NEW YORK · LONDON · SYDNEY · TORONTO

Library of Congress Catalogue Card Number: 78-100319

SBN 471   92568   3

Printed in the United States of America

10   9   8   7   6   5   4   3   2   1

To Fran, Jeremy, and Seth

Series Preface

This series of books is addressed to behavioral scientists concerned with understanding and ameliorating psychological disorders. Its scope should prove pertinent to clinicians and their students in psychology, psychiatry, social work, and other disciplines that deal with problems of human behavior as well as to theoreticians and researchers studying these problems. Although many facets of behavioral science have relevance to psychological disorder, the series concentrates on the three core clinical areas of psychopathology, personality assessment, and psychotherapy.

Each of these clinical areas can be discussed in terms of theoretical foundations that identify directions for further development, empirical data that summarize current knowledge, and practical applications that guide the clinician in his work with patients. The books in this series present scholarly integrations of such theoretical, empirical, and practical approaches to clinical concerns. Some pursue the implications of research findings for the validity of alternative theoretical frameworks or for the utility of various modes of clinical practice; others consider the implication of certain conceptual models for lines of research or for the elaboration of clinical methods; and others encompass a wide range of theoretical, research, and practical issues as they pertain to a specific psychological disturbance, assessment technique, or treatment modality.

University of Rochester   *Irving B. Weiner*
Rochester, New York

Preface

This book is addressed to clinicians, social scientists, and educators who are concerned with identifying psychological disturbance in adolescence and averting its progression to adult psychopathology. The first portion of the book comprises three introductory chapters concerned respectively with theoretical issues in adolescent psychology, normality and abnormality in adolescence, and patterns of adolescent psychopathology. These chapters relate the subject matter of adolescent disturbance to broader concepts of behavioral science; review the complexity of discriminating psychological disturbances from normal developmental phenomena in teenage youngsters; and outline the epidemiology of diagnosed psychopathology in adolescence.

The topics for Chapters 4 to 8 have been chosen from the perspective of the practicing clinician. They do not attempt an encyclopedic coverage of psychopathology, but rather treat in depth those relatively few patterns of psychological disturbance that account for the vast majority of presenting problems in adolescent patients: schizophrenia, depression and suicide, school phobia, academic underachievement, and delinquent behavior. These five chapters review the clinical and experimental literature defining the etiology, psychopathology, and course of each pattern of disturbance; describe and illustrate procedures for assessing their presence and severity; and delineate psychotherapeutic techniques useful in their amelioration.

The final chapter of the book considers general principles of psychotherapy with the disturbed adolescent. The discussion reviews the goals and strategy of adolescent psychotherapy, aspects of initiating, building, and terminating the treatment relationship, and the role of work with parents.

I express my appreciation to Drs. John Romano and Robert J. Haggerty, Chairmen respectively of the Departments of Psychiatry and Pediatrics at the University of Rochester School of Medicine and Dentistry, for their support and encouragement during the writing of this book. I am indebted to Dr. Christopher Hodgman for his many helpful suggestions concerning the manuscript and to my colleagues in the Adolescent Clinic at the

University of Rochester Medical Center, especially Drs. Stanford Friedman and Charles Solky, for their stimulation and clinical comradeship over the years. Finally, I thank Mrs. Patricia Stoffel, Miss Susan Snyder, and Miss Jane Widman for their conscientious and skillful secretarial assistance.

Various copyrighted materials are quoted in the text by the kind permission of Academic Press, Aldine Publishing Company, the American Association on Mental Deficiency, the *American Journal of Orthopsychiatry,* the *American Journal of Public Health,* Appleton-Century-Crofts, the *Archives of General Psychiatry,* Basic Books, Inc., the *British Journal of Psychiatry,* Charles C. Thomas, Publisher, *Daedalus,* Grune and Stratton, Inc., Harper and Row, Publishers, the *International Journal of Psychiatry,* the *International Journal of Psycho-Analysis,* International Universities Press, the *Journal of the American Academy of Child Psychiatry,* the *Journal of the American Psychoanalytic Association,* the *Journal of Nervous and Mental Disease,* Little, Brown and Co., *Medical Clinics of North America, Mental Hygiene,* W. W. Norton and Co., the *Psychiatric Quarterly,* The Ronald Press, Science House, Inc., *Social Casework,* Van Nostrand Reinhold Company, and The Williams and Wilkins Co. Appreciation is also expressed to Sigmund Freud Copyrights Ltd., The Institute of Psycho-Analysis and The Hogarth Press Ltd. for permission to quote from "Mourning and Melancholia" in Volume 14 of the *Standard Edition of the Complete Psychological Works of Sigmund Freud,* revised and edited by James Strachey.

Irving B. Weiner

Rochester, New York
September, 1969

Contents

PSYCHOLOGICAL DISTURBANCE IN ADOLESCENCE

CHAPTER 1

Theoretical Issues in Adolescent Psychology

Problems of youth have concerned parents, educators, philosophers, social scientists, and clinicians since early in man's recorded history. Plato devotes Book III of *The Republic* to the education of youth for solid adult citizenship, and his dialogues portray a broad range of adolescent personalities: Charmides, a temperate youngster whose exemplary physical and personal qualities win him widespread adulation; Lysis, a shy, ingenuous youth who complains that his father forbids him to drive the family chariot although he grants this privilege to their household servants; Meno, a pseudosophisticate whose pretense to full knowledge is readily demolished by penetrating inquiry; and Polus, an impetuous, argumentative boy who scoffs at ideas that differ from his own.

Plato's contemporaries also had much to say about the adolescent personality. Aristotle in his *Rhetoric* instructs his audience in the fickle and unpredictable nature of youth, whom he sees as impulsive, irascible, and impassioned creatures with little capacity to delay gratification or tolerate criticism. Socrates, who paid with his life for his unyielding dedication to teaching the young, raised some startlingly modern concerns about their behavior:

"Children now love luxury. They have bad manners, contempt for authority. They show disrespect for elders and love chatter in place of exercise. Children are now tyrants, not the servants of their households."

Clinicians and scholars are frequently chided for their inadequate knowledge of adolescent phenomena and their insufficient efforts to understand youthful behavior. Anna Freud (1958) labels adolescence the stepchild in psychoanalytic theory, Spiegel (1958) and Rube (1955) lament our static, misleading notions about the teenage years, and Nixon (1961, p. 8) comments that "The dynamics of normal growth in middle to late

1

adolescence constitutes a hiatus in the growing body of knowledge concerning man's psychology." Yet, together with its impressive base in antiquity, the modern development of interest in adolescent problems seriously challenges this imputed ignorance and neglect.

THE DEVELOPMENT OF INTEREST IN ADOLESCENT PROBLEMS

The modern literature of developmental psychology, clinical psychology and psychiatry, and psychoanalysis has paid prominent attention to adolescent problems from its very beginning. The first comprehensive psychology of adolescence was advanced by G. Stanley Hall in two classic volumes published in 1904. Hall's efforts even at this early date were the culmination of years of his own thinking and research and of earlier contributions by his students and contemporaries (see Grinder and Strickland, 1963; Muuss, 1966). These initial psychological studies of adolescence derive from the same period and from many of the same influences as the beginnings of child psychology in general (see Dennis, 1949).

In the clinical area William Healy as early as 1909 established in conjunction with the Chicago courts a Juvenile Psychopathic Institute, forerunner of the current Institute for Juvenile Research. This clinic is often considered the first child-guidance clinic (Reisman, 1966, p. 78), and Healy in 1915 published the first systematic study of psychodynamic factors in juvenile delinquency. These concerns with the needs of troubled adolescents are reasonably contemporaneous with other major historical landmarks of clinical psychology, including the establishment of the first psychological clinic by Lightner Witmer in 1896, the development of the first usable test of intelligence by Binet and Simon in 1905, and the inception of the mental hygiene movement with Beers' (1908) moving account of his experiences as a mental patient in *A Mind That Found Itself.*

As for psychoanalytic theory, Freud included in one of his early works (*Three Essays on the Theory of Sexuality,* 1905) a section concerning the transformation of sexual aims and objects that attends puberty. Freud's discussion of adolescent development in this essay, though considerably less detailed than his analysis of infantile sexuality, preceded by many years his major metapsychological contributions of the second decade of the century and the emergence of his structural theory in the 1920s.

Despite these early and auspicious beginnings, the study of adolescence was not quickly taken up by scholars and clinicians. The next major text on adolescent psychology after Hall's work was written by Hollingworth in 1928. The child-guidance movement did not really burgeon until after World War I (see Garfield, 1965), and no major research studies of adolescent maladjustment were reported until the first of the massive studies of delinquency by Sheldon and Eleanor Glueck appeared in 1934. Psychoanalytic formulations of adolescence did not begin to take shape until the contributions of Aichhorn (1925), Bernfeld (1923, 1927), and Jones (1922) in the 1920s. However, the pace of these developments was certainly no slower than that in many other substantive areas of clinical psychology and psychiatry.

In addition to thus refuting the idea that the history of attention to adolescent behavior is undistinguished, the literature also contradicts current contentions that adolescence is unfathomed and unstudied. Certainly in the area of developmental psychology recent years have seen a proliferation of empirical investigations of adolescent phenomena. Voluminous data concerning adolescents have emerged from such longitudinal studies as the Berkeley, Guidance, and Oakland growth studies at the University of California (see Jones, 1967; Jones, Macfarlane, and Eichorn, 1959) and the Study of Human Development at the Fels Research Institute (Kagan and Moss, 1962).[1]

More recently such extensive surveys of adolescent life patterns as Havighurst and Taba's (1949) *Adolescent Character and Personality,* Hollingshead's (1949) *Elmtown's Youth,* Hathaway and Monachesi's (1963) *Adolescent Personality and Behavior,* Schofield's (1965) *The Sexual Behavior of Young People,* and Douvan and Adelson's (1966) *The Adolescent Experience* have appeared. Beginning with Cole's 1936 *Psychology of Adolescence,* a number of excellent textbooks summarizing theoretical and research studies of adolescent psychology have been published, many in several editions, including those of Ausubel (1954), Cole and Hall (1959), Crow and Crow (1965), Garrison (1965), Horrocks (1962), Hurlock (1967), and Jersild (1963).

With respect to psychoanalytic theory and clinical practice, however, adolescent behavior has not been so fully explicated. Anna Freud (1958) observes that the adolescent's typically strong resistance to the analytic procedure has handicapped direct psychoanalytic efforts to understand adolescent phenomena, whereas attempts to capture the essence of adolescent experience through psychoanalytic work with adults readily turn up the "bare facts" but seldom allow recovery of the essential atmosphere of adolescence. Longitudinal data reported by Rosenthal (1963) confirm sufficient memory gaps to suggest caution in using retrospective data to formulate theories of personality or adolescent development.

Speaking for clinicians, Nixon (1961) offers two explanations for their relative lack of understanding of adolescents. He suggests first that Freud-

---

[1] The history and methodology of these and other major longitudinal studies on adolescent development are summarized by Kagan (1964).

ian emphases on psychosexual development have led psychiatrists to view the attainment of puberty as the last step in the growth of the organism and to overlook subsequent developmental stages between pubescence and adulthood. Second, he comments that most psychiatrists have had little clinical opportunity to observe normal young people.

However cogent these observations, any clinical neglect of disturbed adolescents probably derives most directly from the reluctance of many clinicians to accept adolescent patients. This lack of enthusiasm toward the therapy of adolescents, as well as the discrepancy between expanding developmental knowledge and the relatively meager clinical perspectives concerning adolescence, is emphasized by Holmes (1964, p. 298):

"Although there are many things which the adult finds interesting about *adolescence,* the intensity of his interest tends to vary directly with his distance from the *adolescent.* The psychology of adolescence lends itself admirably to abstract consideration. It has become an increasingly popular subject for articles, books, and panel discussions at professional meetings, but it is still difficult to find someone who is willing to accept an adolescent patient for treatment. Clinical work with disturbed adolescents is, in fact, extremely interesting and rewarding, but it is also an experience which constantly reminds one that there are easier forms of livelihood."

Yet the psychodynamic elusiveness of adolescents and the reluctance of clinicians to engage them should not obscure otherwise significant clinical investments in teenage problems. One-fourth of all persons served by psychiatric outpatient clinics in the United States are between the ages of 10 and 19 (Rosen et al., 1965); adolescent youngsters constitute between 30 and 40% of all patients seen in the psychiatric units in general hospitals in eastern United States (Balser, 1966). Furthermore, the preponderance of developmental over more specifically clinical literature concerning adolescents notwithstanding, many gifted clinicians have addressed themselves in books and journals to numerous aspects of the identification and treatment of behavioral disturbances in young people.

It would appear that the psychodynamic complexity of the adolescent period has at times led to incorrect or overstated conclusions that little is known about adolescence or means of assessing and alleviating its psychological disturbances. Some confusion is reflected in the fact that, beyond a general consensus that adolescence occurs somewhere between childhood and adulthood, the literature reveals widely divergent opinions concerning when adolescence occurs, how it relates to other periods in the life cycle, and what are its normative characteristics.

These differences of opinion generally cluster around five major issues, which can be phrased in the following questions:

1. What are the age limits, if any, of the adolescent period?
2. Is adolescence primarily a biogenetically or a socioculturally determined phenomenon?
3. Is adolescence a unique stage that contrasts sharply with the developmental epochs that precede and follow it or is it rather a relatively unremarkable portion of a continuous growth process?
4. Is adolescence as a distinct developmental phase disappearing or becoming more pronounced in modern society?
5. Is normative adolescence a period of basic psychological stability or an era of crisis, disruption, and maladaptation?

The following overview of these issues will serve to introduce fuller discussion of normality and abnormality in adolescence and of the psychological disturbances that most frequently bring the adolescent to professional attention.

THE DURATION OF ADOLESCENCE

Contrary to popular impressions that adolescence constitutes a clearly demarcated portion of the life cycle, there are sufficiently disparate views on the onset and termination of adolescence to suggest that the very nature of adolescence may preclude a firm definition of its limits. Some writers advance specific, though admittedly approximate, age ranges for adolescence. For Jones (1922) and for Holmes (1964, p. 26) adolescence is the period from age 12 to 18, and for Gardner (1957) it is similarly the age span from 11 or 12 to 17 or 18. Since the beginning of adolescence is usually defined in physiological terms—and its duration and cessation, in psychological terms (Horrocks, 1954, pp. 703–704)—these age ranges can be taken to represent biological sexual maturation at one end and completion of secondary education at the other.

Although these criteria seem simple and logical, they are frequently rejected. Among those who define the onset of adolescence physiologically, some view it as beginning earlier, and others later, than age 12. According to Pearson (1958, p. 19), since the attainment of puberty is only the end point of physiological changes that begin at about age $10\frac{1}{2}$, adolescence should be defined as beginning with these changes. Josselyn (1952) and Stone and Church (1968, p. 436) similarly suggest that, in view of the important influences of physical development on its emotional aspects, adolescence should be regarded as beginning with the prepubertal growth spurt. Hurlock (1967, p. 2), on the other hand, endorses the significance of pubescent growth changes but dates the beginning of adolescence from "sexual maturing," which she ascribes on the average to the 13th year of life for girls and the 14th year for boys.

These differing views raise a number of problems in definition, beyond the question of whether adolescence is to be construed as beginning with pubescent growth changes or with the attainment of puberty. First, it must be recognized that any attempt to affix specific ages to these physical developments is at best inexact. Chronological age is generally a poor indicator of biological age—and especially so at adolescence because of the great individual differences that characterize this developmental period (see Young, 1963).

Second, aside from specific age considerations, the criteria for "puberty" or "sexual maturity" are at best elusive. For girls it is generally agreed that the menarche represents the culmination of pubescence and the attainment of puberty. Yet the evidence suggests that a girl does not become capable of conception until a year or more after her menarche (Mills and Ogle, 1936; Montague, 1946). Hence a biological definition of the onset of female adolescence varies with whether the menarche or fertility is the biological criterion.

The identification of puberty in boys is additionally complicated by the absence of any specific masculine event analogous to the menarche. Kinsey, Pomeroy, and Martin (1948, p. 189) measure male puberty from the first ejaculation, McCandless (1961, p. 278) judges sexual maturity in boys by the appearance of coarse, kinky pubic hair, and Stone and Church (1968, p. 436) consider the appearance of live spermatozoa in the urine as the most reliable index of the culmination of male pubescence. The first two of these criteria, like the menarche, do not necessarily indicate the attainment of procreative capacity, and the third is a rarely observed event.

Furthermore, whatever the biological criterion of puberty that is used, it is clearly erroneous to speak generally of "adolescents" in attempting to delimit the adolescent years. Since girls on the average attain puberty two years earlier than boys (Tanner, 1962), it is necessary to consider separately for the sexes the ages that encompass adolescent phenomena.

In spite of the attractive simplicity of defining the start of adolescence as biological sexual maturation, therefore, this criterion cannot easily be defined. The end of adolescence is also hard to identify. Many writers view adolescence as extending beyond the completion of secondary education. Hurlock (1967, p. 2) prefers to regard the attainment of legal maturity at age 21, with its voting rights and explicit responsibility for one's behavior, as marking the end of adolescence. Gesell and Ilg (1946, p. 10) and Hall (1904) place the end of adolescence in the early twenties, and Adatto (1958) and Pedersen (1961) suggest 25 as the age when adolescence generally passes into adulthood.

For the end as for the beginning of adolescence, both the choice of criteria and the tremendous individual variations in meeting them complicate efforts at age definition. The 20-year-old single male college student who is financially dependent on his parents and undecided on his life goals stands in marked contrast to the 20-year-old high school graduate who is married, a father, and working regularly to support his family. Given the difficulties of specifying the age at which adolescence ends, many writers have instead defined its termination by certain psychological attainments. Speaking within the psychoanalytic framework, Spiegel (1951, p. 380), considers adolescence to end "when the individual finds a nonincestuous love object, and tender as well as sexual drives are directed towards this same object, with the goal of genital sexual gratification, i.e., when sexuality is fully integrated into the personality." Fountain (1961) believes the young person to have reached adulthood when his cathexes of the original oedipal figures have sufficiently diminished in intensity for him to be able to see himself and his world more accurately.

Some authors have described the end of adolescence in the language of their particular conceptual orientations. For Sullivan (1953, p. 297) adolescence extends to "the establishment of a fully human or mature repertory of interpersonal relations, as permitted by available opportunity, personal and cultural." According to Erikson (1956, p. 66), the adolescent process is complete "only when the individual has subordinated his childhood identifications to a new kind of identification, achieved in absorbing sociability and in competitive apprenticeship with and among his age-mates." For Josselyn (1952, p. 5) adolescence "terminates psychologically with the establishment of relatively consistent patterns for dealing with the internal conflicts and demands of reality experienced by the physically mature individual."

In view of the inherent limitations of trying to specify either the physical or the behavioral landmarks of adolescence according to chronological age, it would appear that the duration of adolescence can be reasonably defined only in terms of a psychological process. Within this frame of reference adolescence begins with a youngster's initial psychological reactions to his pubescent physical changes and extends to a reasonable resolution of his personal identity. For some individuals the sexual maturation process may begin in the first decade of life; for some a firm sense of personal identity may never be achieved. For the majority of young people, however, these events will occur largely between the ages of 11 and 21, and it is this age group, with primary emphasis on the teenage youngster, to which this book is devoted.

BIOGENETIC AND SOCIOCULTURAL DETERMINISM

Implicit in any discussion of physical and psychological criteria for defining the duration of adolescence is the relative importance attributed to biogenetic and sociocultural influences on personality development. Ausubel (1958, pp. 22–49), outlining the historical roots of these developmental orientations, traces the biogenetic viewpoint to "preformationistic" and "predeterministic" approaches to the study of man. The preformationistic approach, which derives primarily from theological concepts of man's instantaneous creation, asserts that all of man's basic properties and behavioral capacities exist preformed at birth, never to be altered by interaction with his environment. The predeterministic approach, first clearly stated by Rousseau (1762), regards development as a series of predetermined and internally regulated sequential changes with which the environment can interfere but rarely does.

Sociocultural theories of development, on the other hand, relate to the *tabula rasa* concept of man proposed by John Locke (1960). In Locke's empiricist philosophy experience is the central influence on man's nature; although biogenetic factors may contribute some broad developmental dispositions, the most important determinants of an individual's potentialities, personality patterns, and life course are to be found in environmental factors.

These contrasting views of human development have figured prominently in the study of adolescence. Hall (1904), heavily influenced by Darwin's theory of biological evolution, formulated an essentially evolutionary theory of psychological development based on a "law of recapitulation." According to this "law" individuals develop through predetermined stages from primitiveness to civilized behavior in a manner that re-creates the development of the human race (Vol. I, p. 2). Hall regarded the adolescent era as specifically analogous to the turbulent period in man's history that heralded the beginning of modern civilization: adolescent development, compared with that of childhood, "is less gradual and more saltatory, suggestive of some ancient period of storm and stress when old moorings were broken and a higher level attained" (Vol. I, p. xiii). In this theory personality development is directed by genetically determined physiological factors that are immutable, inevitable, universal, and unaffected by environmental influences.

Freud's (1905) early analysis of childhood development also reflected a strong biogenetic emphasis. Freudian libido theory postulates certain innate drives or sources of energy that unfold in predetermined ways to produce a number of universal psychosexual stages (oral, anal, phallic, genital) and focal conflict areas (e.g., the oedipus complex). As elaborated by Bernfeld (1938), adolescence from the classical psychoanalytic point of view is the adjustment of personality to the biological fact of puberty. Differences among adolescents may be influenced by external circumstances, he continues, but are interpretable primarily in terms of the individual's particular pattern of reaction to the sudden upsurge of libido that accompanies puberty.

Jones (1922) in his early psychoanalytic contribution presented a specifically evolutionary view of adolescent development, although he chose an ontogenetic base for his recapitulation theory rather than the phylogenetic premise used by Hall. In Jones' theory adolescence recapitulates and expands the development of the first five years of life, including five stages of sexual development common to both—diffuse autoerotic, pregenital, genital-narcissistic, homosexual, and heterosexual. Consistently with the view of early fixed determination of personality, Jones asserted that these stages are passed through on different planes by infants and adolescents but in very similar ways in the same individual.

The environmentalist or sociocultural view of personality development began potently to challenge these biogenetic orientations with the advent of John Watson's (1913, 1925) behaviorism and the cultural anthropological studies of the 1920s and 1930s. Watson (1925, p. 82) argued vigorously for a *tabula rasa* view of the neonate:

"Give me a dozen healthy infants, well-formed, and my own specified world to bring them up in and I'll guarantee to take any one at random and train him to become any type of specialist I might select—doctor, lawyer, artist, merchant-chief and, yes, even beggar-man and thief, regardless of his talents, penchants, tendencies, abilities, vocations, and race of his ancestors."

The implications of Watson's behaviorist model for the modifiability of personality directly negate biological, predeterministic interpretations of human development, as do many of the findings of cultural anthropologists. Margaret Mead (1928) in *Coming of Age in Samoa* described a relatively unambiguous society in which children began to assume adult roles and responsibilities at age six or seven and proceeded gradually and uneventfully toward full adult status. The Samoan youngsters displayed none of the distinctly adolescent behavior patterns and developmental stages described by Hall and Freud as biological universals. In subsequent contributions Mead (1930), Benedict (1938), and others further documented the marked intercultural variability of teenage behavior patterns and formulated theories of cultural relativism to account for these differences.

Developmental psychologists have generally interpreted the data of cultural anthropology as signaling the demise of personality theories organized around biological universals. Horrocks (1962, p. 6) considers cross-cultural data to have vitiated evolutionary notions of adolescent development; Hurlock (1966) comments that American adolescents of today are different from those of past generations and from other societies not because of alterations in hereditary endowment but because of cultural differences; and Stone and Church (1968, p. 438) conclude from intersocietal variations in adolescent behavior patterns that "the individual psychology of adolescence can only be grasped against the sociology and social psychology of this age."

Contemporary psychoanalytic theorists have criticized as well the earlier interpretation of adolescence as a simple repetition or new edition of the Oedipus complex. Spiegel (1951) points out that the adolescent has intellectual and physical resources unknown to the child, including ejaculatory capacity, and that puberty is followed not by a latency period but by a stage of sexual activity and competence in which pressing problems of sexual role, ego identity, and social mobility must be confronted. He accordingly stresses the role of experiential factors in adolescent development and sees little necessary predictability of pubertal behavior patterns from those of childhood: "In general, the plentitude, scope and variety of adolescent personality, achievement and interest, contrast impressively with the 'expectedness' of earlier times" (Spiegel, 1951, p. 376). Hartmann, Kris, and Loewenstein (1946) similarly contend that potentialities for personality transformation in adolescence have been underrated in psychoanalytic writings, and Toolan (1960) suggests that attention to the role of early experience in personality formation has led to an underestimation of the influence of later life events, especially those that occur during puberty.

Despite these various arguments and conclusions, however, biogenetic interpretations of adolescent development are by no means out of fashion. The influential contributions of Gesell and his co-workers to the study of human development are very much in the Hall tradition. In *Youth: The Years from Ten to Sixteen* Gesell, Ilg, and Ames (1956) outline a basically evolutionary conception of adolescent development, with predetermined maturational phases unfolding in orderly sequence. Similarly any analysis of adolescent development expressed in the Gesell style of "the typical 12-year-old does so and so" or "the modal 13-year-old becomes such and such" implicitly endorses biological notions of universal unfolding behavior patterns, whatever allowances are made for individual variation and external influence.

Cultural determinism itself has also been challenged on empirical grounds. Kiell (1964) presents numerous personal documents from diverse cultural contexts and historical epochs as evidence that adolescence, in its behavioral as well as physiological aspects, is a universal phenomenon:

"It is my thesis that the great internal turmoil and external disorder of adolescence are universal and only moderately affected by cultural determinants. In spite of many specific differences in content and degree of stress from one culture to another, adolescent development is basically uniform in all societies" (p. 9).

The viability of the biogenetic approach to human development is further illustrated by the contrasting views of Inhelder and Piaget (1958) and of Shapiro (1963). Inhelder and Piaget regard the fundamental problem and distinctive feature of adolescence as being the young person's initial assumption of adult roles and not the physiological fact of his puberty. They accordingly stress that the growth of formal thinking during adolescence and the age at which adolescence occurs depend primarily on social rather than neurological factors (pp. 334–350). Shapiro, however, sees the Inhelder and Piaget observations not as grounds for an environmentalist interpretation of adolescent development, but rather as fitting neatly with a psychoanalytic theory of ego epigenesis. In contrast to their preference for a social interpretation of their observations, he considers the significant cognitive developments in early adolescence to be "sufficiently detailed and of sufficient regularity and generalization to warrant the assumption of autonomous ego development as one of the maturational elements of this phase" (p. 87).

As has been true for many of psychology's finely drawn issues, the biogenetic-sociocultural controversy highlighted in this discussion has lately come to interactional arbitration:

"In summary, we do not believe it is possible to gain a proper understanding of adolescent development, in our own or any other culture, without a full awareness of both the biological changes occurring at this time and also of the cultural influences to which the individual is subjected" (Mussen, Conger, and Kagan, 1963, p. 508).

"In conclusion, then, I would emphasize again that these adolescent children of ours cannot be considered solely from the viewpoint of their internal conflicts and processes, but must on the contrary be considered biosocially, with due emphasis upon the pressures and value systems of the groups that surround them, and with emphasis upon the sometimes sharply conflicting values in the multiple roles that they must assume" (Gardner, 1957, p. 517).

It is doubtful whether any of the predeterminists quoted above would unequivocally reject the influence of experimental factors on personality development, nor would any of the environmentalists completely deny the contribution of constitutional factors to individual differences. In the science of the modern world, when even the path of a beam of light has been demonstrated to depend on its proximity to a gravitational field and on the strength of that field, it seems difficult to justify any clinging to "absolutes" and "universals"; likewise the readily demonstrable fallacies in viewing human beings as organisms of essentially equal potential (see Ausubel, 1958, pp. 47–48) challenge any total commitment to cultural relativism in the study of human behavior. The question therefore is not what is given, what is acquired, and what is a result of interaction between the inborn and the experienced; it is rather the infinitely more complex question of what specific biological or environmental events, or combination thereof, in what degree and under what circumstances, operate to influence a specific pattern of personality development or behavior.

CONTINUITY AND DISCONTINUITY

The question of continuity and discontinuity in adolescent development concerns the extent to which adolescence is a unique, sharply distinct developmental epoch bearing little relationship to child and adult patterns or is rather a relatively smooth transition period between the first and third decades of life. Hall's evolutionary formulation of adolescence was firmly anchored in the first of these alternatives. As he saw it, the biogenetic events that initiate the adolescent's phylogenetic recapitulation suddenly and precipitously sever his ties with his past:

"The child from nine to twelve is well adjusted to his environment and proportionately developed; he represents probably an old and relatively perfected stage of race-maturity, still in some sense and degree feasible in warm climates, which, as we have previously urged, stands for a long-continued one, a terminal stage of human development at some post-simian point. At dawning adolescence this old unity and harmony with nature is broken up; the child is driven from his paradise and must enter upon a long viaticum of ascent, must conquer a higher kingdom of man for himself, break out a new sphere, and evolve a more modern story to his psycho-physical nature" (1904, Vol. II, p. 71).

Hall considered it inevitable that the several years following this disruption of the young person's harmony with nature would be marked by turmoil, uncertainty, and a spectrum of disconcerting and maladaptive behaviors. This period of irascibility and unpredictability must be endured until full adult status has been attained, at which time the turmoil subsides and a new adult figure emerges, a civilized man bearing little resemblance to the unruly adolescent who preceded him. Hall regarded this eventual emergence of the more completely human traits as a "new birth":

"Youth awakes to a new world and understands neither it nor himself. The whole future of life depends on how the new powers now given suddenly and in profusion are husbanded and directed. Character and personality are taking form, but everything is plastic. Self-feeling and ambition are increased and every trait and faculty is liable to exaggeration and excess. It is all a marvelous new birth . . ." (1904, Vol. I, p. xv).

Other advocates of a recapitulative view of adolescent development similarly anticipate major changes in personality organization at puberty. Jones' (1922) psychosexual recapitulation theory presumes a marked pubertal regression toward infancy. Wittels (1949) describes adolescent recapitulation as a major rearrangement of the ego's defenses, with the individual becoming disorganized under the instinctual pressures of puberty and subsequently working to establish a new equilibrium. Rube (1955), comparing the cycle between puberty and leaving the parental home to the cycle between conception and birth, argues that adolescence is clearly a "second birth" rather than any type of developmental transition.

Hollingworth (1928), on the other hand, took strong exception to this "new birth" view of adolescent development. She rejected the inevitability of teenage storm and stress and challenged the belief that entirely new character and personality traits begin to form at adolescence. She maintained instead that developmental changes during adolescence are continuous and gradual:

"The child grows by imperceptible degrees into the adolescent, and the adolescent turns by gradual degrees into the adult. . . . [The] widespread myth that every child is a changeling, who at puberty comes forth as a different personality, is doubtless a survival in folklore of the ceremonial rebirth, which constituted the formal initiation of our savage ancestors into manhood and womanhood" (pp. 1 and 17).

There are considerable longitudinal data to support Hollingworth's insistence on a continuous, transitional view of development. The most dramatic and consistent finding of the Study of Human Development at the Fels Research Institute was that many of the behaviors exhibited by children between ages six and ten, and even a few between ages three and six, are moderately good predictors of theoretically related behaviors during their adulthood (Kagan and Moss, 1962, p. 226). Each of the following adult behavior patterns was found to be related to reasonably analogous behavioral dispositions during the early school years: passive withdrawal from stressful situations, dependency on family, ease of anger arousal, involvement in intellectual mastery, social-interaction anxiety, sex-role identification, and pattern of sexual behavior.

Bronson (1966) also reports reasonably continuous patterns of behavior organization from childhood to adolescence. Using as her data repeated ratings of a wide variety of behaviors shown by children in the California Guidance Study (Macfarlane, 1938) between the age of 5 and 16, she describes particular persistence and centrality over this whole developmental span and for both sexes of behaviors in the three broad areas of withdrawal-expressiveness, reactivity-placidity, and passivity-dominance. Furthermore from follow-up studies of these same subjects at age 30 Bronson (1967, p. 817) concludes, "A very long-range continuity of development becomes apparent when the focus is on . . . characteristic response tendencies."

Other longitudinal studies investigating the validity of adolescent personality patterns in predicting adult behavior have challenged the view that the adolescent bears little similarity to his adult self. Symonds and Jensen (1961) report a follow-up study of men and women who were interviewed and examined with projective tests during junior or senior high school and again as adults 13 years later. These subjects displayed a high degree of consistency over the 13-year interval with respect to their general personality characteristics, nervous signs, hobbies, and attitudes. Furthermore, although they could not predict their adult attitudes toward interpersonal relationships from their adolescent attitudes, Symonds and Jensen found that their subjects' later attitudes toward sex had been anticipated in their adolescent fantasies.

Tuddenham (1959) compared the adolescent personality rating of subjects in the Oakland Growth Study (Jones, 1938, 1939) with their ratings as adults, 13 to 19 years later. All but 8 of 106 stability coefficients that he determined for these data were positive, and the average stability coefficients over the personality variables he explored were .27 for male and .24 for female subjects. However, it should be noted that, just as Symonds found aspects of the adult personality that could not be predicted from adolescent attitudes, Tuddenham's low average stability coefficients reflect large portions of adult personality variance unaccounted for by predictions from adolescent data.

Further evidence that adolescence is more a period of gradual transition than of discontinuous personality reorganization has come from a number of studies employing repetitive projective testing. Ames (1966) reports an extensive Rorschach study in which several hundred subjects ranging in age from 2 to 102 were examined on three successive occasions. Among her groups of boys and girls seen first at age 2, 5, 8, 11, or 14 and retested one and two years later, there was generally increasing stability in the Rorschach response from one age interval to the next, with fewer changes over the 11 to 13 and 14 to 16 age periods than over the younger ages. It is significant that she observed a conspicuous degree of constancy as early as the age 8 to 10 period.

Hertz and Baker (1941) similarly conclude from Rorschach data obtained from adolescents tested at age 12 and retested at 15 that certain traits show a moderate degree of stability during this period of life. However, they add, some changes toward introversiveness and increased emotional adaptability and stability usually occur between ages 12 and 15. Elsewhere Hertz (1960), reviewing in detail several longitudinal Rorschach studies of adolescents, emphasizes the gradual rather than precipitous nature of personality changes during adolescence:

"In general, studies of children in the second decade point to marked growth toward intellectual and emotional maturity with gradual expansion of personality, increase in ego strength and increased intellectual adaptability to the thinking of the group. Their functioning approaches that which is anticipated of the normal adult, although there is still evidence of instability, lack of inner organization, and even some confusion" (p. 52).

In agreement with these data, most current writers view adolescence neither as an unremarkable period that is completely continuous with childhood behavior patterns and predictive of adult personality nor as a seething cauldron having little relationship to, or continuity with, the calm latency preceding or the civilized adulthood following it. As with the question of biogenetic and sociocultural influences, the central question is not either-or, but rather which adolescence behavior patterns are continuous with those of other life periods and which are unique to adolescence. The particular pitfalls of an exclusive storm and stress conception of adolescence are elaborated on later in this chapter (see p. 21) and in Chapter 2.

ADOLESCENCE IN MODERN SOCIETY

Social scientists vary widely in their interpretation of the impact of modern society on the adolescent era. In *The Vanishing Adolescent* Edgar Friedenberg (1959) postulates an essential incompatibility between modern society and adolescence as a unique developmental period. In his view adolescent identity formation proceeds mainly through conflict with society. Since modern technological society emphasizes conformity and institutionalization, idealizes the organization man, and disparages the very individuality and conflict on which adolescent self-definition depends, he continues, it is bitterly hostile and destructive to the positive goals of adolescence:

"We do not tolerate in our adolescents a firm sense of their own identity, or the impassioned, if transitory, commitments through which different identities can be tried and accepted or rejected. We are deathly afraid they will get a record that will count against them in later life—as, indeed, they will. School counselors compile it continuously and record strong commitment as an aberration. We do not tolerate intimacy in young adults; parents and teachers fear going steady or homosexuality, as the occasion appears to warrant, and cripple the young with their fears. Fraternities and sororities are decried and put down as antidemocratic unless they transform themselves into good-natured service clubs open to all comers" (Friedenberg, 1966, p. 307).

Friedenberg concludes that modern society is ceasing to foster "real," struggling adolescents and instead is turning out conformist youngsters homogeneously identified with school and other institutional values. Since individuality cannot develop without conflict, and since our adolescents are being enjoined from conflict, "adolescence, as a developmental process, is becoming obsolete" (Friedenberg, 1959, p. 133).

Kenneth Keniston (1962, 1965), on the other hand, argues in *The Uncommitted: Alienated Youth in American Society* that modern society, far from fostering homogeneity and a premature closure of identity seeking in adolescents, is rather serving increasingly to alienate youth from adult value systems. He maintains that a technological society, because of its chronic social change and fragmentation, holds neither clarity nor attraction for its young people:

"They view the adult world they expect to enter with a subtle distrust, a lack of high expectations, hopes, or dreams, and an often unstated feeling that they will have to "settle" for less than they would hope for if they let themselves hope . . . . Essentially, they recognize that adulthood is a relatively cold, demanding, specialized, and abstracted world where "meaningful" work is so scarce they do not even ask for it. . . . The adult world, then, as seen from within the youth culture, inspires neither enthusiasm nor deep commitment" (1965, pp. 396–398).

Thus where Friedenberg perceives in today's youth a pubertal simulation of maturity through a nonconflictual allegiance to societal values, Keniston sees them as struggling through their adolescence, without commitment, with a disaffection from adulthood, and with a limited sense of what they are. From the first point of view the impact of modern society is to attenuate and abbreviate any identity crisis, whereas from the second it is to intensify and prolong it.

Whereas Friedenberg sees adolescence disappearing as a distinct phase of the life cycle, Keniston (1965, p. 394) predicts that youth will increasingly have "a special culture of its own, with characteristics that are those of neither childhood or adulthood." Where Friedenberg sees the process of adolescent self-definition becoming obsolete, Keniston (1965, p. 400) regards the differences he perceives between the youth culture and adult society as providing an opportunity for "experimentation in the service of unconscious choice, exposure to experience for the sake of selection, and trial commitment in the interest of future self-definition."

Despite their divergence, both these views of contemporary adolescence have received impressive empirical support. Douvan and Adelson (1966, pp. 353–354) conclude from an extensive interview study of over 3,000 teenage boys and girls that traditional adolescence may, as Friedenberg maintains, be a disappearing phenomenon. Their findings confirmed in particular the notions of "homogenization" and limited experimentation in self-definition among American adolescents: "In the normative response to adolescence, however, we more commonly find an avoidance of inner and outer conflict, premature identity consolidation, ego and ideological constriction, and a general unwillingness to take psychic risks" (p. 351). As defined by their data, the typical adolescent is stereotyped in his thinking, conforming in his behavior, resistive to conflict and change, averse to identity diffusion, and willing to settle for "a modest resynthesis of the ego." Douvan and Adelson do not believe that the peer group plays any pervasive role in these developments and report that their boys and girls varied considerably in the extent of their peer-group allegiance and in their utilization of peer ties.

Elkin and Westley (1955) also minimize the significance of any peer-group culture for adolescent development. They investigated a suburban community and found more continuity than discontinuity in socialization, few sharp conflicts between parents and their adolescent children, and no serious overt problems of occupational choice or emancipation from authority figures. They conclude that, although elements of a youth culture may exist in middle class communities, they are less influential than patterns of family authority and guidance. From their point of view "adolescent culture" is for practical purposes a mythical concept.

Strong exception to such a benign view of adolescent culture is voiced by Coleman (1961), whose data are consistent with Keniston's description of alienated youth. In *The Adolescent Society* Coleman infers from a study of several thousand high school students that the modern adolescent is experiencing a marginal existence between childhood and adulthood that requires him to look increasingly to his peers for his rewards and values. Far from becoming prematurely assimilated into adult society, Coleman continues, today's adolescents have developed their own teenage subculture, replete with its own terminology, language, and standards, all of which contribute to distinctly adolescent personality patterns:

"He is 'cut off' from the rest of society, forced inward toward his own age group, made to carry out his whole social life with others his own age. With his fellows, he comes to constitute a small society, one that has most of its important interactions within itself, and maintains only a few threads of connection with the outside adult society" (p. 3).

Clinicians and social scientists generally agree on the existence of a prominent youth culture. Eisenberg (1965) maintains that, since societal demands determine the complexity of adult roles, increasing technological sophistication in a society tends to prolong the adolescence experienced by its youth. Especially in the absence of puberty rites to signify maturation, he adds, modern society is producing an increasingly lengthy and confused struggle to attain adult status. Blos (1962, p. 204) similarly comments that modern society progressively tends to decrease the ritualization of adolescence and adolescent roles and to place a heavy burden of self-determination on the adolescent's shoulders: "The vacuum of institutionalized adolescence in Western society thus allows . . . a high degree of personality differentiation and individuation, since there are no obligatory models." Sherif and Sherif (1965) assert that, to the extent that adolescence is a prolonged period of transition unmarked by clear procedures for progressing to adult status and responsibilities, it produces a "dilemma" in response to which young people turn for support to their agemates:

"Hence, like any individuals during a period of prolonged problems for which common effort may provide comfort or solution, adolescents tend toward group formation. Although adolescents may live in what is called a 'mass society,' they do have a social life that is far more patterned than adults are willing to believe" (p. 5).

Although the majority of behavioral scientists appear to agree with Coleman about the existence of a significant youth culture (see Gottlieb, 1965; Gottlieb and Ramsey, 1964, pp. 29–33), it remains unclear whether adolescents should be regarded as a vanishing species or as an increasingly distinct subculture. First, any discussion of this issue requires some definition of what constitutes a youth culture, and there is little consensus on such a definition. According to Berger (1963, p. 396), the existence of a subculture can be defined only by distinctive life styles, "which are to a great extent self-generated, autonomous, having institutional and territorial resources capable of sustaining it in crisis and insulating it from pressures from without." Schwartz and Merten (1967), on the other hand, hold that the essence of a youth culture can reside solely in the distinctive language and terminology in which it casts its norms, standards, and values, regardless of whether there is anything distinctive about the norms, standards, and themselves:

"The normative integrity, coherence, and identity of a subculture is not always based upon estrangement from the larger culture nor does it always reside in social organizations which resist integration into the larger society" (p. 468).

Second, as Gottlieb (1965) points out, most investigators have assessed the subculture hypothesis only in terms of the degree of difference they could observe between adolescents and other age groups; that is, the deviation of adolescent values or behavior patterns from some norm has been taken as evidence of a youth culture, and nondeviation has been regarded as presumptive evidence that no such subculture exists. The problem with this approach, Gottlieb notes, is that it is completely relative to the particular adolescents and the specific values and behavior patterns involved: given knowledge of the adolescent group to be studied and the normative standards to be investigated, the results of any such research are virtually predictable.

Thus some of the contradictions in views of the existence and role of a youth culture may reflect sampling differences. Keniston's experience was largely with a college population, whereas Elkin and Westley's survey was restricted to 14- and 15-years-olds. Although both the Coleman and the Douvan and Adelson studies involved large, carefully stratified samples and a broad band of behavioral and attitudinal variables, furthermore, Douvan and Adelson utilized intensive interviewing as their major investigative tool, whereas Coleman relied primarily on questionnaire data with only informal interviewing of selected subjects. Only additional work can determine what influence these sampling and methodological differences may have had on the data obtained.

Third, findings that appear to demonstrate the existence of a significant youth culture do not indicate how much of the culture has been generated by adolescents in genuine response to a complex, ambiguous society and how much has been artificially imposed on young people by the society's advertising onslaught. The adolescent is widely recognized as a major consumer, and lucrative rewards await the entertainer, manufacturer, or promoter who can create a teenage fad. Gottlieb and Ramsey (1964, pp. 33–39) review the vulnerability of adolescents to fashions in clothing, music, reading, language, and extracurricular activities promoted in the popular media as what is "in" for all youngsters who are "with it."

To complicate the situation further various writers disagree sharply concerning the merits of a youth culture for personality development. Friedenberg and Keniston both stress the adolescent's need for a period of freedom from premature commitment to adult roles and responsibilities, during which he can work toward self-definition by experimentation. Coleman, on the other hand, decries a youth culture that is unfettered by adult restrictions and aspirations. In his opinion the adolescent culture is a frivolous society that stresses such superficial values as personal attractiveness, social and athletic success, and material assets at the expense of serious attention to academic attainment and the formulation of meaningful life goals. He pleads for educational policies that will reduce the pervasive influence of the adolescent society on teenagers and "bring the adolescents back into the home," to a state where "each boy and girl responds principally to his parents' demands" (see Coleman, 1961, Chapter XI).

Coleman therefore appears to advocate the very submission to adult values that Friedenberg abhors in his view of the modern adolescent. The adolescent Friedenberg would like to see, freed from premature identity consolidation and enmeshed in a peer-group arena for self-confrontation and experimentation with identities, is regarded by Coleman (1961, p. 311) as "disturbing to one concerned with the ability of an open society to raise its children today and in the future."

These issues border closely on the question of whether normative, optimal adolescence is a time of crisis, confusion, rebellion, and alienation or rather an era of reasonably steady, stable development and smooth progression to adult values and behavior patterns. Certainly there is no question that adolescents confront developmental tasks unique to their time of life, and clinical experience consistently proves the folly of regarding teenagers either as big children or young adults. In this sense, then, it is important to recognize that adolescence does demonstrate distinctive personality patterns.

On the other hand, there is no necessary uniformity in these distinctive patterns from one youngster to the next, and even values and behaviors shared by groups of youngsters may be highly variable between the groups in relation to their modal age, sex, social class, and the like. Thus it would seem erroneous to speak of any single "youth culture." Furthermore, to the extent that the notion of multiple "youth cultures" implies major gaps between the adolescent and adult generations, the evidence reviewed in the next section seriously challenges the existence of anything more than a superficial adolescent society.

DISRUPTION AND STABILITY IN ADOLESCENCE

As already noted, the pioneering contributions of G. Stanley Hall (1904) depicted adolescence as an era of inevitable turmoil in which the major predictable feature of a young person's behavior is his unpredictability:

"The 'teens' are emotionally unstable and pathic. It is the age of natural inebriation without the need of intoxicants, which made Plato define youth as spiritual drunkenness. It is a natural impulse to experience hot and perfervid psychic states, and it is characterized by emotionalism. . . . We see here the instability and fluctuations now so characteristic. The emotions develop by contrast and reaction into the opposite" (Vol. II, pp. 74–75).

Hall further explicated several antithetical traits that he believed to define normal adolescence: alternations of eagerness, zest, enthusiasm, and intellectual curiosity with apathy, inertia, and cultivated indifference; oscillations between pleasure and pain and euphoria and melancholy; periods of both extreme egoism and abject humility; alternating selfishness and altruism, conservatism and radicalism, and gregariousness and seclusiveness; changes from exquisite sensitiveness to imperturbability, hard-heartedness, and cruelty; vacillations between knowing and doing and between the ascendance of sense and intellect; and the juxtaposition of wisdom and folly (Vol. II, pp. 75–88).

Although subsequent cultural anthropological data challenged the inevitability of adolescent turmoil as described by Hall (see pp. 9–10), later psychoanalytic interpretations of adolescence strongly supported his views, at least with respect to Western civilization. Perhaps foremost among psychoanalytic writers in her influence on contemporary thinking about adolescent development is Anna Freud (1936), whose description of normal adolescence is strikingly similar to Hall's:

"Adolescents are excessively egoistic, regarding themselves as the centre of the universe and the sole object of interest, and yet at no time in later life are they capable of so much self-sacrifice and devotion. They form the most passionate love-relations, only to break them off as abruptly as they began them. On the one hand they throw themselves enthusiastically into the life of the community and, on the other, they have an overpowering longing for solitude. They oscillate between blind submission to some self-chosen leader and defiant rebellion against any and every authority. They are selfish and materially-minded and at the same time full of lofty idealism. They are ascetic but will suddenly plunge into in-

stinctual indulgence of the most primitive character. At times their behaviour to other people is rough and inconsiderate, yet they themselves
are extremely touchy. Their moods veer between light-hearted optimism
and the blackest pessimism. Sometimes they will work with indefatigable
enthusiasm and at other times they are sluggish and apathetic" (pp.
149–150).

Elsewhere Anna Freud (1958) affirms her belief that these adolescent
upheavals are nothing more than external indications that normal developmental internal adjustments are in progress: "Adolescence constitutes by
definition an interruption of peaceful growth which resembles in appearance a variety of other emotional upsets and structural upheavals"
(p. 267). Among psychoanalytic writers endorsing Anna Freud's position,
Geleerd (1957) considers that, since adolescence is a physiologically
troubled state,[2] a certain amount of psychological disturbance is normal:
"Personally I would feel greater concern for the adolescent who causes
no trouble and feels no disturbance" (p. 267). Geleerd (1961) further
maintains that a partial regression to an undifferentiated phase of object
relationships, accompanied by increased ego vulnerability and sensitivity
to trauma, is not only a normal but a necessary aspect of adolescent
maturation.

Spiegel (1951, 1961) comments on the resemblance of adolescence
to some psychotic episodes and reports that observations of adolescents
over any period of time normally reveal alternating phases of chaos and
consolidation. Harley (1961) discusses at length the role in normal adolescent development of the dissolution of psychic structures that have been
built up during childhood and consolidated during latency. According
to Eissler (1958, p. 224), "Although puberty may take many courses,
we think predominantly of stormy and unpredictable behavior marked
by mood swings and melancholy." Fountain (1961) asserts that adolescents can be distinguished from adults by their intensity and volatility
of feeling, need for frequent and immediate gratification, ineffective reality
testing, and failure of self-criticism.

Other psychoanalytic contributors have focused specifically on the manner in which certain adolescent modes of dealing with conflicts and frustrations normally lead to inconsistent and maladaptive behavior patterns. Bern-

---

[2] Although physiological instability in normal adolescents has been inferred by
several investigators, Eichorn and McKee (1958) consider available data inadequate
to justify such a conclusion. In their study of 100 adolescent boys and girls, on
whom physiological measures were taken every six months from age 11.5 to 17.5
years, they found no evidence of a temporary period of heightened physiological
variability for girls and only a slight indication for boys.

feld (1938) categorized adolescents according to their preference for rebellious or compliant modes of responding to environmental demands. The strictly rebellious adolescent, according to Bernfeld, disregards prohibitions, seeks immediate gratification of his needs, and struggles against all obstacles, self-righteously seeking to overcome them by any means possible. The strictly compliant adolescent, in contrast, settles all problems by repressing them and, at the expense of transient neurotic symptoms and persistently childish affective responses, frequently passes an uneventful adolescence. For Bernfeld various sequential combinations and permutations of these reactive modes define the majority of personality types observed in adolescents.

Ackerman (1958, p. 116) has more recently expressed a similar view of adolescent personality:

"The behavior of adolescents today is bipolar. They tend to seek identity at one of two poles: conformity or delinquency. At one extreme occur the weird explosive acts that lean toward crime. At the other extreme emerges a kind of caricature of cautious, monotonous, conforming behavior."

Ackerman (1962) believes that mild and transitory manifestations of many undesirable personality traits normally characterize contemporary adolescents, including the following: antisocial behavior, especially in acts of violence; sexual promiscuity; a quest for kicks but also for a "safe" existence; overconformity with peers; withdrawal with a loss of faith, disillusionment and despair, lack of adventuresomeness, and loss of spark; disorientation in relations with family and community; and increased vulnerability to mental breakdown. In his opinion all of these difficulties are attributable to the turbulence and instability of the modern family, which he sees as providing the adolescent few of the types of intrafamilial relationships optimal for emotional growth. Pearson (1958) in *Adolescence and the Conflict of Generations* also develops the theme that adolescents today face a serious struggle for maturity because of the older generation's lack of sympathy or understanding and general resistance to their attaining adulthood.

Thus these writers posit either that adolescence is inevitably a period of disruption and maladaptive behavior or that modern civilized environment makes it so. These views have somewhat different implications for individual and social action. To assume that in adolescence disruption is inevitable is to advocate the tolerance, patience, and forebearance in the face of adolescent idiosyncracies originally encouraged by Hall. To trace adolescent turmoil to modifiable environmental circumstances, on the other hand, is to champion a search for social psychological means of redressing the plight of youth.

The latter attitude is implicit in a paper by Hurlock (1966), who attributes a host of negative developments in modal adolescent behavior to increasingly progressive and permissive child-rearing practices. In a sweeping indictment of modern youth she castigates him for his peer conformity; preoccupation with status symbols; irresponsibility; antiwork and anti-intellectual attitudes; disregard for manners, grooming, and virginity; disrespect for older generations; criticism and debunking of those in authority; disregard for rules and laws; and unrealistic levels of aspiration.

The writings of Ackerman, Hurlock, Coleman, and others of a similar persuasion convey a clarion call for a return to the "good old days." This yearning for the way youth used to be bears a disconcerting resemblance to the Socratic plaint quoted on page 1. Things seemed little improved in Shakespeare's time:

"I would there were no age between ten and three-and-twenty, or that youth would sleep out the rest; for there is nothing in the between but getting wenches with child, wronging the ancientry, stealing, fighting" (*The Winter's Tale,* Act III, Scene iii).

More pertinent to the modern era, however, is the following impression of the adolescent dilemma:

"Modern life is hard, and in many respects, increasingly so, on youth. Home, school, church, fail to recognize its nature and needs and, perhaps most of all, its perils. . . . Never has youth been exposed to such dangers of both perversion and arrest as in our own land and day. Increasing urban life with its temptations, prematurities, sedentary occupations, and passive stimuli just when an active, objective life is most needed, early emancipations and a lessening sense for both duty and discipline, the haste to know and do all befitting man's estate before its time, the mad rush for sudden wealth and the reckless fashions set by its gilded youth— all these lack some of the regulatives they still have in older lands with more conservative traditions."

These timely views were voiced by Hall in 1904 (Vol. I, pp. xiv–xvi). Their vintage raises the question of how good indeed were the "good old days." Furthermore, if the adolescents of Hall's day exhibited many of the personality characteristics that are viewed with alarm by current writers, is not the idea of progressive adolescent decadence a myth? Kelley (1962, p. 4), for one, writing from many years' experience as an educator, disputes vigorously the belief that youth has gone to the dogs: "The overall evidence, however, is that youth as a whole behave better than they ever did." And if the decadence idea is after all a myth, is it possible that the whole notion of normative adolescent turmoil and misbehavior, both then and now, is also a myth?

At issue, then, is the oft-stated conviction that adolescence is, or is progressively becoming, an era of disruption during which young people wage undeclared warfare against their parents and other authorities, reject adult values, plunge into sexual promiscuity, pursue transient and super-ficial interests, and undergo a state of psychological disequilibrium that borders on psychopathology. In fact, a heavy weight of contrary data and opinion argue strongly that these views, whenever generalized to the adolescent population, are indeed a myth.

The Conflict of Generations

With regard first to the frequently deplored conflict of generations, most empirical studies have consistently failed to demonstrate that adoles-cents and parents are at loggerheads and that there is a prevailing at-mosphere of mutual disrespect, derogation, and disaffection, as depicted in generation-conflict interpretations of adolescence. According to Berger (1963, p. 395), "There is absolutely no good body of data on adolescents, Coleman's included, which indicates the existence of a really deviant sys-tem of norms which govern adolescent life." Schwartz and Merten (1967, p. 458) likewise find no basis in the literature for inferring increasing generational conflict: "In fact, the traditional cycle of intense intergenera-tional conflict followed by reconciliation when the younger generation takes its place in society seems less common today than in the past."

Impressive data that contradict the notion of a generation conflict be-tween adolescents and their parents are reported by Meissner (1965), Hess and Goldblatt (1957), and Offer, Sabshin, and Marcus (1965). Meissner describes a questionnaire study in which 1278 thirteen- to eigh-teen-year-old high school boys generally expressed positive views toward their parents. Only 15% of the boys felt that their parents were overly strict, and 74% indicated that they were proud of their parents and en-joyed having them meet their friends. Although among the older teenagers there was a pattern of increasing resistance to parental control and influ-ence, there was also increased acceptance of the principle of parental authority and growing respect for parental jugment. Thus the "resistance" pattern appeared to represent a gradual and essential disengagement from parental influence rather than any rebelliousness. Furthermore, despite some dissatisfaction with home life that increased with age, 89% of Meiss-ner's teenage subjects reported being happy in their homes and 84% re-ported spending half or more of their leisure time there.

Hess and Goldblatt interviewed 32 teenage boys and girls and their families and had them complete a series of ratings on trait adjectives representing socially desirable aspects of character and personality. The youngsters completed the rating scales to describe the average teenager, the average adult, the average teenager from the adult viewpoint, and the average adult from the adult viewpoint; the parents similarly made ratings from several different viewpoints. Although these adolescents believed that the average adult has a generalized tendency to depreciate teenagers, and the adults believed that teenagers have unrealistically high opinions of themselves, in fact both the adolescents and parents in the study expressed mildly favorable opinions of teenagers. Furthermore, although the parents anticipated that teenagers would have a selective tendency to undervalue adults, these adolescents tended to idealize adults, expressing much higher opinions of adults than did the adults themselves.

Offer, Sabshin, and Marcus (1965) conducted a series of depth interviews with 84 fourteen- to sixteen-year-old boys carefully chosen as typical of freshmen boys in two high schools. They found these modal adolescents generally to have good capacity for object relations with adults, to demonstrate little of the intense conflict with parental values reported elsewhere, to view their fathers as reliable and knowledgeable and their mothers as understanding and sympathetic, and to feel a part of the larger cultural environment. Offer (1967) reports that repeated interviews with 73 of these boys over a three-year period continued to demonstrate positive family relationships, significant sharing of their parent's values, and basic satisfaction with the home environment.

These congruent data from questionnaires, interview-rating scales, and depth clinical interviews, when taken together with the already noted findings of Douvan and Adelson (1966) and Elkin and Westley (1955), seriously challenge the usual descriptions of generation conflict in adolescence. Yet, as noted in the section "Adolescents in Modern Society," there is widespread conviction among social scientists of the existence of a youth culture that is at odds with adult values, and any observer of the current American scene is bombarded with evidence of teenage fads, interests, tastes, and heroes that have little appeal for the majority of adults.

It would appear that the apparent pervasiveness of some uniquely teenage values, from which many observers have inferred a significant adolescent culture and corresponding generation conflict, is a relatively superficial phenomenon that obscures an underlying normative pattern of family accord. Douvan and Adelson suggest in this regard that normal adolescents share with their parents a common core of values concerning the major aspects of living but discharge normal familial tensions through marked disagreements on relatively trivial issues. Thus parents and their teenage children may basically love and respect one another and agree on fundamental standards of conduct and decency but vigorously dispute appropriate hair and skirt lengths, the charm of rock music and dancing, and the use of the family car (Douvan and Adelson, 1966, p. 352). Bandura and Walters (1959, p. 372) express a similar view of the existence of both unique teenage values and of empirical contradictions of basic generation conflict:

"The view that adolescence is a period of rebellion is often supported by references to superficial and external signs of nonconformity such as the adolescent's fondness for unorthodox clothing, mannerisms, and language. Too often his fundamental and deep-seated acceptance of parental values is thus overlooked."

Sexual Values and Behavior

The area of sexual behavior has provided especially fertile ground for the inference of disparity in values between adolescents and adults. As noted on page 24 and reflected in numerous "Sunday Supplements," the presumed sexual decadence of our youth is feared by some to herald the demise of our civilization. As in the case of generation conflict, however, social science data stamp such gloomy prophecies as unfounded. Emphasizing the important distinction between endorsed values and actual behavior, Bell (1966) and Reiss (1960, p. 233; 1966) document that, although the last 40 years have seen changes in attitudes toward premarital sexual behavior to match actual behavioral changes occurring in the 1920s, available evidence indicates no significant changes in the frequency of premarital petting or intercourse over the past 40 years.

Some attitudinal differences toward sexual behavior, apparently consistent with generation conflict, are demonstrated in studies by Reiss (1964) and Bell and Buerkle (1961), in which adults expressed more conservative views on the acceptability of premarital petting and sexual intercourse than high school and college students. However, a closer look at the data reveals that, when 217 college girls in the Bell and Buerkle study were asked their opinion of intercourse by engaged couples, only 17% considered it "right in many situations," with the remaining 83% viewing it as either "generally wrong" or "very wrong"; 87% of these girls considered it "generally wrong" or "very wrong" not to be virginal at marriage. Bell and Buerkle furthermore report that discrepant sexual attitudes between these college girls and their mothers had emerged only during the late college years, whereas prior to this time they had had very similar attitudes toward virginity.

As for actual sexual behavior, it is not difficult to unearth the following type of assertion, unencumbered by documentary citations or evidence:

"Statistical inquiries as well as news reports indicate an increasing incidence of adolescent premarital intercourse. It has become a perfunctory aspect of the dating system" (Glassberg, 1965, p. 190).

Yet Offer (1967) reports that in the group of modal adolescent boys that he followed intensively for three years only 5% had had sexual intercourse by the time they were halfway through their junior year of high school. Eighty percent of these boys confided that they approved of premarital intercourse, but only after high school. Contrary to popular opinion, furthermore, the rate of illegitimate births in the United States during the period 1938 to 1957 increased less among 15- to 19-year-old girls than among women in any other child-bearing age group (Vincent, 1961).

In other relevant work Schofield (1965) reports an extensive study of over 1800 fifteen- to nineteen-year-old boys and girls selected from several areas of London and representing a broad socioeconomic spectrum. His voluminous data, gathered by experienced and well-trained interviewers employing a carefully developed interview schedule, generally demonstrate that rampant sexuality among youth exists only in fantasy. Of his 15- to 17-year-olds, only 11% of the boys and 6% of the girls reported having had sexual intercourse; among the 17- to 19-year-olds the proportions of sexually experienced rose only to 30% for the boys and 16% for the girls (pp. 29–31). Thus for the sample as a whole four-fifths of the boys and almost nine-tenths of the girls had not had sexual intercourse.

As far as even older adolescents are concerned, available data indicate that free love on the college campus is similarly mythical. According to reports by Ehrmann (1959), Freedman (1965), and Grinder and Schmitt (1966), depth interview and questionnaire studies on university campuses indicate that approximately only 15 to 20% of freshman through senior girls have experienced sexual intercourse. Halleck (1967) has recently reviewed evidence that college students hold increasingly liberal attitudes toward sex and particularly toward sexual activity among couples who intend to marry but firmly reject casual sexuality or any wish to become members of a promiscuous society.

Areas of Interest and Concern

The frivolity that is frequently attributed to youth also rests on shaky empirical grounds, despite the large and varied sample from which Coleman (1961) concludes that the chief concerns of high school students are athletic prowess, car ownership, and father's occupation among boys and clothes, social success, and physical beauty among girls. Contrasting with Coleman's data is the work of three separate investigators who asked high school students to rank order their concerns about 15 issues generally considered to be problems for adolescents. This list was given to 1641 students by Symonds (1936), 1165 students by Harris (1959), and 600 students by Kaczkowski (1962). These samples included several states and a variety of high school settings.

In all three studies the adolescents uniformly rated study habits high among their areas of concern; in the Harris study in fact study habits were ranked the leading concern by both boys and girls. Although problems involving money were also highly ranked in the three studies, these adolescents additionally reported considerable concern about the philosophy of life and about personal and moral qualities. The Kaczkowski study revealed increasing attention to philosophical issues over the high school years, with problems related to the philosophy of the life ranked second in importance by the senior boys and third by the senior girls. Although concern about personal attractiveness was generally high among the girls, Harris reports a significant decrease in the importance of physical attractiveness as rated by his female subjects compared with those of Symonds 20 years earlier. For both boys and girls and at all ages concerns about recreation rated at or near the bottom of the list.

The major findings of these three investigators are confirmed in numerous other studies. Adams (1964, 1966) asked 4,000 ten- to nineteen-year-old boys and girls from over 30 different schools to report which personal problems caused them greatest difficulty. Listed most frequently by both boys and girls (35 and 23%, respectively) was concern about academic achievement. Sports and recreation problems—including the use of leisure time, learning to drive, and athletics—were in contrast mentioned by only 4% of the boys and 2% of the girls.

Meissner (1961) in his study of 1278 high school boys and Abel and Gingles (1965) in a survey of 2500 ninth- and tenth-grade girls also found that school problems constituted their subjects' primary source of worry. In the latter study, for example, 52% of the girls expressed concern about their study habits, whereas problems involving physical appearance were indicated by 46%, wanting to be more popular by 43%, and wishing for a more pleasing personality by 34%. As for what is valued by teenagers, Keislar (1953) found prestige among 353 tenth-grade students to correlate .58 and .63 with school marks among boys and girls, respectively, .55 and .69 with effort in school work, and .60 and .74 with cooperation with teachers; sociability, at .50 and .43, was somewhat less important to prestige, and occupation of father correlated only .21 with prestige among boys and only .19 among girls. Havighurst and Taba (1949) indicate that school grades correlated more highly (.74) with character reputation among 16-year-olds than any of the other variables in their extensive study.

Offer, Sabshin, and Marcus (1965) asked their subjects to indicate the three most difficult problems an adolescent has to overcome during the high school years and found the area of vocational and educational goals mentioned most frequently. Garrison (1966), after studying 465 high school boys and girls, concludes: "The large percentage of students showing a concern about world conditions and atomic war attests to the seriousness of high school boys and girls about world affairs" (p. 248).

The frivolous adolescent—unconcerned about his studies, interested more in popularity than intellect, and detached from the problems and values of adult society—simply does not appear as typical among the several thousand teenagers sampled in the above studies. His purported frivolity thus appears to be as mythical as his alienation and promiscuity.

Normal Adolescence and Borderline Psychopathology

Finally relevant to the case for adolescent disruption is the supposition that adolescents will normatively manifest a degree of storm, stress, and unpredictability barely distinguishable from psychopathologic states. The accuracy of this expectation is considered at length in Chapter 2, which deals with the nature of normality and abnormality in adolescence. At this point, however, it is pertinent to mention briefly some of the evidence contradicting the notion that the normal adolescent is by definition a psychological cripple.

The most extensive work relevant to this question is the already mentioned study by Douvan and Adelson (1966). Their detailed investigation of over 3000 adolescents revealed little of the turmoil, conflict, and instability that are attributed by some to normal adolescence. Rather, their data delineated a somewhat staid, conservative adolescent, one who neither displays nor seeks turmoil and conflict. Douvan and Adelson even express concern that modern adolescents do not demonstrate more of "the passions, the restlessness, the vivacity of adolescence" they would see as contributing to optimal emotional maturation.

Several other writers comment on the conservatism they have observed to be characteristic of adolescents. Ross and Johnson (1949, pp. 149–150), express their impressions of the adolescent growth process as follows:

"The basic characteristic of the normal adolescent is conservatism. Some people may take exception to this, emphasizing that this period is one of revolt and indiscretion. To be sure, the normal adolescent's chief emotional problem is to achieve emancipation from childish ties to the parents. This is a gradual emancipation, however, not an amputation or violent revolt."

Elsewhere Johnson and Burke (1955) reaffirm the conviction that adolescence is not necessarily an emotionally volatile age but rather "a very conservative age unless misguided adults interfere with or disrupt a fine balance" (p. 558). Offer, Sabshin, and Marcus (1965) similarly report that the adolescents they studied, though concerned about control and mastery of their impulses, were generally constrained and conservative in their behavior.

Just as these reports challenge the anticipation of excess and exaggeration in adolescents, other data fail to confirm the notion that instability and inadequate ego resources are hallmarks of normal adolescence. Engel (1959), comparing self-descriptive ratings made by eight- and tenth-grade students and repeated by them two years later, was able to demonstrate relative stability of the self-concept over these teenage years. As summarized by Hertz (1960, p. 54), extensive normative Rorschach studies indicate that adolescents for the most part have many adaptive strengths for coping with new experiences, display adequate controls, and are able to direct their energies into effective and socially adequate channels. Rorschach findings of Ames, Metraux, and Walker (1959, pp. 24–28) specifically demonstrate consistently good reality-testing capacity over the adolescent years as reflected in accurate perceptions and endorsement of conventional modes of response.

These data support the view expressed many years ago by Kanner (1941, pp. 515 and 525) that the many demands, conflicts, and quandaries that confront adolescents do not necessarily induce psychological incapacitation:

"A combination of innate soundness, wholesome childhood, and guidance from understanding elders helps most adolescents to feel their way safely through the groping and floundering which often precede maturation. The majority tread or fight their way through adolescence with reasonable efficiency and emerge with some kind of serviceable solution of their problems. They are helped by their ability to make use of their assets without being stumped by the obstacles. . . ."

The Mystique of Adolescence

It is interesting finally to speculate on the origin of the myth of the normatively turbulent and unstable adolescence. Adelson (1964) in a paper entitled "The Mystique of Adolescence" points out that two caricatured images of the adolescent have emerged in recent years: the adolescent as *visionary-victim*—a noble, martyred figure, pure in moral vision but betrayed, exploited, and neglected by the adult world, to whose corruption he falls passive victim; and the adolescent as *victimizer*—a cruel, sinister, amoral person who wreaks destruction and sorrow on innocent victims powerless to combat him.

Adelson attributes this mystique to the inordinate attention given to two conspicuous but atypical groups of adolescents whose behaviors represent exceptional solutions to adolescent developmental crises. The *visionary-victim* adolescent corresponds to the sensitive, articulate, intense, intelligent, upper middle class adolescent patient on whom much of the psychoanalytic theory of adolescence is based, whereas the *victimizer* adolescent is the delinquent whose escapades are recounted in the popular media. Adelson concludes that the descriptions in the literature of the turbulent adolescent bear little relation to the large majority of teenagers whose behavior attracts little notoriety:

"In all likelihood, the degree of tension and disorder has always been more apparent than real. It is always more likely that passion, defiance, and suffering will capture the fancy, and that the amiable, colorless forms of adaptation will be ignored" (p. 4).

The problems inherent in generalizing from patient to general populations have been demonstrated in many contexts and certainly could account for the views held in some quarters that adolescence is generally an unstable, borderline psychopathologic time of life. A pertinent illustration of such fallacious overgeneralization is reported in Halleck's (1967) already cited paper on college sexual behavior. Halleck found that of 107 unmarried coeds in treatment with private psychiatrists in a university community, 86% had had premarital sexual relations, a fact apparently justifying an impression of widespread promiscuity among youth. However, this figure contrasted sharply with his findings that only 22% of a representative sample of coeds at the university had engaged in premarital intercourse. He concludes that, although psychiatric patients may be promiscuous, most of the population is not, and he appropriately cautions against overgeneralizations from clinical experience.

This caution is also raised by Gardner (1957, p. 509) in the following pertinent remarks:

"I think it also is extremely important for us to bear in mind that we are dealing here with a "95 and 5 percent" problem-proposition in that we are compelled to agree that 95 percent of our adolescents in present-day American society develop, albeit with some heartaches, into reasonably healthy and reasonably well adjusted adults. When evaluating the positive and negative influences of society as a whole upon them, one cannot establish conclusions based solely, or even predominantly, upon the factors allegedly determining the disabilities of the 5 percent."

The following two chapters elaborate the normative implications of adolescent development for psychological stability and disruption and consider in greater detail the patterns of normal and abnormal behavior that are most frequently observed in adolescent youngsters.

REFERENCES

Abel, H., and Gingles, R. Identifying problems of adolescent girls. *Journal of Educational Research,* **58**:389–391, 1965.

Ackerman, N. W. *The Psychodynamics of Family Life.* New York: Basic Books, 1958.

Ackerman, N. W. Adolescent problems: A symptom of family disorder. *Family Process,* **1**:202–213, 1962.

Adams, J. F. Adolescent personal problems as a function of age and sex. *Journal of Genetic Psychology,* **104**:207–214, 1964.

Adams, J. F. Adolescents' identification of personal and national problems. *Adolescence,* **1**:240–250, 1966.

Adatto, C. P. Ego reintegration observed in analysis of late adolescents. *International Journal of Psychoanalysis,* **39**:172–177, 1958.

Adelson, J. The mystique of adolescence. *Psychiatry,* **27**:1–5, 1964.

Aichhorn, A. (1925). *Wayward Youth.* New York: Viking, 1935.

Ames, L. B. Changes in Rorschach response throughout the human life span. *Genetic Psychology Monographs,* **74**:89–125, 1966.

Ames, L. B., Metraux, R. W., and Walker, R. N. *Adolescent Rorschach Responses.* New York: Hoeber-Harper, 1961.

Aristotle. *Treatise on Rhetoric.* Translated by T. Hobbes. Oxford: D. A. Talboy, 1833. Book II, Chapter XII.

Ausubel, D. P. *Theory and Problems of Adolescent Development.* New York: Grune and Stratton, 1954.

Ausubel, D. P. *Theory and Problems of Child Development.* New York: Grune and Stratton, 1958.

Balser, B. H. A new recognition of adolescents. *American Journal of Psychiatry,* **122**:1281–1282, 1966.

Bandura, A., and Walters, R. H. *Adolescent Aggression: A Study of the Influence of Child-Training Practices and Family Interrelationships.* New York: Ronald, 1959.

Beers, C. W. *A Mind That Found Itself.* New York: Longmans Green, 1908.

Bell, R. R. Parent-child conflict in sexual values. *Journal of Social Issues,* **22**:34–44, 1966.

Bell, R. R., and Buerkle, J. V. Mother and daughter attitudes to premarital sexual behavior. *Marriage and Family Living,* **23**:390–392, 1961.

Benedict, R. Continuities and discontinuities in cultural conditioning. *Psychiatry*, 1:161–167, 1938.

Berger, B. Adolescence and beyond. *Social Problems*, 10:394–408, 1963.

Bernfeld, S. Über eine typische form der männlichen Pubertät (A typical form of male puberty). *Imago*, 9:169–188, 1923.

Bernfeld, S. Die heutige Psychologie der Pubertät (Present-day psychology of puberty). *Imago*, 13:1–56, 1927.

Bernfeld, S. Types of adolescence. *Psychonanalytic Quarterly*, 7:243–253, 1938.

Blos, P. *On Adolescence: A Psychoanalytic Interpretation.* New York: Free Press of Glencoe, 1962.

Bronson, W. C. Central orientations: A study of behavior organization from childhood to adolescence. *Child Development*, 37:125–155, 1966.

Bronson, W. C. Adult derivatives of emotnal expressiveness and reactivity-control: Developmental continuities from childhood to adulthood. *Child Development*, 38:801–817, 1967.

Cole, L. *Psychology of Adolescence.* New York: Farrar and Rinehart, 1936.

Cole, L. W., and Hall, I. N. *Psychology of Adolescence,* 5th edition. New York: Rinehart, 1959.

Coleman, J. S. *The Adolescent Society.* New York: Free Press of Glencoe, 1961.

Crow, L. D., and Crow, A. *Adolescent Development and Adjustment,* 2nd edition. New York: McGraw-Hill, 1965.

Dennis, W. Historical beginnings of child psychology. *Psychological Bulletin*, 46:224–235, 1949.

Douvan, E., and Adelson, J. *The Adolescent Experience.* New York: Wiley, 1966.

Ehrmann, W. *Premarital Dating Behavior.* New York: Holt, 1959.

Eichorn, D. H., and McKee, J. P. Physiological instability during adolescence. *Child Development*, 29:255–268, 1958.

Eisenberg, L. A developmental approach to adolescence. *Children*, 12:131–135, 1965.

Eissler, K. R. Notes on problems of technique in the psychoanalytic treatment of adolescents. *Psychoanalytic Study of the Child*, 13:223–254, 1958.

Elkin, F., and Westley, W. A. The myth of adolescent culture. *American Sociological Review*, 20:680–684, 1955.

Engel, M. The stability of the self-concept in adolescence. *Journal of Abnormal and Social Psychology*, 58:211–215, 1959.

Erikson, E. H. The probem of ego identity. *Journal of the American Psychoanalytic Association*, 4:56–121, 1956.

Fountain, G. Adolescent into adult: An inquiry. *Journal of the American Psychoanalytic Association*, 9:417–433, 1961.

Freedman, M. B. The sexual behavior of American college women. *Merrill Palmer Quarterly*, 11:33–48, 1965.

Freud, A. (1936). *The Ego and the Mechanisms of Defence.* New York: International Universities Press, 1946.

Freud, A. Adolescence. *Psychoanalytic Study of the Child,* **13**:255–278, 1958.

Freud, S. (1905). Three essays on the theory of sexuality. *Standard Edition,* Vol. VII. London: Hogarth, 1953, pp. 125–243.

Friedenberg, E. Z. *The Vanishing Adolescent.* Boston: Beacon, 1959.

Friedenberg, E. Z. Discussion of Erik Erikson's "Eight stages of man." *International Journal of Psychiatry,* **2**:306–307, 1966.

Gardner, G. E. Present-day society and the adolescent. *American Journal of Orthopsychiatry,* **27**:508–517, 1957.

Garfield, S. L. Historical introduction. In B. B. Wolman, ed., *Handbook of Clinical Psychology.* New York: McGraw-Hill, 1965.

Garrison, K. C. *Psychology of Adolescence,* 6th edition. Englewood Cliffs, N.J.: Prentice-Hall, 1965.

Garrison, K. C. A study of the aspirations and concerns of ninth-grade pupils from the public schools of Georgia. *Journal of Social Psychology,* **69**:245–252, 1966.

Geleerd, E. R. Some aspects of psychoanalytic technique in adolescence. *Psychoanalytic Study of the Child,* **12**:263–283, 1957.

Geleerd, E. R. Some aspects of ego vicissitudes in adolescence. *Journal of the American Psychoanalytic Association,* **9**:394–405, 1961.

Gesell, A. L., and Ilg, F. L. *The Child from Five to Ten.* New York: Harper, 1946.

Gesell, A. L., Ilg, F. L., and Ames, L. B. *Youth: The Years from Ten to Sixteen.* New York: Harper, 1956.

Glassberg, B. Y. Sexual behavior patterns in contemporary youth culture: Implications for later marriage. *Journal of Marriage and the Family,* **27**:190–192, 1965.

Glueck, S., and Glueck, E. T. *One Thousand Delinquents: Their Treatment by Court and Clinic.* Cambridge, Mass.: Harvard University Press, 1934.

Gottlieb, D. Youth subculture: Variations on a general theme. In M. Sherif and C. W. Sherif, eds., *Problems of Youth: Transition to Adulthood in a Changing World.* Chicago: Aldine, 1965, pp. 28–45.

Gottlieb, D., and Ramsey, C. E. *The American Adolescent.* Homewood, Ill.: Dorsey, 1964.

Grinder, R. E., and Schmitt, S. S. Coeds and contraceptive information. *Journal of Marriage and the Family,* **28**:471–479, 1966.

Grinder, R. E., and Strickland, C. E. G. Stanley Hall and the social significance of adolescence. In R. E. Grinder, ed., *Studies in Adolescence.* New York: Macmillan, 1963, pp. 3–16.

Hall, G. S. *Adolescence: Its Psychology and Its Relations to Physiology, Anthropology, Sociology, Sex, Crime, Religion, and Education,* Vols. I and II. New York: D. Appleton, 1904.

Halleck, S. L. Sex and mental health on the campus. *Journal of the American Medical Association,* **200**:684–690, 1967.

Harley, M. Some observations on the relationship between genitality and structural development at adolescence. *Journal of the American Psychoanalytic Association,* **9**:434–460, 1961.

Harris, D. B. Sex differences in the life problems and interest of adolescents, 1935 and 1957. *Child Development,* **30**:453–459, 1959.

Hartmann, H., Kris, E., and Loewenstein, R. M. Comments on the formation of psychic structure. *Psychoanalytic Study of the Child,* **2**:11–38, 1946.

Hathaway, S. R., and Monachesi, E. D. *Adolescent Personality and Behavior.* Minneapolis, Minn.: University of Minnesota Press, 1963.

Havighurst, R. J., and Taba, H. *Adolescent Character and Personality.* New York: Wiley, 1949.

Healy, W. H. *The Individual Delinquent: A Textbook of Diagnosis and Prognosis for All Concerned in Understanding Offenders.* Boston: Little, 1915.

Hertz, M. R. The Rorschach in adolescence. In A. I. Rabin and M. R. Haworth, eds., *Projective Techniques with Children.* New York: Grune and Stratton, 1960, pp. 29–60.

Hertz, M. R., and Baker, E. Personality changes in adolescence. *Rorschach Research Exchange,* **5**:30, 1941.

Hess, R. D., and Goldblatt, I. The status of adolescents in American society: A problem in social identity. *Child Development,* **28**:459–468, 1957.

Hollingshead, A. B. *Elmtown's youth.* New York: Wiley, 1949.

Hollingworth, L. S. *The Psychology of the Adolescent.* New York: D. Appleton, 1928.

Holmes, D. J. *The Adolescent in Psychotherapy.* Boston: Little, Brown, 1964.

Horrocks, J. E. The adolescent. In L. Carmichael, ed., *Manual of Child Psychology,* 2nd edition. New York: Wiley, 1954, pp. 697–734.

Horrocks, J. E. *The Psychlogy of Adolescence,* 2nd edition. Boston: Houghton-Mifflin, 1962.

Hurlock, E. B. American adolescents today—a new species. *Adolescence,* **1**:7–21, 1966.

Hurlock, E. B. *Adolescent Development,* 3rd edition. New York: McGraw-Hill, 1967.

Inhelder, B., and Piaget, J. *The Growth of Logical Thinking from Childhood to Adolescence.* New York: Basic Books, 1958.

Jersild, A. T. *The Psychology of Adolescence,* 2nd edition. New York: Macmillan, 1963.

Johnson, A. M., and Burke, E. C. Parental permissiveness and fostering in child rearing and their relationship to juvenile delinquency. *Proceedings of Staff Meetings, Mayo Clinic,* **30**:557–565, 1955.

Jones, E. Some problems of adolescence. *British Journal of Psychology,* **13**:41–47, 1922.

Jones, H. E. The California Adolescent Growth Study. *Journal of Educational Research,* **31**:561–567, 1938.

Jones, H. E. Procedures of the Adolescent Growth Study. *Journal of Consulting Psychology,* **3**:177–180, 1939.

Jones, H. E., Macfarlane, J. W., and Eichorn, D. H. A progress report on growth studies at the University of California. *Vita Humana,* **3**:17–31, 1959.

Jones, M. C. A report on three growth studies at the University of California. *The Gerontologist*, **7**:49–54, 1967.

Josselyn, I. M. *The Adolescent and His World*. New York: Family Service Association of America, 1952.

Kaczkowski, H. Sex and age differences in the life problems of adolescents. *Journal of Psychological Studies*, **13**:165–169, 1962.

Kagan, J. American longitudinal research in psychological development. *Child Development*, **35**:1–32, 1964.

Kagan, J., and Moss, H. A. *Birth to Maturity: A Study in Psychological Development*. New York: Wiley, 1962.

Kanner, L. Mental disturbances in adolescents. *Medical Clinics of North America*, **25**:515–527, 1941.

Keislar, E. R. A distinction between social acceptance and prestige among adolescents. *Child Development*, **24**:275–283, 1953.

Kelley, E. C. *In Defense of Youth*. Englewood Cliffs. N.J.: Prentice-Hall, 1962.

Keniston, K. Social change and youth in America. *Daedalus*, **91**:145–171, 1962.

Keniston, K. *The Uncommitted: Alienated Youth in American Society*. New York: Harcourt, Brace, and World, 1965.

Kiell, N. *The Universal Experience of Adolescence*. New York: International Universities Press, 1964.

Kinsey, A. C., Pomeroy, W. B., and Martin, C. F. *Sexual Behavior in the Human Male*. Philadelphia: Saunders, 1948.

Locke, J. (1690). *An Essay Concerning Human Understanding*. New York: Dover, 1959.

McCandless, B. R. *Children and Adolescents: Behavior and Development*. New York: Holt, Rinehart, and Winston, 1961.

Macfarlane, J. W. Studies in child guidance: I. Methodology of data collection and organization. *Monographs of the Society for Research in Child Development*, **3**:1–254, 1938.

Mead, M. *Coming of Age in Samoa*. New York: Morrow, 1928.

Mead, M. Adolescence in primitive and modern society. In F. V. Calverton and S. D. Schmalhausen, eds., *The New Generation: A Symposium*. New York: Macauley, 1930, pp. 169–188.

Meissner, W. W. Some indications of the sources of anxiety in adolescent boys. *Journal of Genetic Psychology*, **99**:65–73, 1961.

Meissner, W. W. Parental interaction of the adolescent boy. *Journal of Genetic Psychology*, **107**:225–233, 1965.

Mills, C. A., and Ogle, C. Physiologic sterility of adolescence. *Human Biology*, **8**:607–615, 1936.

Montague, M. F. A. Adolescent sterility in the human female. *Human Fertility*, **11**:33–41, 1946.

Mussen, P. H., Conger, J. J., and Kagan, J. *Child Development and Personality*, 2nd edition. New York: Harper and Row, 1963.

Muuss, R. E. Theories of adolescent development—their philosophical and historical roots. *Adolescence,* 1:22–44, 1966.

Nixon, R. E. An approach to the dynamics of growth in adolescence. *Psychiatry,* 24:18–31, 1961.

Offer, D. Normal adolescents: Interview strategy and selected results. *Archives of General Psychiatry,* 17:285–290, 1967.

Offer, D., Sabshin M., and Marcus, D. Clinical evaluation of normal adolescents. *American Journal of Psychiatry,* 121:864–872, 1965.

Pearson, G. H. J. *Adolescence and the Conflict of Generations.* New York: Norton, 1958.

Pederson, S. Personality formation in adolescence and its impact upon the psycho-analytical treatment of adults. *International Journal of Psycho-Analysis,* 42:381–388, 1961.

Plato. *The Works of . . . .* Translated by B. Jowett. New York: Dial, 1938, 4 vols.

Reisman, J. M. *The Development of Clinical Psychology.* New York: Appleton-Century-Crofts, 1966.

Reiss, I. L. *Premarital Sexual Standards in America.* Glencoe, Ill.: Free Press, 1960.

Reiss, I. L. The scaling of premartial sexual permissiveness. *Journal of Marriage and the Family,* 26:188–198, 1964.

Reiss, I. L. The sexual renaissance: A summary and analysis. *Journal of Social Issues,* 22:123–137, 1966.

Rosen, B. M., Bahn, A. K., Shellow, R., and Bower, E. M. Adolescent patients served in outpatient psychiatric clinics. *American Journal of Public Health,* 55:1563–1577, 1965.

Rosenthal, I. Reliability of retrospective reports of adolescence. *Journal of Consulting Psychology,* 27:189–198, 1963.

Ross, H., and Johnson, A. M. Psychiatric interpretation of the growth process. Part II. Latency and adolescence. *Social Casework,* 30:148–154, 1949.

Rousseau, J. J. (1762). *Emile.* Translated by B. Foxley. London: J. M. Dent, 1911.

Rube, P. Is there a problem of adolescence? *American Journal of Psychotherapy,* 9:503–509, 1955.

Schofield, M. *The Sexual Behavior of Young People.* Boston: Little, Brown, 1965.

Schwartz, G., and Merten, D. The language of adolescence: An anthropological approach to the youth culture. *American Journal of Sociology,* 72:453–468, 1967.

Shapiro, R. L. Adolescence and the psychology of the age. *Psychiatry,* 26:77–87, 1963.

Sherif, M., and Sherif, C. W. Problems of youth in transition. In M. Sherif and C. W. Sherif, eds., *Problems of Youth: Transition to Adulthood in a Changing World.* Chicago: Aldine, 1965, pp. 1–12.

Spiegel, L. A. A review of contributions to a psychoanalytic theory of adolescence. *Psychoanalytic Study of the Child,* 6:375–393, 1951.

Spiegel, L. A. Comments on the psychoanalytic psychology of the adolescent. *Psychoanalytic Study of the Child*, **13**:296–308, 1958.

Spiegel, L. A. Disorder and consolidation in adolescence. *Journal of the American Psychoanalytic Association*, **9**:406–417, 1961.

Stone, L. J., and Church, J. *Childhood and Adolescence*, 2nd edition. New York: Random House, 1968.

Sullivan, H. S. *The Interpersonal Theory of Psychiatry*. New York: Norton, 1953.

Symonds, P. M. Sex differences in the life interests and problems of adolescents. *School and Society*, **43**:751–752, 1936.

Symonds, P. M. *Adolescent Fantasy*. New York: Columbia University Press, 1949.

Symonds, P. M., and Jensen, A. R. *From Adolescent to Adult*. New York: Columbia University Press, 1961.

Tanner, J. M. *Growth at Adolescence*, 2nd edition. Springfield, Ill.: Thomas, 1962.

Toolan, J. M. Changes in personality structure during adolescence. In J. H. Masserman, ed., *Science and Psychoanalysis*. Vol. III. *Psychoanalysis and Human Values*. New York: Grune and Stratton, 1960, pp. 189–200.

Tuddenham, R. D. The constancy of personality ratings over two decades. *Genetic Psychology Monographs*, **60**:3–29, 1959.

Vincent, C. E. *Unmarried Mothers*. New York: Free Press of Glencoe, 1961.

Watson, J. B. Psychology as the behaviorist views it. *Psychological Review*, **20**:158–177, 1913.

Watson, J. B. *Behaviorism*. New York: Norton, 1925.

Wittels, F. The ego of the adolescent. In K. R. Eissler, ed., *Searchlights on Delinquency*. New York: International Universities Press, 1949, pp. 256–262.

Young, H. B. Ageing and adolescence. *Developmental Medicine and Child Neurology*, **5**:451–460, 1963.

CHAPTER 2

Normality and Abnormality in Adolescence

The identification of psychological disturbance proceeds from comparisons between observed behavior patterns and explicit criteria of normality and abnormality. Diagnostic assessments of teenage patients accordingly rest largely with the extent of personality disruption considered commensurate with normal adolescent development. As noted in Chapter 1 (see pp. 21–33), the question of whether adolescence is normally a period of psychological stability or instability has provoked a wide range of opinion.

Expanding on the preceding discussion in Chapter 1, this chapter first elaborates views of normal adolescence as a disturbed state. Subsequent sections of the chapter then review additional data that challenge this assertion by demonstrating (a) that normative adolescence is not characterized by indices of psychological incapacity, (b) that marked adolescent turmoil reflects deviant rather than normative adjustment, and (c) that most symptom formation in adolescents constitutes psychopathology that should not be taken lightly.

VIEWS OF NORMAL ADOLESCENCE AS A DISTURBED STATE

Descriptions of normal adolescence as a disturbed state generally comprise two related expectations: first, that normal adolescent development will be characterized by distressing, turbulent, and unpredictable thoughts, feelings, and actions; and second, that as a consequence of such storm and stress adolescents will normatively display symptoms that in an adult would suggest definitive psychopathology. These expectations derive primarily from psychoanalytic conceptualizations of adolescence, and the writings of Anna Freud, Geleerd, Spiegel, Harley, Eissler, and Fountain cited in Chapter 1 illustrate the conviction of most psychoanalytic clinicians that the normal adolescent is at least transiently a disturbed, maladjusted person. Ackerman (1958, pp. 227–228) specifies this impression of normative adolescence as follows:

"The fluidity of the adolescent's self-image, his changing aims and aspirations, his sex drives, his unstable powers of repression, his struggle to readapt his childhood standards of right and wrong to the needs of maturity bring into sharp focus every conflict, past and present, that he has failed to solve. The protective coloring of the personality is stripped off, and the deeper emotional currents are laid bare."

Several writers share Geleerd's already noted opinion (see p. 22) that psychological disturbance is so much a normal concomitant of adolescence that its absence is a cause for concern. Beres (1961) suggests that the adolescent who does not experience a state of flux and uncertainty is likely to have suffered a premature crystallization of his response patterns that may presage serious psychopathology. Anna Freud (1958) contends that teenagers who remain "good children" and fail to show outer evidence of inner unrest are displaying deviant development. In her view such children are responding to their impulses with excessive, crippling defenses that impede normal maturational processes. These sentiments are endorsed by Lindemann (1964, p. 407) in the following comment:

"We have learned to become equally concerned about those adolescents who show no evidence of disturbance and retain the patterns of allegiance, obedience to common family goals, and unmarred achievement throughout the puberty period. We know that such persons are likely to become profoundly disturbed at a later time when adult behavior is unquestionably demanded."

Some interesting empirical data that are apparently consistent with these views are reported by Spivack (1957), who compared child-rearing attitudes of adolescents in a residential treatment setting with those of nonpatient controls. The disturbed adolescents expressed significantly more restrictive controlling attitudes toward child rearing than the nonpatient group. One possible inference from this finding is that emotionally disturbed adolescents feel stronger needs for parental imposition of external controls and for conformity to their perception of parental values than do nondisturbed adolescents. Spivack accordingly hypothesizes that rebellious behavior may be less characteristic of emotionally disturbed than of normal adolescents, which implies that the absence of rebellion may sometimes indicate emotional disturbance in young people.

The companion expectation that normal adolescent turmoil will be reflected in symptoms of apparent psychopathology has been advanced by a number of clinicians; for example, Josselyn (1954) maintains that, although ego capacity at adolescence is greater than at any earlier age, the formidable tasks that confront the adolescent ego are likely to drain its resources:

"The behavior of the adolescent is typical of that of individuals, of whatever age, who have not found an adequate integrative pattern with which to reconcile their own impulses, the demands of conscience, and the demands of reality. Adolescence, as is equally true of the neuroses and psychoses, is characterized by relative failure of the ego. Demands placed upon it have caused a strain it cannot meet" (p. 225).

Josselyn concludes that the characteristic syndrome of adolescence is "ego exhaustion," a state of inadequate resources resulting from the ego's tilting with excessive demands. She clearly differentiates this state of relative ego failure from psychopathology: "The normal adolescent is inevitably a mixed-up person, but not at all in the sense of being a psychologically sick person" (Josselyn, 1959, p. 43). Finally, she asserts that most adolescents, in spite of their apparent instability, actually have sufficient inherent personality strengths to emerge from their confusion as relatively healthy adults.

Such a conception of normal adolescence implies that many apparently disturbed behavior patterns resembling adult psychopathology are in adolescents benign and transient phenomena that do not require professional attention. Gardner (1947, pp. 529 and 540) expresses this interpretation of adolescent behavior in the following remarks:

"It is my feeling and my experience that 90 percent of the so-called 'problems' of adolescents have to do with *normal* reactions or *normal phases* through which the adolescent passes in his journey toward adulthood. . . . My main therapeutic approach to the parents of adolescents . . . is the tried and true phrase of the men of the ancient church who, when beset by the unpredictable and seemingly uncontrollable, comforted themselves and one another with the words, 'It will pass. It will pass.' "

The Identity Crisis

Among specific patterns of adolescent disruption that have been defined as normal developmental concomitants, the one most prominent in the literature is the identity crisis. The role of identity formation in adolescent development was first explicated by Erikson (1950, pp. 227–228), who shares Hall's concern that adolescents are precipitously cast off from their former moorings (see p. 12.) Erikson considers pubescent development and the advent of genital maturity to disrupt "all samenesses and continuities relied on earlier." It is therefore incumbent on the adolescent to establish bridges between his previously cultivated roles and skills and his prospective adult roles and responsibilities. In his quest for a new sense of sameness and continuity the young person must refight many of the battles of his earlier years, Erikson continues, and these necessary battles constitute the normatively observed identity crisis.

Erikson (1956, pp. 66–68) later elaborated the specific implications of the concept of *ego identity* for adolescent development:

"This period [adolescence] can be viewed as a *psychosocial moratorium* during which the individual through free role experimentation may find a niche in some section of his society, a niche which is firmly defined and yet seems to be uniquely made for him. In finding it the young adult gains an assured sense of inner continuity and social sameness which will bridge what he *was* as a child and what he is *about to become,* and will reconcile his *conception of himself* and his *community's recognition* of him. . . . *Identity formation,* finally, begins where the usefulness of identification ends. It arises from the selective repudiation and mutual assimilation of childhood identifications, and their absorption in a new configuration, which in turn, is dependent on the process by which a *society . . . identifies the young individual,* recognizing him as somebody who had to become the way he is, and who, being the way he is, is taken for granted."

Erikson ascribes a number of apparently maladaptive reaction patterns to the role diffusion that accompanies identity crisis, including labile and unpredictable behavior, lack of commitment, semideliberate experimentation with dangerous or deviant behavior, and experimentation with fantasy and introspection, the latter involving conscious awareness of many thoughts and impulses ordinarily repressed by adults. Yet he maintains that such phenomena, although indicative of major psychopathology when they occur in adults, are normative and healthy in adolescents:

"Adolescence is not an affliction but a *normative crisis* . . . in which only fluid defenses can overcome a sense of victimization by inner and outer demands, and in which only trial and error can lead to the most felicitous avenues of action and self-expression" (Erikson, 1956, pp. 72–73).

Many clinicians stress the particular significance of an identity crisis among late adolescents, especially those who attend college. In Erikson's (1959, p. 75) view a college education, by artificially postponing the establishment of identity, leads to conspicuously acute identity crises and fosters "extended childishness even as it cultivates certain forms of one-sided precocity." Blos (1946) likewise comments on the collegiate postponement of adulthood, which he sees as contributing to a "protracted adolescence" among college students. According to Blos virtually every college student suffers at one time or another from problems created by the artificial prolongation of his maturation.

Nixon (1961, 1966) shares the belief that all late adolescents experience crises in relation to their attitudes toward independence and sexuality; their feelings toward parents, peers, siblings, and themselves; and their definitions of their interests and motivations. He further contends that college students who do not at some time or other evince such concerns are specifically denying them, and he interprets such denials as indicating a maladaptive incapacity for self-cognition. In basic agreement with Erikson, Nixon argues that introspection is the essential business of middle and late adolescence, and he includes among criteria for psychological normality in adolescents (a) the current or previous questioning of some of the principles by which they were brought up and (b) a visible degree of conscious recognition of anxiety in regard to their self-awareness.

The normative appearance of identity crises in late adolescence is also postulated by Gardner (1959) and Spiegel (1961). Gardner maintains that a temporary stage of role diffusion is an inevitable concomitant of adolescence (p. 872). Spiegel considers disturbances in the sense of self to exist in nearly all adolescents, except for those in whom a severely fixed obsessive-compulsive character structure resists the loosening effect of adolescence. He cautions that apparent freedom from such normative disturbances may be due to their cryptic nature and the adolescent's capacity for symptom absorption; hence the psychological instabilities of normal adolescents may at times be demonstrable only by detailed, persistent, and sophisticated questioning.

Empirical work by Marcia (1966) provides some noteworthy construct validation for several hypothesized patterns of *identity status,* which are alternative modes of reacting to the presumably normative late-adolescent identity crisis. Focusing on the presence of crisis and commitment in the areas of occupation and ideology, Marcia proposes that late adolescents can be assigned to one of four identity statuses. Two of these statuses, *identity achievement* and *identity diffusion,* are reaction patterns originally described by Erikson as polar outcomes of the identity crisis. Identity achievement is defined by the prior experience of a crisis period and current commitment to an occupation and an ideology. The young person with identity achievement has chosen an occupation from among several previously considered possibilities and has reevaluated and resolved his past beliefs in a manner that leaves him free to act. Identity diffusion is identified by lack of commitment, regardless of whether or not a crisis period has occurred. The person with identity diffusion is undecided and unconcerned about an occupation and uninterested or undiscriminating in regard to ideological matters.

The other two identity statuses formulated by Marcia, *moratorium* and *foreclosure,* are intermediate between achievement and diffusion. The moratorium is defined by an ongoing crisis period in which the young person is actively struggling to make commitments but has not yet achieved a clear and satisfying self-definition. Foreclosure has occurred when a person, without having experienced any overt identity crisis, already embraces specific commitments, usually those intended or prepared for him by others.

Marcia used individual interviews to assign 86 male college students in approximately equal numbers to these four identity statuses. He was subsequently able to confirm significant differences among these groups on measures of concept attainment, goal-setting behavior, and authoritarianism consistent with theoretical conceptions of ego identity. The identity-achievement subjects demonstrated significantly better concept attainment than the other three groups, who were of comparable intelligence, and the foreclosure group differed significantly from the others (a) in their firm authoritarian values and (b) in their tendency to set unrealistically high goals for themselves and to maintain these goals even in the face of failure.

In a later study of 72 male college students Marcia (1967) confirmed the particularly strong endorsement of authoritarianism among identity-foreclosure subjects. He additionally found foreclosure and identity-diffusion subjects to be significantly more vulnerable to experimental manipulations of their self-esteem than identity-achievement and moratorium groups.

Some further empirical confirmation of the identity-diffusion construct is reported by Bronson (1959), who inferred from the literature that persons in a state of identity diffusion, in contrast to those having a stable sense of self, should (a) be less certain about the relationship between their past and current notions of self, (b) show a higher degree of internal tension or anxiety, (c) be less certain of their dominant personal characteristics, and (d) fluctuate more in their feelings about themselves. Using interview and semantic differential techniques to rate 46 college students on these four hypothesized characteristics of ego diffusion, Bronson found consistently significant intercorrelations among them; that is, the presence of a high score on any one of the four dimensions was associated with a high score on each of the others, which lends additional construct validity to the notion of identity diffusion.

Before concluding this discussion of the identity crisis as an example of normative adolescent disturbance, it should be noted that Erikson, Blos, and the other major contributors in this area do indicate limits beyond which the extent of identity diffusion in adolescents must be considered pathological. Erikson (1956, pp. 77–88) describes acute identity diffusion as a serious clinical syndrome that shares many features with borderline schizophrenia (see Knight, 1953; Weiner, 1966, pp. 398–407), including the following:

1. Incapacity for personal intimacy, with resulting isolation, stereotyped interpersonal relationships, and frenzied quests for intimacy with improbable partners.

2. Diffusion of time perspective, with disbelief in the possibility that time may bring change.

3. Diffusion of industry, with inability to concentrate, self-destructive preoccupation with narrow activities, and an abhorrence of competitiveness.

4. The choice of a negative identity, expressed through utter disdain for roles commensurate with family and community standards of desirability and propriety.

Blos (1954) comments at length on "prolonged adolescence," a condition first described by Bernfeld (1923), which refers to an abnormal persistence of the identity crisis. In prolonged adolescence the individual clings to the turmoil and uncertainty of adolescence and stringently avoids the finality of choices that normally mark their demise. Such flight from commitment and abstention from decision-making characterize the contemporary "hippie" who would "turn on" and "drop out." For some young people such adolescent phenomena eventually give way to productive social and vocational goals. For others, however, the pattern of prolonged adolescence extends far beyond any of the age ranges usually associated with the adolescent period and for practical purposes becomes adult psychopathology.

Modern fiction provides some superb examples of pathologically prolonged identity crises. In Arthur Miller's *Death of a Salesman* Biff at age 34 confesses, "I just can't take hold, Mom, I can't take hold of some kind of a life." Lenny, the antihero of Romain Gary's *The Ski Bum,* opts for total detachment from family, country, love, and work; to a girlfriend of the moment he says, "Trudi, when two people begin to stick together for good they end up by having jobs, kids, homes, cars, problems, and that's no love no longer, that's living. We don't want that."

THE ADAPTIVE NATURE OF NORMATIVE ADOLESCENCE

Contrary to these influential views that adolescence is normally and normatively a disturbed state, considerable data suggest that the modal teenager is a reasonably well-adjusted individual whose daily functioning is minimally marred by psychological incapacity. Before considering these data, it should be noted that the words "normal" and "normative" have been rather loosely employed thus far. It is indicated at this point to review briefly the concept of "normality" and to specify the relevance of the research findings to be presented.

Definitions of Normality

Contributions to the definition of normality have been thoroughly reviewed by Offer and Sabshin (1963, 1966; see also Sabshin, 1967), who outline four major perspectives on normality: (a) normality as *health,* (b) normality as *utopia,* (c) normality as *average,* and (d) normality as *process.* Normality as health refers to a reasonable rather than an optimal state of functioning and is defined by the absence of manifest pathology. This perspective on normality is stated by Romano (1950, p. 411) as follows:

"Health, in a positive sense, consists in the capacity of the organism to maintain a balance in which it may be reasonably free of undue pain, discomfort, disability or limitation of action including social capacity."

Normality as utopia, in contrast, defines normality as optimal functioning, an ideal state of complete self-knowledge and full self-actualization that is seldom if ever realized. From this perspective *normality* is "a term to denote a limit to which real people approximate in various degrees," and the completely normal person is largely hypothetical (Money-Kyrle, 1952, p. 234).

Normality as average is a statistical perspective according to which the normative, or most common, behaviors among a defined group are considered normal for that group, and deviations from modal patterns, in any direction, constitute abnormality. The major test of normality from this perspective is stated by Linton (1956, p. 63):

"Relative normality . . . is a matter of the individual's adjustment to the cultural milieu and of the degree to which his personality configuration approaches the basic personality of his society."

In contrast to the cross-sectional nature of these three perspectives, normality as process is a longitudinal interpretation of behavior. From the process point of view only the successful unfolding of developmental phases and the adaptive handling of sequential developmental tasks can adequately define normality; at any single point in time the most accurate estimation of normality may come from any one of the three other criteria, depending on the particular age, sex, and circumstances of the person being evaluated.

Offer and Sabshin relate the "health," "utopia," and "average" perspectives to medical, psychoanalytic, and social psychological interpretations of normality, respectively, but they refrain from weighing the relative validity of these perspectives. Definitions of normality, like definitions in general, can of course not be adjudged right or wrong on the basis of argument or evidence. The merit of a definition lies in its clarity and utility. Hence the appropriate emphasis for the present discussion must be on a clinically meaningful and useful concept of normality against which psychological disturbance can be evaluated.

The perspective on normality most useful to the practicing clinician would seem to be that of normality as health. To define normality otherwise poses difficult clinical problems. Normality as utopia implies that everyone is psychologically disturbed, more or less. From this perspective the clinician is hard put to identify the particular circumstances that require or justify his professional attention, unless he takes the debatable stance that everyone is more or less in need of psychotherapy.

Health as average implies that the gifted as well as the retarded, the creative as well as the unproductive, and the extremely happy as well as the despondent are psychologically disturbed. It also implies that people manifesting irrational or maladaptive behavior in the context of an extreme situation or mass panic are responding normally, because theirs is the modal response in the given circumstance. Relying on the average as an index of normality, the clinician would not bother to treat victims of an epidemic or endemic condition, whatever its consequences, because they would be "normal." From the clinical point of view it is unwarranted automatically to interpret modal behavior as behavior that does not call for professional assistance.

Yet judgments about normality cannot be completely independent of the context in which behavior occurs. Few would disagree that ritual suicidal behavior has different implications for psychological disturbance in Japan and the United States, primarily because of the different sociocultural values attached to such behavior in the two countries. However, it is possible to encompass the import of sociocultural relativism within the normality-as-health perspective. As Romano and others propose, "health" criteria for normality can be defined to include adequate capacity for social interaction, which implies that the individual is in relative harmony with his immediate society. At the same time, by focusing on freedom from pain, discomfort, and disability, the health perspective of normality avoids the error of labeling as abnormal an individual who calmly meets an emergency or crisis that is unnerving most of those around him.

Those writers who consider normal adolescence to be a disturbed state might interpret the normality-as-health definition as tantamount in adolescents to a definition of normality as utopia; in this framework most adolescents are believed to experience psychological turbulence and distress and hence to be psychologically disturbed. As noted on p. 48, however, there is considerable evidence to suggest that normative adolescence is not a state of psychological disturbance. In other words, the *normative,* or *modal,* adolescent appears also to be a psychologically *normal* adolescent.

This assertion is supported by normative studies, which have assessed the behavior patterns of teenagers randomly chosen from large populations, and also by studies of normal adolescents, which have examined the behavior and experiences of youngsters previously screened for major maladjustments or psychopathology. As reviewed below, both lines of research tend to contradict the notion of psychological disturbance as a widespread or adaptive concomitant of adolescence.

Psychological Patterns of Normative Adolescents

This section focuses on four major, clinically relevant studies of normative adolescent behavior and will not attempt to outline the general psychology of adolescence. The several texts mentioned on page 3 provide extensive surveys of adolescent psychology, and for briefer overviews of adolescence the reader is referred to chapters by Blanchard (1944), Dennis (1946), Horrocks (1954), McCandless (1961), Mussen, Conger, and Kagan (1963, Chapters 13–15), and Stone and Church (1968, Chapters 10 and 11).

The most ambitious recent survey of normative adolescent behavior patterns is the work of Douvan and Adelson (1966), whose salient findings have been noted in Chapter 1 (see pp. 17, 27, and 30). It is pertinent to reemphasize here the considerable breadth and corresponding import of their research design. They and their staff worked with some 3500 adolescents, of whom over 3000 were eventually studied with detailed interviews and questionnaires. These youngsters were carefully chosen to yield a stratified sample representative of virtually the entire United States population of school-age boys from 14 to 16 years old and school-age girls in grades 6 through 13 (see Douvan and Adelson, 1966, pp. 451–457).

Stressing that the merit of their survey technique lies in allowing study of the middle majority of adolescents, Douvan and Adelson conclude that the behavior patterns of normative adolescents contradict the traditional picture of psychological turbulence defined for this age group in the earlier literature. Their data strongly suggest that it is only the adolescent at the extremes who "responds to the instinctual and psychosocial upheaval of puberty by disorder, by failures of ego-synthesis, and by a tendency to abandon earlier values and object attachments" (Douvan and Adelson, 1966, p. 351).

A similarly extensive normative study is reported by Hathaway and Monachesi (1963), who administered the Minnesota Multiphasic Personality Inventory (MMPI) to a Minnesota-wide sample of over 11,000 ninth-grade students. Hathaway and Monachesi found these adolescents' MMPI profiles on the average to demonstrate fewer neurotic but more sociopathic and psychotic features than are normatively observed among adults, and they infer that normal personality occurs less frequently among adolescents than adults (p. 39).

Yet their data also clearly illustrate that personality maladjustment, even as judged from adult norms, is far from modal among adolescents. According to their frequency tables for pathologically elevated scores on the nine clinical scales of the MMPI, scores in the traditional maladjustment range ($T = 70$) for the adolescents' three highest scales occurred at the following rates: for the Psychopathic scale 182 per 1000 among the boys and 199 per 1000 among the girls; for Schizophrenia 186 and 102 per 1000 for boys and girls, respectively; and for Hypomania 210 and 174 per 1000 for boys and girls, respectively (pp. 119–121). In other words, maladjustment as assessed by pathologically elevated scores on any one of their three highest MMPI scales characterized only between 10 and 20% of the adolescents studied by Hathaway and Monachesi.

Intensive studies of individual subjects tend to confirm good adjustment among normative adolescents. Offer, Sabshin, and Marcus (1965) employed pretesting procedures to select 106 boys who were "modal" among their freshmen classmates at two suburban high schools, one drawing its students primarily from mobile middle class and lower middle class families and the other representing a stable upper middle class population. Offer and Sabshin (1966, p. 151) report that repetitive interviewing, psychological testing, and family studies with 84 of these boys identified the modal adolescent boy as (a) being almost completely free from psychopathology, severe physical deficits, or severe physical illness; (b) having mastered previous developmental tasks without serious setbacks; (c) being able to experience affects flexibly and to achieve reasonably successful resolutions of his conflicts; (d) having relatively good object relationships with adults; and (e) feeling a part of a larger cultural environment and being aware of its norms and values.

With specific regard to the normative incidence of psychological disturbance, Offer (1967) reports that the initial studies and a three-year follow-up of these 106 boys revealed serious behavior problems in only three cases and moderately severe emotional problems, including chronic delinquency and prominent character disorder, in only seven others. This 9% incidence of marked psychopathology in the modal high school boys approximates a 12% incidence of clinical disturbance observed among college freshmen boys by Smith, Hansell, and English (1963) and Weiss, Segal, and Sokol (1965). Both of these normative rates of disturbance are considerably smaller than analogous figures for modal adults. Srole et al. (1962, p. 342) found a 23.4% incidence of psychological impairment due to marked, severe, or incapacitating symptoms in a large representative sample of 20- to 59-year-old adults living at home in midtown Manhattan.

A report by Masterson et al. (1966; see also Masterson, 1967a, pp. 137–144) provides a similar basis for comparing the normative incidence of psychopathology in nonpatient adolescents and adults. Masterson et al. assessed symptom patterns in 101 nonpatient adolescents chosen as controls in a study of adolescents accepted for evaluation at the Payne Whitney Clinic. Defining symptom patterns to include even mild manifestations of anxiety or depression, Masterson et al. found only 17% of these nonpatient adolescents to be completely free from symptoms; however, only 20% of this group demonstrated moderate or severe impairments of school and/or social functioning.

This 20% incidence of moderate or severe impairment among nonpatient adolescents approximates the 23.4% incidence for adults noted by Srole et al. The 17% incidence of symptom-free adolescents also corresponds closely to the Srole et al. data, which list 18.5% of the normative adults as free from symptoms (p. 342). Thus among adolescents and adults alike about 60% of persons demonstrate subclinical forms of symptom formation and the remaining 40% are equally divided between symptom-free and moderately or severely impaired groups. These data clearly indicate that adolescents in general are no more likely than other segments of the population to display features of psychological maladjustment.

Psychological Patterns of Normal Adolescents

The above studies of normative adolescents are complemented by several investigations of behavior patterns in adolescents previously identified as psychologically normal or competent. Westley (1958) and his colleagues selected for study 20 college freshmen who had demonstrated good social and academic adjustment and relative freedom from psychiatric symptoms. These normal late adolescents were found to manifest an impressive array of psychologically adaptive characteristics—including capacity for love and trust of others, an inherent sense of autonomy based on healthy self-esteem, freedom of action based on a satisfactorily developed conscience, adequate capacity to work for mastery within individual limitations of ability, a sense of ego identity, and acceptance and enjoyment of sexual impulses (see Epstein, 1958).

Grinker (1962) similarly studied a group of 65 college freshman males who had displayed no psychotic, neurotic, or disabling personality traits and for whom he suggests the label "homoclites," meaning people who follow the common rule. In clinical interviews these "homoclites" generally evinced effective coping devices; a high degree of ethics, morality, and honesty; good capacity for adequate human relationships; little heterosexual experimentation; fairly strong impulse control; and a realistic self-image *achieved without identity crisis*.

Equally compelling evidence of adequate coping behaviors and minimal turbulence among normal adolescents has emerged from several studies by Silber, Coelho, and their co-workers of competent high school and college students. Silber, Hamburg, Coelho, Murphey, Rosenberg, and Pearlin (1961) initially selected 15 senior boys and girls whose high school careers had been marked by academic success, close interpersonal relationships with peers, and active participation in social groups. In repeated individual interviews Silber et al. observed that these competent adolescents employ a number of effective coping behaviors, reach out for new experience, deal actively with challenge, and find considerable enjoyment in the sense of mastery.

Silber et al. (1961, p. 365) also noted considerable industriousness and productivity among their subjects and correspondingly little of the adolescent conservatism and conflict avoidance reported by Douvan and Adelson (see p. 30):

"The active search for manageable levels of challenge in newness is more characteristic of the coping behavior of competent adolescents than a stabilized adaptation to the environment with maximal reduction of tension."

In subsequent work Silber, Coelho, Murphey, Hamburg, Pearlin, and Rosenberg (1961) and Coelho, Hamburg, and Murphey (1963) explored these adolescents' decisions about college and their adjustment during their first college year. They found a continuing pattern of effective coping techniques for dealing with the social and academic challenges of the transition from high school to college, and they reaffirmed their impression of active and energetic confrontation of developmental tasks by these young people:

"As part of their general coping strategies most of these students, covering a fairly wide range of mental ability, were typically active in exploring problem-solving opportunities and used them in a way that reinforced their self-image as effective doers, working toward valued goals" (Coelho et al., 1963, p. 442).

It may be that the divergence between these findings and the conservative picture of normative adolescents painted by Douvan and Adelson is primarily a function of the superiority of the Silber and Coelho adolescents, whose attainments are clearly above average. In this regard, Offer and Sabshin (1966, p. 145) suggest that the data of Silber et al. and Coelho et al. describing psychological mechanisms used by high school students in the transition to college may be incomplete. Specifically they recommend further research to determine whether such superior students are broadly well adjusted or whether their competence in the transition from high school to college is achieved at the expense of overcompensation in such other areas as sexual adjustment and interpersonal relationships.

Although additional clinical studies of normal adolescents are certainly needed, existing work by Havighurst and Schoeppe tends to obviate Offer and Sabshin's particular concern. Schoeppe and Havighurst (1952) evaluated the status of a group of adolescents in reference to the following nine developmental tasks outlined by Havighurst (1951) as central to adolescent adjustment:

1. Accepting one's physique and sexual role.
2. Establishing new peer relationships.
3. Attaining emotional independence of parents.
4. Achieving assurance of economic independence.
5. Choosing and preparing for an occupation.
6. Developing intellectual skills and concepts necessary for civic competence.
7. Acquiring socially responsible behavior patterns.
8. Preparing for marriage and family life.
9. Building conscious values that are harmonious with one's environment.

Schoeppe and Havighurst found clear positive relationships between good achievement on any one of these tasks and good performance on the others. Their data justify the expectation that the competent adolescents studied by Silber et al. matched their adaptive transition from high school to college with equally adaptive modes of coping with interpersonal relationships and other aspects of adjustment. Such an expectation is consistent with the widely acknowledged findings of the Terman *Genetic Studies of Genius* (see Terman and Oden, 1951), which demonstrated superior personal, professional, and social attainments in the later lives of intellectually gifted children.

The consistent findings of the studies by Westley, by Grinker, and by Silber et al. strongly suggest that, contrary to generalizations from restricted clinical samples, there is little basis for anticipating psychological disruption and maladaptive behavior in normal adolescents. The following remarks of Horrocks (1954, p. 700) appear to be well substantiated by available data:

"If the environment is such that the adolescent can gradually be inducted into experiences for which he is prepared and with which he is able to cope, if he is allowed to assume responsibility and play a mature role when he is ready to do so, and if there is a real effort on the part of adults to accept his interests and, where possible, to meet his needs, the adolescent will find his transition into maturity comparatively smooth and uncomplicated."

ADOLESCENT TURMOIL AS A REFLECTION OF DEVIANT ADJUSTMENT

The conceptualization of adolescence as a normatively disturbed state is challenged not only by evidence that the modal adolescent does not display prominent psychological turmoil but also by empirical indications that a turbulent adolescence, when it does occur, reflects deviant and not normative adjustment. As noted on page 43, interpretations of adolescence as a normatively turbulent developmental period frequently emphasize the identity crisis. The following discussion is accordingly focused on research findings in three areas relevant to identity formation: intrafamilial relationships, identification patterns, and self-image consistency.

Intrafamilial Relationships

Numerous studies reveal that adolescents who experience or report marked conflict with, or alienation from, their families tend also to demonstrate impaired psychological adjustment. Reviewing early research on relationships between adolescents and their parents, Partridge (1939) concluded that good adjustment during adolescence is typically accompanied by intimate and confidential relationships with parents, whereas boys and girls who are unable to establish and maintain harmonious and confidential relationships with their parents are much more likely to be demonstrably maladjusted. In another early contribution Stott (1940) reported a negative relationship between adjustment and criticism of parents, with those adolescents who were most critical of their parents displaying the poorest adjustment on personality tests.

These early results have been confirmed in later, more intensive investigations by Peck (1958) and Marcus et al. (1966). Peck conducted repetitive interviews, sociometric analyses, and projective test examinations with 34 ten- to eighteen-year-old adolescents and their families and found a positive relation between several measures of ego strength in these youngsters and a family life characterized by stable consistency and reciprocal warmth, trust, and approval. Conversely, indices of intrafamilial disharmony were associated with evidence of immature, irrational, and socially maladaptive behavior in the adolescent.

Marcus et al. found that the families of adolescents with diagnosed psychopathology were markedly less able to communicate with each other than were families of nonpatient controls. Relative to the nonpatient adolescents, the disturbed youngsters had greater difficulty in understanding their parents' expectations for them, and their parents in turn had greater difficulty in understanding their youngsters' descriptions of themselves. Thus a pattern of poor or impeded intrafamilial communication was directly related to the existence of psychological maladjustment in the adolescent. Interestingly, nondisturbed siblings of the patient group were found to communicate with their parents better than their disturbed siblings, but not as well as the controls.

A similar relationship between turbulent intrafamilial relationships and relatively impaired adjustment has been demonstrated even within essentially normal or superior adolescents. Among the competent adolescents studied by Silber et al. (see p. 000), the youngsters who demonstrated better developed autonomy and capacity for relatedness also indicated stronger patterns of identification with their parents and greater experience of their parents' confidence in them (Murphey et al., 1963). Those who expressed relatively less clarity about their parents' values and less feeling of parental confidence in them, on the other hand, also tended to display relatively limited autonomy and relatedness. The narrow range of adolescent behavior within which these important relationships occurred—that is, within a preselected group of competent youngsters—emphasizes the extent to which any disturbances of intrafamilial relationships, far from being a normal concomitant of adolescent development, may accompany and reflect adjustment difficulties.

Although focused on phenomenology rather than etiology, this discussion of the relationship between familial disharmony and adolescent maladjustment bears generally on the question of whether parameters of family interaction influence personality patterns and psychopathologic tendencies.

The widely held view that family experiences exert a major impact on personality development has been challenged in a review by Frank (1965, p. 201):

"We end this survey by concluding that we have not been able to find any unique factors in the family of the schizophrenic which distinguishes it from the family of controls, who are ostensibly free from evidence of patterns of gross psychopathology. In short, we end by stating that the assumption that the family is *the* factor in the development of personality has not been validated."

If Frank is correct, it may be misleading to infer from some observed correlations between family conflict and adolescent maladjustment that adolescent turmoil is deviant behavior. However, other researchers have challenged Frank's conclusion and affirmed the relevance of intrafamilial relationship patterns to personality and behavioral variables; for example, in a series of important studies focused specifically on adolescent subjects Heilbrun and his coworkers have demonstrated significant relationships between perceived parental behavior and adjustment. In summarizing these experiments Heilbrun (1966) points out methodological weaknesses in many of the negative studies cited by Frank and concludes:

"Accordingly, a relationship between perceived maternal control and psychological disturbance had been established with a standard procedure in both sexes of offspring and in both seriously disturbed and relatively normal populations" (p. 159).

Such relationships between maternal behavior and adjustment have been confirmed in both early and late adolescent groups. Vogel and Lauterbach (1963) compared the intrafamilial patterns of approximately 14-year-old behaviorally disturbed and normal adolescent boys and found that the behavior-problem adolescents tended more than the controls to perceive their mothers as controlling and as "physically controlling." Nikelly (1967) reports significant differences in the perception of their mothers between college students receiving psychotherapy and nonpatient controls, with the treatment group regarding their mothers as being more selfish and demanding, more pampering and overprotective, and less tolerant and less concerned for their welfare. Other studies by Heilbrun and his students have established relationships between intrafamilial patterns and a variety of attitudinal and performance variables:

"More precisely, the accrued experimental evidence supports the importance of the late adolescent's perception of the mother's child-rearing behavior as a mediating factor in his cognitive and motivational behavior within a social context" (Heilbrun, Harrell, and Gillard, 1967, pp. 277–278).

Taken together these studies appear to justify the conclusions (a) that an adolescent's actual or perceived relationship to his parents is significantly related to his personality style in general and to his adjustment level in particular, and (b) that actual or perceived conflict, disharmony, and mutual dissatisfaction in relation to their parents tend in adolescents to be associated with deviant rather than adaptive adjustment.

Identification Patterns

As a further challenge to the interpretation of turbulent family relationships as a normal adolescent phenomenon a number of studies suggest that weak parental identification in adolescents is associated with psychological maladjustment. Gray (1959) assessed the adjustment and the perceived similarity to their parents of a group of fifth- to eighth-grade students and found that the boys in her sample who displayed the strongest identification with their fathers were also the better adjusted boys. For the girls, however, her data yielded the opposite result: those who considered themselves more like their mothers tended to be those who were rated less favorably by their peers on measures relating to adjustment.

Several writers have commented on the apparently different implications of parental identification in early adolescent boys and girls. Lynn (1959) attributes these differences to the impact on developing young girls of cultural emphases on masculine activities and prerogatives; he postulates that with age boys become relatively more firmly identified with the masculine role, whereas girls become less firmly identified with the feminine role. In a similar vein Webb (1963) reviews a number of studies suggesting that adjustment in early adolescence is enhanced by masculine sex-role preferences in boys but by flexible sex-role preferences in girls. Although Webb's own comparisons between social acceptance and the femininity scale of the California Personality Inventory yielded somewhat inconsistent results, he did find a positive relationship between high anxiety and high femininity among ninth-grade girls.

Gray (1959), however, does not regard these differences between boys and girls as negating the general relationship between weak parental identification and poor adjustment. She cites extrapolations from earlier studies by Tryon (1939) and Tuddenham (1951) indicating that the general devaluation of feminine characteristics observed among junior high school girls gives way to a reendorsement of femininity and feminine-role models when the girls reach age 14 or 15. Hence, she concludes, lack of identification with the mother would be expected to be associated with poor social adjustment among middle and late adolescent girls, just as weak paternal identification has negative implications for adjustment among boys.

Cross-cultural data reported by Abramson (1961) lend support to Gray's conclusion. In studying 16- and 17-year-old girls and their mothers in a South African village undergoing rapid changes in its traditional patterns he found a direct relationship between emotional disturbance and mother-daughter discrepancies in attitudes, regardless of the direction of the discrepancy. That is, the daughters of mothers who were clinging to traditional ways suffered disturbance to the extent they were rejecting traditional patterns in favor of more modern attitudes; conversely, where the mothers were relatively modern, daughters who remained relatively traditional gave more evidence of emotional disturbance than those who shared with their mothers the move toward new patterns.

As for middle adolescent boys, Cava and Raush (1952) found a direct relationship between perceived dissimilarity from their fathers and the amount of conflict shown by projective tests among high school senior boys. At the late adolescent level Sopchak (1952) confirmed the importance of parental identification for the adjustment of college students of both sexes. He asked his subjects to complete the Minnesota Multiphasic Personality Inventory (MMPI) for themselves and also as they thought both their mothers and fathers would. For both males and females he found a close association between low perceived identification with parents, as measured by dissimilar MMPI profiles, and MMPI indices of abnormality.

Sopchak also reports, however, that failure to identify with the father was more closely associated with abnormal tendencies than failure to identify with the mother *for both sexes.* In his female subjects in fact the degree of identification with mother was positively correlated with certain types of abnormality. This finding appears to be consistent with the already noted suggestion of Lynn and Webb that masculine cultural emphases account for some relationship in girls between strong feminine identifications and adjustment difficulties.

Another possible interpretation of the coincidence of strong maternal identification and patterns of abnormality in some late adolescent girls is proposed in work by Heilbrun and McKinley (1962) and Heilbrun (1964). They divided 108 college girls into relatively poor and relatively good adjustment groups on the basis of their MMPI profiles. The relatively poorly adjusted group, in relation to the better adjusted girls, were found to perceive their mothers as significantly more authoritarian and controlling and as significantly more inclined to reject their homemaking role. At the same time these relatively poorly adjusted girls themselves demonstrated more masculine personality patterns than did their better adjusted peers.

Additional measures administered to 48 of these subjects revealed that the relatively maladjusted girls perceived themselves as more similar to their mothers than did the relatively well adjusted girls. Heilbrun (1964) concludes from these studies that the association between maladjustment and maternal identification in his subjects derived from the extent to which the relatively maladjusted girls (a) perceived their mothers as masculine and authoritarian and (b) achieved identification with them at the price of a maladaptive rejection of feminine roles.

In other words, a late adolescent girl who strongly identifies with her mother may experience adjustment difficulties either because of hyperfeminine orientations at variance with generally masculine cultural values or because of excessive masculinity adopted from her mother, which also impedes smooth social adjustment. Further consideration of these or other alternative explanations for the Sopchak and Heilbrun findings would require a more precise definition of masculine and feminine values and a more extensive review of research on the identification process than is relevant to the present discussion. As they stand, however, these studies do indicate that, although an adolescent's strong identification with the parent of the same sex may not always ensure his good adjustment, particularly if the parent identified with has adjustment problems of his own, the failure to establish and/or report parental identifications of some sort is likely to be associated with psychological disturbance and not with normal development.

In concluding this section it is important to note that many of the above studies are subject to the criticism raised by Child (1954, p. 163) that measures of *perceived* similarity may indicate only a youngster's *projected* similarity to his parents and not necessarily any *actual* similarity to them. This possibility notwithstanding, available data from direct studies of identification patterns support the already cited research. Payne and Mussen (1956) compared independent responses to a personality questionnaire by 11th and 12th grade boys and by their parents. For these boys identification with father, as measured by actual similarity of father and son responses, was positively related to the boys' masculinity of attitudes, their perception of the father as a rewarding and affectionate person, and their degree of calmness and friendliness as rated by their teachers.

In a later study of 12th grade boys Mussen (1961) confirmed a significant positive relationship between masculine interests, thematic portrayal of the father as a positive and rewarding figure, and good adjustment. He concludes that masculine identification and a positive attitude toward the father in adolescent boys are associated with a degree of contentment, relaxation, happiness, calmness, and smooth social functioning that is not found in the absence of a good father-son relationship. Studying boys of Italian descent in both Italy and in the United States Mussen, Young, Gaddini, and Morante (1963) further demonstrated that a strong identification with father, based on an affectionate relationship with him, is conducive to the establishment of good personal and social adjustment in adolescent boys; boys with weaker identifications, on the other hand, are likely to have fewer friends, to feel less competent to deal with environmental circumstances, and to feel less socially secure and independent.

In a discussion of such weak identificatory patterns Greenson (1954) suggests that an adolescent's failure to manifest strong parental identification may in part result from an active struggle against identification. He outlines a number of neurotic concerns that can contribute to a resistance to identification, including fears of competing with the same-sex parent or being rejected by the opposite-sex parent. Without speculating further here on the maladaptive orientations that may interfere with parental identification in the adolescent boy or girl, it certainly appears justified to reemphasize the indications from available data that a teenage pattern of negative attitudes toward parents and reluctance to emulate them or acknowledge similarities to them is an index of psychological disturbance and not of normal adolescent development.

Consistency of Self-Image

In opposition to the view that role diffusion and experimentation with identities is a normative and adaptive characteristic of late adolescence, several studies demonstrate that, even within populations of relatively healthy college students, inconsistent self-images tend to be associated with psychological maladjustment. For example, Cartwright (1957) asked students with psychoneurotic difficulties who were applying to a university counseling center and nonclient controls to complete three Q-sort measures in which they described themselves as they were with each of three important people in their lives. She found (a) that the clients displayed more variability among these sortings than the controls and (b) that on retesting clients who were considered to have had a successful treatment course showed greater change toward increased consistency of self-description than did the less successfully treated clients. In a replication and extension of this study Cartwright (1961) confirmed both lower self-consistency in clients than in controls and increasing self-consistency in clients in the course of successful psychotherapy.

Block (1961) similarly asked college students to characterize their own behavior with eight other people by rank-ordering a list of self-descriptive adjectives eight times. Interpersonal consistency as indicated by these self-descriptions correlated significantly (.52) with maladjustment as measured by the Psychoneuroticism scale of the California Personality Inventory. Interestingly, Block failed to confirm his hypothesis that persons with relatively little role variability would also display adjustment difficulties.

These indications that inconsistent self-images and prominent role experimentation may reflect psychological disturbance rather than normative adolescent development are supported in studies by Heilbrun and Goodstein (1961) and by Heilbrun (1963) of relationships between social values and social behavior. Heilbrun and Goodstein had college students complete the Edwards Personality Preference Scale first to describe themselves and again two months later in terms of the social desirability they attached to the scale items. Significantly more of the students who demonstrated relatively large discrepancies between their estimates of social desirability and their own behavior subsequently requested counseling for adjustment difficulties; in fact none of the group with relatively little such discrepancy (i.e., below the median value for the sample) appeared at the university counseling center during the follow-up period of the study. Heilbrun repeated this measure of social-behavior consistency with a group of college students who were also given the MMPI. He found significant differences in adjustment between the upper and lower quartiles of his sample: the students who showed the lowest correlation between behaviors endorsed as desirable and behaviors reported as self-characteristic appeared to be more schizoid and more anxious than the students who showed high self-consistency.

In sum these research findings in the areas of intrafamilial relationships, identification patterns, and consistency of self-image strongly suggest that the adolescent who gets along poorly with his family and is unable or unwilling to identify with his parents and their values is not a normal youngster demonstrating developmental vagaries common to his age group. Rather, together with the late adolescent who is still frequently varying the role he plays in relation to other people, he is likely to be suffering adjustment disturbances.

PSYCHOPATHOLOGIC IMPLICATIONS OF SYMPTOM FORMATION IN ADOLESCENTS

Contrary to impressions that apparent symptom formation in adolescents is a normal, transient, self-limited, and spontaneously remitting phenomenon (see pp. 41–43), accumulating evidence suggests that symptoms of psychological disturbance warrant as much concern and professional attention in adolescents as they do in adults. Some clinicians take an intermediate position on this issue by stressing developmental history rather than presenting symptoms in distinguishing normal from abnormal behavior in adolescents: "It is only when a developmental reconstruction can be made in the course of diagnosis and therapy that a clear distinction between pathology and the normal adolescent process can be attempted" (Sprince, 1964, p. 103). Yet, despite the unquestionable importance of historical data in assessing the specific nature and severity of a psychological disturbance, symptom formation alone is often grounds for diagnosing psychopathology in the teenage youngster and instituting appropriate treatment.

In documenting this assertion it is important to note that various writers have used the term "serious" somewhat differently in their discussions of symptom formation in adolescents. For some "not serious" means "not psychopathologic" and "not requiring diagnostic assessment or treatment"; for others "not serious" indicates only (a) that a given constellation of symptoms in an adolescent may reflect a lesser degree of disturbance than it would in an adult and (b) that the disturbance present may accordingly be more amenable to conservative treatment procedures than it would in the older person.

The latter interpretation of "serious" is expressed by Gallagher and Harris (1964, p. 67), who state that, although adolescents may display as transient phenomena symptoms that in an adult would be diagnostic of severe and chronic disturbance, such symptoms nevertheless demand expert attention when they arise. Gillespie and Lay (1936, p. 1129) similarly regard adolescent symptoms as developmental rather than established disturbances of function but stress the importance of undoing such "faulty tendencies" before unretraceable lines of deviant development are established.

Contemporary clinical and research findings, as reviewed below, do not challenge this latter position regarding adolescent symptomatology. They do, however, strongly contradict the belief that psychological symptoms in adolescents can for the most part be ignored, at least with respect to professional assistance, in the expectation that the young person will grow out of them.

The Symptomatic Adolescent Research Project

The currently most extensive data concerning the implications of symptom formation in adolescents have emerged from the Symptomatic Adolescent Research Project, conducted by Masterson and his co-workers at the Payne Whitney Clinic (summarized in Masterson, 1967a, 1968), which seriously challenges a benign view of adolescent symptom formation. The project began with a detailed evaluation of 101 twelve- to eighteen-year-old boys and girls seen consecutively as patients at the Payne Whitney Clinic and 101 carefully matched (age, grade, sex, race, religion, and type of school attended) controls who had never been seen for psychological evaluation or psychotherapy. Case records, interviews, questionnaires, and home visits provided the raw data for the study, which focused on establishing the frequency of various symptom patterns in the patient and control groups (Masterson et al., 1966; see p. 52).

Masterson et al. found psychiatric symptoms to be fairly common among their nonpatient controls: approximately 65% presented anxiety symptoms and 41% gave evidence of some depressive phenomena. As noted on page 52, however, the incidence of moderate or severe psychological impairment among these adolescents closely approximates findings for normative adults. Furthermore Masterson et al. had little difficulty in discriminating the patients from the control group on the basis of their symptom patterns. In the first place the patient group demonstrated far more frequent symptoms than did the controls. Despite the controls' high incidence of anxiety and depression, the patients still exceeded them in overall incidence of symptom patterns by a 50% margin.

Second, several symptom patterns that occurred frequently among the patients were rarely present in the controls. Seventeen percent of the controls presented no symptom patterns at all, and for another 54% anxiety or depression was the principal symptom picture. In contrast, only 4% of the patients failed to demonstrate some symptoms, and anxiety or depression as the principal symptom accounted for but another 33% of this group. On the other hand, 17% of the patients but only 5% of the controls manifested acting-out behavior as the principal symptom pattern; schizophrenia was the principal picture in 16% of the patients but in only 4% of the controls; and principal symptom patterns of hypochondriasis, hysterical personality disorder, conversion reaction, or psychophysiologic reaction characterized 15% of the patients but did not occur at all in the controls.

These data suggest that, when symptom patterns occur in adolescents, particularly symptoms other than anxiety and depression, they represent psychological disturbance and warrant professional attention. Unfortunately such an inference from the findings by Masterson et al. is attenuated by the fact that they defined their experimental and control groups according to patient-nonpatient status. The varying circumstances that determine who becomes a patient confound attempts to define relatively well-adjusted and relatively poorly adjusted samples solely on the basis of patient status.

Recognizing this problem, Masterson and Washburne (1966) reevaluated the adolescents in the project to select a "psychiatrically ill" group from among the patients and a "relatively healthy" group from among the nonpatients. They then studied the symptom patterns and functioning impairments evinced by these newly defined disturbed and healthy groups. Their findings were entirely consistent with the earlier report by Masterson et al. and even more strongly suggest (a) a much greater incidence of symptom patterns among disturbed than among healthy adolescents and (b) the special likelihood that symptoms other than anxiety and depression are indicative of psychopathology in adolescents.

A problematic feature of the Masterson and Washburne study, however, is that the criteria they used to establish the "psychiatrically ill" and "relatively healthy" groups were identical to the variables they were investigating—namely, incidence of symptoms and impairment of social and academic functioning. Because of this contamination of their independent and dependent variables, the authors have demonstrated merely that the adolescents who were judged to have more, or more severe, symptoms and/or greater impairments of functioning (the "psychiatrically ill") turn out to display more symptomatology and greater impairment than those who were judged to be relatively healthy.

Despite this difficulty with design, the Masterson and Washburne report contains valuable data that are not affected by such contamination of variables. Although the disturbed and nondisturbed groups were defined independently of their family backgrounds, for example, Masterson and Washburne observed marked differences between them in their familial interaction patterns. The "relatively healthy" youngsters tended to come from relatively benign home environments in which both parents were present and shared accepting, constructive attitudes toward their teenage children. These healthy adolescents in turn displayed a positive regard for their parents and their siblings, and their intrafamilial conflicts tended to center around such superficial matters as dress, hours, allowance, and dating. This observed restriction of disputes to fairly mundane matters corresponds to the normative adolescent patterns noted by Douvan and Adelson (see p. 27).

The "psychiatrically ill" adolescents, on the other hand, were frequently enmeshed in relatively unsatisfactory, unrewarding familial interactions. Their parents were likely to be absent or to be manifesting their own psychopathology through domineering, rejecting, or oversolicitous relationships with their children. These disturbed youngsters were commonly in marked and chronic conflict with their parents, and these conflicts usually involved long-standing, fundamental issues rather than such day-to-day practical matters as dress or dating. Thus the Masterson and Washburne data appear to demonstrate distinct clustering of marked symptom formation, impaired school and social functioning, and a turbulent family situation on the one hand, and relative freedom from symptoms, minimal functioning impairment, and smooth, rewarding family relationships on the other.

Masterson (1967b) was able to reevaluate 72 of the 101 adolescent patients in the project 2½ years after the original study and again 5 years after the study, when their average age was 21. In the follow-up interviews the subjects were rated for minimal, mild, moderate, and severe psychological impairment. Although more than half the group had received some sort of treatment subsequent to their initial evaluation, Masterson found that 62% of them demonstrated moderate or severe impairment at the five-year follow-up. In other words, approximately two-thirds of these adolescent patients clearly did not grow out of their difficulties. Furthermore, of the 27 subjects only minimally or mildly impaired at follow-up, most continued to show some symptomatology (such as anxiety, depression, or mild phobic complaints), and Masterson concluded that those who had been helped by treatment or who had improved spontaneously had found ways of dealing better with their conflicts but had not fully resolved them. Masterson does not delineate further the relationship between psychotherapy and improvement, although he does note that 16 of the 30 adolescents in the sample treated at the Payne Whitney Clinic were improved at follow-up.

This compelling evidence of persistent psychopathology in disturbed adolescents firmly buttresses Masterson's three main arguments:

1. There is no common picture of "adolescent turmoil" simulating major psychopathology.

2. There is no basis for blandly assuming that an adolescent will "grow out of" most adjustment difficulties he manifests.

3. The indiscriminate application of "adolescent turmoil" and "he'll-grow-out-of-it" notions to symptomatic adolescents runs the grave risk of discouraging the professional attention that may be necessary to avert serious psychological disturbance:

"The symptomatic adolescent is believed to step to a different drummer only temporarily under the surge of the adolescent growth process. However, the music to which these adolescents stepped was not a transient melody orchestrated by growth and development but a persistent and pervasive symphony arranged by psychiatric illness. Its somber cadence pursued these patients through their adolescent years into adulthood. Adolescence was but a way station in a long history of psychiatric illness that began in childhood and followed its own inexorable course—a course only temporarily colored by the developmental state of adolescence. The decisive influence was psychiatric illness, not 'adolescent turmoil' " (Masterson, 1967b, p. 1343).

Psychological Symptoms in College Students

The psychopathologic implications of symptom formation have in part been demonstrated among college students as well as among younger adolescents. In a paper entitled "The Happy College Student Myth" Selzer (1960) advances the same view of "adolescent turmoil" among late adolescent patients as Masterson propounds for 12- to 18-year-olds. Selzer challenges reports from college health centers that minimize the extent of psychological disturbance among student patients. Too often, he suggests, the clinician's busy schedule and the student's youth and academic prowess combine to abbreviate diagnostic evaluations. As a result, he continues, euphemistic, superficial, or wastebasket diagnoses—of which "adolescent turmoil" and "adolescent adjustment reaction" are prime examples—are assigned to student patients with inordinate frequency.

Selzer concludes from his experience at the University of Michigan Mental Hygiene Clinic that the patients applying there are diagnostically comparable to patients seen in any public psychiatric clinic. He found an incidence of fewer than 10% of adjustment reactions in a sample of over 500 student patients, which corresponds closely to the 15% incidence of transient situational personality disturbance observed in adult outpatient clinics (*Outpatient Psychiatric Clinics,* 1966, pp. 6–7). On the other hand, over 80% of Selzer's sample were clearly diagnosable in the three major categories of psychoneurosis, personality disorder, and schizophrenia. Similar data are reported from Boston University, where Swartz, Posin, and Kaye (1958) found that 78% of all students seeking psychiatric help over a four-year period presented emotional problems of long duration, full-blown neuroses, or character disorders.

Yet Selzer does not intend to imply that psychopathology is particularly common or widespread among college students. Indeed he reports that the yearly patient load at the Mental Hygiene Clinic comprises but 8% of the University of Michigan student body. This incidence rate approximates the experience of most campus clinics: surveys by Gundle and Kraft (1956), Whittington (1963, p. 28), and Wilms (1965) indicate that the average yearly rate of students seen in the mental health units of American colleges and universities is 5% of the student population. What Selzer does emphasize is that emotional disorders experienced by college students are *not* largely situational or transient and are no less serious than similar difficulties occurring in the rest of the population.

Thus late adolescents whose symptoms or adjustment difficulties bring them to professional attention are likely to be suffering from psychopathology that warrants such attention, rather than from transient developmental phenomena that will pass with time. Masterson (1967a, p. 158), who would emphatically endorse such a conclusion, stresses that the clinician's diagnostic dilemma does not lie in whether a seriously troubled youngster is psychologically disturbed or is merely experiencing an adolescent adjustment reaction; the youngster is in all likelihood disturbed, and the major challenge is in making an exact clinical diagnosis of his disturbance. Offer (1966, p. 1247) similarly asserts, "We should . . . realize that an adolescent in severe turmoil is disturbed and will most probably continue to be disturbed later in life unless he is treated psychotherapeutically."

It is interesting to note that, although these conclusions derive from recently emerging data and are often presented as corrective to earlier extrapolations from psychoanalytic experience, they in fact merely turn back the clock to views expressed early in this century. The following comments by Burr in a 1905 paper, "Insanity at Puberty," adroitly summarize the data of the 1960s:

"Any mental abnormality occurring during the developmental period is of importance, however trifling it may seem in itself, as indicating mental instability or a tendency toward deviation from the normal, which under proper education may be corrected, but which if left uncorrected will certainly lead to disaster in the future" (p. 36).

In summary, then, studies of normative and normal samples of adolescents demonstrate that adolescents in general are no more likely than other segments of the population to display features of psychopathology and that there is little basis for anticipating psychological disruption and maladaptive behavior in normal adolescents. Furthermore, investigations of intrafamilial relationships, identification patterns, and self-image consistency reveal that, contrary to hypotheses derived from the notion of the normative identity crisis, those adolescents who get along poorly with their families, are unable or unwilling to identify with their parents and with parental values, and frequently alter the role they play in relation to others are likely to be deviant youngsters and not normal young people demonstrating developmental vagaries common to their age group. Finally, accumulating evidence suggests that symptoms of psychological disturbance warrant concern and professional attention as much in adolescents as they do in adults and for the most part cannot be ignored in the expectation that the young person will in time grow out of them.

REFERENCES

Abramson, J. H. Observations on the health of adolescent girls in relation to cultural change. *Psychosomatic Medicine,* **23**:156–165, 1961.

Ackerman, N. W. *The Psychodynamics of Family Life.* New York: Basic Books, 1958.

Beres, D. Character formation. In S. Lorand and H. I. Schneer, eds., *Adolescents: Psychoanalytic Approach to Problems and Therapy*. New York: Hoeber, 1961, pp. 1–9.

Bernfeld, S. Über eine typische form der männlichen Pubertät. (A typical form of male puberty.) *Imago,* 9:169–188, 1923.

Blanchard, P. Adolescent experience in relation to personality and behavior. In J. McV. Hunt, ed., *Personality and the Behavior Disorders,* Vol. II. New York: Ronald, 1944, pp. 691–713.

Block, J. Ego identity, role variability and adjustment. *Journal of Consulting Psychology,* 25:392–397, 1961.

Blos, P. Psychological counseling of college students. *American Journal of Orthopsychiatry,* 16:571–580, 1946.

Blos, P. Prolonged adolescence: The formulation of a syndrome and its therapeutic implication. *American Journal of Orthopsychiatry,* 24:733–742, 1954.

Bronson, G. W. Identity diffusion in late adolescents. *Journal of Abnormal and Social Psychology,* 59:414–417, 1959.

Burr, C. W. Insanity at puberty. *Journal of the American Medical Association,* 45:36–39, 1905

Cartwright, R. D. Effects of psychotherapy on self-consistency. *Journal of Counseling Psychology,* 21:15–22, 1957.

Cartwright, R. D. The effects of psychotherapy on self-consistency: A replication and extension. *Journal of Consulting Psychology,* 25:376–382, 1961.

Cava, E. L., and Raush, H. L. Identification and the adolescent boy's perception of his father. *Journal of Abnormal and Social Psychology,* 47:855–856, 1952.

Child, I. L. Personality. *Annual Review of Psychology,* 5:149–170, 1954.

Coelho, G. V., Hamburg, D. A., and Murphey, E. B. Coping strategies in a new learning environment. *Archives of General Psychiatry,* 9:433–443, 1963.

Dennis, W. The adolescent. In L. Carmichael, ed., *Manual of Child Psychology,* 1st edition. New York: Wiley, 1946, pp. 633–666.

Douvan, E., and Adelson, J. *The Adolescent Experience.* New York: Wiley, 1966.

Epstein, N. B. Concepts of normality or evaluation of emotional health. *Behavioral Science,* 3:335–343, 1958.

Erikson, E. H. *Childhood and Society,* 1st edition. New York: Norton, 1950.

Erikson, E. H. The problem of ego identity. *Journal of the American Psychoanalytic Association,* 4:56–121, 1956.

Erikson, E H. Late adolescence. In D. H. Funkenstein, ed., *The Student and Mental Health.* Cambridge, Mass.: World Federation for Mental Health, 1959, pp. 66–106.

Frank, G. H. The role of the family in the development of psychopathology. *Psychological Bulletin,* 64:191–205, 1965.

Freud, A. Adolescence. *Psychoanalytic Study of the Child,* 13:255–278, 1958.

Gallagher, J. R., and Harris, H. I. *Emotional Problems of Adolescents,* revised edition. New York: Oxford University Press, 1964.

Gardner, G. E. The mental health of normal adolescents. *Mental Hygiene,* **31**:529–540, 1947.

Gardner, G. E. Psychiatric problems of adolescents. In S. Arieti, ed., *American Handbook of Psychiatry,* Vol. I. New York: Basic Books, 1959, pp. 870–892:

Gillespie, R. D., and Lay, R. A. Q. Prognosis of psychological disturbances in childhood and adolescence. *Lancet,* **1**:1129–1131, 1936.

Gray, S. W. Perceived similarity to parents and adjustment. *Child Development,* **30**:97–107, 1959.

Greenson, R. R. The struggle against identification. *Journal of the American Psychoanalytic Association,* **2**:200–217, 1954.

Grinker, R. R. "Mentally healthy" young males (homoclites). *Archives of General Psychiatry,* **6**:405–453, 1962.

Gundle, S., and Kraft, A. Mental health programs in American colleges and universities. *Bulletin of the Menninger Clinic,* **20**:57–69, 1956.

Hathaway, S. R., and Monachesi, E. D. *Adolescent Personality and Behavior.* Minneapolis, Minn.: University of Minnesota Press, 1963.

Havighurst, R. J. *Developmental Tasks and Education.* New York: Longmans, Green, 1951.

Heilbrun, A. B. Social value: Social behavior inconsistency and early signs of psychopathology in adolescence. *Child Development,* **34**:187–194, 1963.

Heilbrun, A. B. Perceived maternal attitudes, masculinity-femininity of the maternal model, and identification as related to incipient psychopathology in adolescent girls. *Journal of General Psychology,* **70**:33–40, 1964.

Heilbrun, A. B. Perceived maternal child-rearing patterns and subsequent deviance in adolescence. *Adolescence,* **1**:152–178, 1966.

Heilbrun, A. B., and Goodstein, L. D. Consistency between social desirability ratings and item endorsement as a function of psychopathology. *Psychological Reports,* **8**:69–70, 1961.

Heilbrun, A. B., Harrell, S. N., and Gillard, B. J. Perceived maternal child-rearing patterns and the effects of social nonreaction upon achievement motivation. *Child Development,* **38**:267–281, 1967.

Heilbrun, A. B., and McKinley, R. A. Perception of maternal child-bearing attitudes, personality of the perceiver, and incipient psychopathology. *Child Development,* **33**:73–83, 1962.

Horrocks, J. E. The adolescent. In L. Carmichael, ed., *Manual of Child Psychology,* 2nd edition New York: Wiley, 1954, pp. 697–734.

Josselyn, I. M. The ego in adolescence. *American Journal of Orthopsychiatry,* **24**:223–227, 1954.

Josselyn, I. M. Psychological changes in adolescence. *Children,* **6**:43–47, 1959.

Knight, R. P. Borderline states. *Bulletin of the Menninger Clinic,* **17**:1–12, 1953.

Lindemann, E. Adolescent behavior as a community concern. *American Journal of Psychotherapy,* **18**:405–417, 1964.

Linton, R. *Culture and Mental Disorders.* Springfield, Ill.: Thomas, 1956.

Lynn, D. B. A note on sex differences in the development of masculine and feminine identification. *Psychological Review,* **66**:126–135, 1959.

McCandless, B. R. *Children and Adolescents: Behavior and Development.* New York: Holt, Rinehart, and Winston, 1961.

Marcia, J. E. Development and validation of ego-identity status. *Journal of Personality and Social Psychology,* **3**:551–558, 1966.

Marcia, J. E. Ego identity status: Relationship to change in self-esteem, "general maladjustment," and authoritarianism. *Journal of Personality,* **35**:119–133, 1967.

Marcus, D., Offer, D., Blatt, S., and Gratch, G. A clinical approach to the understanding of normal and pathologic adolescence. *Archives of General Psychiatry,* **15**:569–576, 1966.

Masterson, J. F. *The Psychiatric Dilemma of Adolescence.* Boston: Little, Brown, 1967a.

Masterson, J. F. The symptomatic adolescent five years later: He didn't grow out of it. *American Journal of Psychiatry,* **123**:1338–1345, 1967b.

Masterson, J. F. The psychiatric significance of adolescent turmoil. *American Journal of Psychiatry,* **124,**1549–1554, 1968.

Masterson, J. F., Corrigan, E. M., Kofkin, M. I., and Wallenstein, H. G. The symptomatic adolescent: Comparing patients with controls. Presented to the American Orthopsychiatric Association, 1966.

Masterson, J. F., and Washburne, A. The symptomatic adolescent: Psychiatric illness or adolescent turmoil? *American Journal of Psychiatry,* **122**:1240–1248, 1966.

Money-Kyrle, R. E. Psycho-analysis and ethics. *International Journal of Psycho-Analysis,* **33**:225–234, 1952.

Murphey, E. B., Silber, E., Coelho, G. V., Hamburg, D. A., and Greenberg, I. Development of autonomy and parent-child interaction in late adolescence. *American Journal of Orthopsychiatry,* **33**:643–652, 1963.

Mussen, P. H. Some antecendents and consequents of masculine sex-typing in adolescent boys. *Psychological Monographs,* **75** (Whole No. 506), 1961.

Mussen, P. H., Conger, J. J., and Kagan, J. *Child Development and Personality,* 2nd edition. New York: Harper and Row, 1963.

Mussen, P. H., Young, H. B., Gaddini, R., and Morante, L. The influence of father-son relationships on adolescent personality and attitudes. *Journal of Child Psychology and Psychiatry,* **4**:3–16, 1963.

Nikelly, A. G. Maternal indulgence and maladjustment in adolescents. *Journal of Clinical Psychology,* **23**:148–150, 1967.

Nixon, R. E. An approach to the dynamics of growth in adolescence. *Psychiatry,* **24**:18–31, 1961.

Nixon, R. E. Psychological normality in adolescence. *Adolescence,* **1**:211–223, 1966.

Offer, D. Discussion of Masterson and Washburne's "The symptomatic adolescent: Psychiatric illness or adolescent turmoil?" *American Journal of Psychiatry,* **122**:1246–1248, 1966.

Offer, D. Normal adolescents: Interview strategy and selected results. *Archives of General Psychiatry,* 17:285–290, 1967.

Offer, D., and Sabshin, M. The psychiatrist and the normal adolescent. *Archives of General Psychiatry,* 9:427–432, 1963.

Offer, D., and Sabshin, M. *Normality: Theoretical and Clinical Concepts of Mental Health.* New York: Basic Books, 1966.

Offer, D., Sabshin, M., and Marcus, D. Clinical evaluation of normal adolescents. *American Journal of Psychiatry,* 121:864–872, 1965.

Outpatient Psychiatric Clinics: Special Statistical Report, 1961. Bethesda, Md.: National Institute of Mental Health, 1963.

Partridge, E. DeA. (1939) Social psychology of adolescence. Cited by P. Blanchard, Adolescent experience in relation to personality and behavior. In J. McV. Hunt, ed., *Personality and the Behavior Disorders,* Vol. II. New York: Ronald, 1944, pp. 691–713.

Payne, D. E., and Mussen, P. H. Parent-child relations and father identification among adolescent boys. *Journal of Abnormal and Social Psychology,* 52:358–362, 1956.

Peck, R. F. Family patterns correlated with adolescent personality structure. *Journal of Abnormal and Social Psychology,* 57:347–350, 1958.

Romano, J. Basic orientation and education of the medical student. *Journal of the American Medical Association,* 143:409–412, 1950.

Sabshin, M. Psychiatric perspectives on normality. *Archives of General Psychiatry,* 17:258–264, 1967.

Schoeppe, A., and Havighurst, R. J. A validation of development and adjustment hypotheses of adolescence. *Journal of Educational Psychology,* 43:339–353, 1952.

Selzer, M. L. The happy college student myth. *Archives of General Psychiatry,* 2:131–136, 1960.

Silber, E., Coelho, G. V., Murphey, E. B., Hamburg, D. A., Pearlin, L. I., and Rosenberg, M. Competent adolescents coping with college decisions. *Archives of General Psychiatry,* 5:517–527, 1961.

Silber, E., Hamburg, D. A., Coelho, G. V., Murphey, E. B., Rosenberg, M., and Pearlin, L. I. Adaptive behavior in competent adolescents: Coping with the anticipation of college. *Archives of General Psychiatry* 5:354–365, 1961.

Smith, W. G., Hansell, N., and English, J. T. Psychiatric disorder in a college population. *Archives of General Psychiatry,* 9:351–361, 1963.

Sopchak, A. Parental "identification" and "tendency toward disorders" as measured by the Minnesota Multiphasic Personality Inventory. *Journal of Abnormal and Social Psychology,* 47:159–165, 1952.

Spiegel, L. A. Identity and adolescence. In S. Lorand and H. I. Schneer, eds., *Adolescents: Psychoanalytic Approach to Problems and Therapy.* New York: Hoeber, 1961, pp. 10–18.

Spivack, G. Child-rearing attitudes of emotionally disturbed adolescents. *Journal of Consulting Psychology,* 21:178, 1957.

Sprince, M. P. A contribution to the study of homosexuality in adolescence. *Journal of Child Psychology and Psychiatry,* **5**:103–117, 1964.

Srole, L., Langner, T. S., Michael, S. T., Opler, M. K., and Rennie, T. A. C. *Mental Health in the Metropolis: The Midtown Manhattan Study.* New York: McGraw-Hill, 1962.

Stone, L. J., and Church, J. *Childhood and Adolescence,* 2nd edition. New York: Random House, 1968.

Stott, L. H. Adolescents' dislikes regarding parental behavior and their significance. *Journal of Genetic Psychology,* **57**:393–414, 1940.

Swartz, J., Posin, H. I., and Kaye, A. Psychiatric problems in an urban university. *Mental Hygiene,* **42**:224–228, 1958.

Terman, L. M., and Oden, M. H. The Stanford studies of the gifted. In P. Witty, ed., *The Gifted Child.* New York: Heath, 1951, pp. 20–37.

Tryon, C. M. Evaluations of adolescent personality by adolescents. *Monographs of the Society for Research in Child Development,* **4** (Whole No. 4), 1939.

Tuddenham, R. D. Studies in reputation. III. Correlates of popularity among elementary school children. *Journal of Educational Psychology,* **42**:257–276, 1951.

Vogel, W., and Lauterbach, C. G. Relationships between normal and disturbed sons' percepts of their parents' behavior, and personality attributes of the parents and sons. *Journal of Clinical Psychology,* **19**:52–56, 1963.

Webb, A. P. Sex-role preference and adjustment in early adolescents. *Child Development,* **34**:609–618, 1963.

Weiner, I. B. *Psychodiagnosis in Schizophrenia.* New York: Wiley, 1966.

Weiss, R. J., Segal, B. E., and Sokol, R. Epidemiology of emotional disturbance in a men's college. *Journal of Nervous and Mental Disease,* **141**:240–250, 1965.

Westley, W. A. Emotionally healthy adolescents and their family backgrounds. In I. Goldstein, ed., *The Family in Contemporary Society.* New York: International Universities Press, 1958.

Whittington, H. G. *Psychiatry on the College Campus.* New York: International Universities Press, 1963.

Wilms, J. H. How much for mental health? *Journal of the American College Health Association,* **13**:422–430, 1965.

CHAPTER 3

Patterns of Psychopathology in Adolescence

Efforts to classify adolescent psychopathology have been challenged by arguments (a) that traditional diagnostic classification is generally an unrealiable and useless procedure and (b) that conventional diagnostic labels are particularly ill-suited to describe the psychological disturbances of adolescents. This chapter compares these arguments with the positive case for pursuing diagnostic classification and then reviews epidemiologic data and clinical reports that delineate the major patterns of psychopathology in adolescence.

CLASSIFICATION OF PSYCHOLOGICAL DISTURBANCE

The diagnostic classification of psychological disturbance, although widely employed in research and clinical practice, has come under heavy attack on both conceptual and empirical grounds. Menninger, Mayman, and Pruyser (1963, Chapters 2 and 3), in a particularly resolute conceptual indictment of traditional diagnosis, have emphasized undesirable nomothetic tendencies intrinsic to all classification schemes: the reification of abstract conceptions of various disorders at the expense of describing the unique behavior patterns manifested by an individual patient; the drawing of global conclusions concerning a patient's difficulties from only minimal similarities between his behavior and the behaviors attributed to a particular syndrome; and the inattention to complex, contradictory phenomena to allow a narrow focus on signs and symptoms that can readily be subsumed within a preconceived nosologic category. Menninger et al. reject diagnostic categories in favor of a proposed unitary concept: "Instead of putting so much emphasis on different kinds of clinical pictures of illness, we propose to think of all forms of mental illness as being essentially the same in quality, and differing in quantity" (p. 32).

Empirical work has additionally questioned the reliability and validity of many traditional diagnostic labels. A number of studies suggest that clinicians have difficulty agreeing on diagnostic impressions, that diagnoses are not notably consistent over time, and that diagnostic labeling has not been particularly helpful in predicting various parameters of psychological disturbance (see Zubin, 1967, pp. 380–394).

Yet many clinicians and researchers regard the potential merits of diagnostic classification as far outweighing its current limitations. Shakow (1966), for one, argues vigorously that the problems inherent in diagnostic categorizations do not preclude their effective clinical utilization. In his view these inherent difficulties will in time yield to increasingly sophisticated and self-critical efforts to study and implement the diagnostic process. He protests any movement to discard classification, which he considers "essential to the objective investigation which is the core of the scientific method," and he maintains that "the systematic study and thought exerted in these past and present attempts at categorization have resulted in advances in our knowledge of mental disorders and will, I believe, continue to provide valuable new insights in the field of psychopathology" (pp. 150 and 151). Eisenberg (1967, pp. 179–180) similarly endorses the quest for adequate nosology:

"That the establishment of a valid and reliable scheme of classification is difficult is no argument against the attempt. We are not here concerned with an obsessional exercise in pigeon-holing patients purely for the convenience of statistical clerks. What is at stake is our ability to recognize and differentiate clinical syndromes, the specification of which will be necessary for effective research on causes and for meaningful attempts to evaluate treatment."

As for empirical critiques of diagnostic classification, Beck (1962) has pointed out that many of the studies reporting diagnostic unreliability have failed to provide an adequate test of the nomenclature itself. Specifically, Ward et al. (1962) demonstrated that fully one-third of the diagnostic disagreements they observed in an empirical study were attributable to variabilities among the diagnosticians, particularly with respect to their capacities to elicit covert material and identify the predominant pathology in mixed pictures. Of the remaining two-third of disagreements, many could be ascribed to requirements for impractically fine or unnecessarily forced decisions, such as having to discriminate psychophysiological from conversion reaction or neurotic symptoms from personality disorder, when both were present. It would thus appear that many empirically demonstrated deficiencies of the diagnostic process could be eliminated by improved training of diagnosticians and relatively minor alterations in the specificity of traditional nomenclature (see also Lehmann, 1967).

Other writers have admitted dissatisfaction with diagnostic labels but agreed with Shakow that formal classification is an essential clinical function that warrants continued research efforts; for example, Nathan (1967) acknowledges the empirical data on which criticisms of traditional diagnostic labels are based (Chapter II) but devotes the remainder of a recent book to developing improved methods of collecting and evaluating behavior descriptions to yield relevant and valid diagnoses of psychopathology:

"The fundamental premise of this book is that clinically relevant and reliable diagnostic procedures for valid behavioral diagnosis can and ultimately will be specified. . . . Lending urgency to efforts to implement this premise is a view of the history of diagnosis that maintains that specification of a set of objective and reliable procedures to diagnose (describe and differentiate) an illness is often a necessary precursor to its successful treatment" (p. 3).

Issues concerning the comparative merit of traditional and revised diagnostic procedures are beyond the scope of this discussion. The present author has previously aired his conviction that adequate classification is essential to fruitful scientific investigation and effective clinical practice (see Weiner, 1966). It is difficult for him to conceive how the origin, course, and indicated treatment of diverse psychological disturbances can be explored without first labeling what these disturbances are. Accordingly, the subsequent chapters of this book emphasize careful diagnostic study as a basic aspect of efforts to aid the troubled teenager.

Diagnostic Classification of Adolescents: Objections

Many writers who take little issue with the diagnostic process in general have objected strenuously to efforts to impose on adolescents the nosological concepts that are traditionally applied to disturbed adults. These objections for the most part derive from the already discussed (see pp. 41–43) view that adolescence is normatively a turbulent, unpredictable time of life in which apparently psychopathologic behavior may occur as transient developmental phenomena. From the postulate that normal adolescent turmoil commonly produces transient symptomatology it follows that any actual emotional disturbance in an adolescent is so likely to be rendered vague, ill-defined, and unstable by the impact of adolescent turmoil that efforts at diagnostic classification are futile. The diagnostic evaluation of adolescents within this frame of reference has consequently focused not on differential diagnosis but primarily on attempts to estimate the eventual outcome of an observed disturbance.

Among prominent spokesmen for this point of view, Ackerman (1958, pp. 231–232) in particular has stressed the extent to which adolescent turmoil obfuscates traditional diagnostic distinctions:

"Regardless of the type of pathology that emerges in adolescence, the typical symptoms of each psychiatric entity are significantly affected by the total dynamic movement characteristic of adolescence. It is therefore an imperative necessity to discern the course and ultimate destination of such movement. . . . But differential diagnosis in the adolescent era presents great difficulties. It is highly complicated by the infinitely changing facades of personality that are characteristic of this period. . . . The task of diagnosis is complicated by the essential fluidity of adolescent personality which imparts relatively ambiguous outlines to all psychiatric entities. In the final analysis, the test of the relative accuracy of clinical diagnosis is the ability to predict successfully the course of future behavior."

Laufer (1965) similarly argues that accurate differential diagnosis of adolescent disturbance requires careful assessment of the interplay between basic pathology and adolescent dynamics. In his view the clinical evaluation of adolescents therefore has much more in common with that of children than of adults. Whereas adults can be assessed solely according to the outcomes of their internalized conflicts, he continues, the problems of adolescents and children represent complex interactions of pathological and developmental processes. He agrees with Ackerman that the necessary distinction between transitory and pathological phenomena in disturbed adolescents is little aided by traditional diagnoses:

"We try to determine whether there already is a deadlock or whether the disturbance represents a temporary defensive measure. In this sense, the psychiatric categories used to describe adult pathology are not suitable in the classification of adolescent disturbances" (p. 120).

Concerns about the appropriateness and utility of diagnostic classification in clinical work with adolescents are by no means limited to these psychoanalytic writers. On the basis of their experience with teenage patients in a state-hospital setting, Edwalds and Dimitri (1959, p. 615) conclude, "At best, diagnostic categories for the adolescent patient are unsatisfactory, since patterns of illness are rarely stable in this age group." Taking a broad behavioral science view, Miller (1962, p. 211) asserts that the clinical diagnosis of adolescent disturbances is difficult because "we have few reliable constants of a physical or psychological nature which would permit us to construct a model for matching the individual against such constants or scales."

Miller's conclusions would seem to overlook the vast and expanding body of normative data concerning the adolescent's physical growth (e.g., Jones, 1949; Tanner, 1962), personality patterns (e.g., Douvan and Adelson, 1966; Havighust and Taba, 1949), sexual attitudes and behavior (e.g., Reiss, 1967; Schofield, 1965), and psychological test performance (e.g., Ames, Metraux, and Walker, 1959; Hathaway and Monachesi, 1963). However, the availability of such data does not alter the fact that diagnostic labeling of adolescents is deprecated in many influential quarters as an inexact and inappropriate procedure that contributes little to clinical work.

Diagnostic Classification of Adolescents: The Positive Case

In polar opposition to the above views in a number of writers staunchly aver (a) that adequate diagnosis of disturbed adolescents is so necessary to their treatment that it must be undertaken whatever its difficulties, (b) that the apparent diagnostic dilemmas posed by adolescent symptom patterns can be resolved by appropriate attention to the patient's history, and (c) that the difficulty imputed to discriminating adolescent psychopathology from normative adolescent phenomena constitutes an erroneous inference from psychoanalytic conceptualizations of adolescence and is not substantiated by empirical data.

Concerning therapeutic intervention, Hamilton (1947, pp. 249–250) among others stresses that adequate treatment planning for disturbed adolescents requires a number of careful diagnostic distinctions, such as whether the patient's unresolved problems are more likely to be expressed in autoplastic (neurotic symptom formation) or alloplastic (acting-out behavior) solutions. As for the utilization of historical data to resolve otherwise perplexing diagnostic pictures in adolescent patients, Finch (1960, Chapter 15) considers the history of preadolescent development among the most important diagnostic criteria in evaluating a symptomatic adolescent. A history of previously adequate personality adjustment in a relatively normal environment minimizes the likelihood of serious emotional disturbance in the adolescent patient and suggests that his symptom formation may be relatively temporary and transient; conversely, evidence of repeated or pervasive emotional problems during his earlier years increases the probability that an adolescent patient's presenting difficulties reflect persistent, diagnosable psychopathology.

Selzer (1960) advocates a similar approach in the diagnostic assessment of college students. He views chronicity as the essential criterion of whether a college student's complaints are more likely to represent a self-limited "adjustment reaction" or a psychopathologic reaction: "A student of college age who chronically retains adolescent attitudes and reactions to the detriment of his emotional, social, and academic life is probably ill—and not merely an (adolescent) adjustment problem" (p. 133).

Masterson (1967a,b) presents an empirical rebuttal of notions that the fluctuating symptomatology of disturbed adolescents precludes any stable clinical picture and that the impact of adolescent turmoil blurs any distinctive diagnostic features in adolescent patients. His data are based on 101 adolescents admitted to the Payne Whitney clinic, 65 of whom were reevaluated $2\frac{1}{2}$ years later and 72 of whom were studied 5 years after their initial contact (see pp. 63–66). Concerning the postulated symptom fluctuation of disturbed adolescents, he draws the following conclusion:

"Some symptom patterns disappear, some increase in incidence, others diminish in intensity to a subclinical level, while still others show a remarkable degree of persistence. . . . We can say that at three different points in their lives (age sixteen, age eighteen, and age twenty-one) these patients showed remarkable persistence in many of their symptom patterns. . . . The clinical picture of these adolescents as they progress through and emerge from adolescence not only tends toward clearer differentiation of diagnostic category but also shows persistence of many symptom patterns" (Masterson, 1967a, p. 117).

As for the role of adolescent turmoil in the disturbances of these adolescent patients, Masterson and his co-workers came to the following clinical judgment during the several years of their study:

"We found that adolescent turmoil was at most an incidental factor subordinate to that of psychiatric illness in the onset, course, and outcome of the various conditions of our patients. . . . The decisive influence was psychiatric illness, not adolescent turmoil. The latter exerted its effect primarily by exacerbating and giving its own coloring to preexistent pathology. . . . Although we must continue to view adolescent turmoil as a universal psychodynamic factor, its clinical psychiatric effects are surely far less significant than was previously thought. It plays a role subordinate to that of psychiatric illness in the sick and it is not so pronounced an influence as to blur the substantial differences between healthy and sick" (Masterson, 1967a, pp. 157–159).

Thus the Masterson data appear clearly to negate the diagnostic dilemma imputed to adolescence. The problems of diagnosing disturbed adolescents lie not in discriminating between adjustment reactions and diagnosable psychopathology, he contends, but only in determining which particular form of psychopathology a disturbed adolescent is experiencing. Although allowing that adolescent turmoil may operate to impede diagnostic differentiation among various categories of psychopathology, he finds little basis for clinical uncertainty as to what represents normal adolescent variability and what represents psychopathology. Spivack, Haimes, and Spotts (1967), reporting a factor-analytic study of rated behavior problems in several hundred normal and disturbed adolescents, have recently provided additional support for continuing efforts to classify adolescent psychopathology:

"The present results also indicate that behavior dimensions, once reliably measured, may be used to elaborate upon current diagnostic work, as well as to serve as a means through which, via periodic re-ratings, determination can be made of the necessity for change in diagnosis and remedial program. . . . Once this is accomplished, it will not only be possible to apply such a tool as a means of diagnosis and assessment in remedial and rehabilitation programs but also as a tool through which we may obtain deeper understanding of the meaning of adolescent symptomatology. . . ." (p. 77).

EPIDEMIOLOGY OF ADOLESCENT PSYCHOPATHOLOGY

The only major epidemiological survey of diagnosed adolescent psychopathology is reported by Rosen et al. (1965), who collated state-prepared tabulations on all 10- to 19-year-old patients terminated from 788 psychiatric clinics in 1962. Of some 54,000 adolescents included in their survey, roughly 3% were considered to be "without mental disorder" and another 20% were for unspecified reasons undiagnosed. Table 1 compares the incidence of major diagnostic categories among the remaining approximately 42,000 diagnosed adolescent patients with the nosologic distribution of 78,000 adults terminated from United States psychiatric clinics in 1961 (*Outpatient Psychiatric Clinics,* 1963).

Perhaps the most striking aspect of these data is the emergence of transient situational personality disorder as the most common diagnosis in adolescent patients in United States clinics. Although recorded for only some 5% of the adult patients, this category accounts for more than one-third of the adolescents who were diagnosed. Such a predominance of situational diagnosis contrasts sharply with the conclusion drawn in Chapter 2 that psychological disturbances in adolescents brought to professional attention are seldom temporary or transient phenomena (see pp. 62–68). However, there are reasons to believe that the discrepancy between the reported frequency of situational disturbances in the Rosen et al. study and the previously inferred unimportance of such diagnoses is more apparent than real.

Table 1. Diagnoses of Adolescent and Adult Patients Terminated from Psychiatric Clinics[a]

Diagnostic Category	Adolescents[b]		Adults[c]	
	Males	Females	Males	Females
Acute and chronic brain disorders	4.7	3.6	6.6	3.7
Mental deficiency	10.3	10.3	2.2	1.7
Psychotic disorders:	5.7	7.5	24.1	29.4
Schizophrenia	5.6	7.2	20.8	22.8
Other	0.1	0.3	3.3	6.6
Psychoneurotic disorders:	11.4	18.0	20.0	31.9
Anxiety reaction	5.3	6.1	8.0	10.0
Depressive reaction	1.8	4.3	6.9	14.1
Obsessive-compulsive reaction	1.2	1.0	1.7	1.8
Other	3.1	6.6	3.4	5.1
Personality disorders:	30.6	23.7	40.9	25.1
Passive-aggressive personality	11.6	7.2	12.5	8.5
Sociopathic personality[d]	4.8	2.9	4.9	1.2
Schizoid personality	4.3	3.1	4.3	2.6
Emotionally unstable personality	2.3	3.9	2.1	3.6
Inadequate personality	1.4	1.8	3.4	2.3
Other	6.2[e]	4.8[e]	13.7[f]	6.9
Transient situational personality disorder	36.9	36.3	4.3	6.0

[a] Expressed as percentage of total.

[b] From Rosen et al. (1965, pp. 1566–1567), based on 26,254 male and 15,242 female adolescents.

[c] From *Outpatient Psychiatric Clinics* (1963, pp. 150–151), based on 33,046 male and 49,966 female adults.

[d] Includes antisocial reaction, dissocial reaction, and sexual deviation.

[e] Primarily special symptom reaction, including learning disturbance.

[f] Includes 6.2% incidence of alcohol addiction.

First, since the data of Rosen et al. are drawn solely from outpatient clinics, they do not reflect patterns of psychopathology among adolescents who require hospitalization. Among some 19,000 ten- to nineteen-year-old patients admitted to state, county, and private mental hospitals and to psychiatric units of general hospitals in 1966, psychotic disorder was diagnosed in 26.3%, psychoneurotic or personality disorder in 33.1%, and transient situational personality disorder in only 22.1% (*Patients in Mental Institutions,* 1966, Part II, pp. 10–11; and Part III, pp. 38–39).

Studies of samples of adolescents consecutively admitted to psychiatric inpatient units have also yielded a nosologic distribution weighted more toward serious psychopathology, and with correspondingly less emphasis on transient situational personality disorders, than in the clinic survey of Rosen et al. Warren (1965) found a 10% incidence of psychotic disorders among the boys and 17% among the girls in one such study, Annesley (1961) noted diagnosed psychotic disorders in 23% of the boys and 28% of the girls in another, and Larsen (1964) observed psychotic disorders in 27% of both the boys and the girls in a third. Nicklin and Toolan (1959) report a 58% incidence of diagnosed psychotic disorders among admissions to the Bellevue adolescent unit during 1957. In all of these studies the remaining adolescent patients were classified mostly as having some brain dysfunction or as manifesting some specific variety of psychoneurotic, personality, or behavior disturbance, and transient situational reactions were conspicuously infrequent.

Although these diagnostic differences between clinic and inpatient settings may derive entirely from corresponding differences in the actual psychological status of the adolescent patients treated there, it is well known that many factors other than the nature and extent of a psychological disturbance determine who becomes a hospitalized patient (see Hollingshead and Redlich, 1958, Chapters 9 and 10). It may be that clinic reports overemphasize the prevalence of situational reactions among disturbed adolescents not only because clinics see the relatively less disturbed segment of the adolescent patient population but also because they approach the diagnostic process with frames of reference that differ from those common to inpatient settings.

Hospital personnel, because of their orientation toward relatively severe psychological disturbance, may be more inclined than clinic staffs to disregard the possibility of transient situational relations in the patients they see; conversely, the clinic psychologist or psychiatrist may lean toward diagnoses that are less serious than those of his hospital colleagues, perhaps describing as transient reactions the same behavior problems that would be considered major personality disturbances if the youngsters displaying them were admitted to a hospital.

The report of Rosen et al. in fact contains some data to support the hypothesis that transient situational personality disorders as diagnosed in many clinics resemble disturbances requiring professional attention more than temporary, self-limiting upsets. Approximately 50% of the adolescent clinic patients who were assigned the diagnosis of transient situational personality disorder were subsequently seen in treatment, and this 50% incidence of treatment in cases of "situational reaction" was roughly identical to the treatment incidence reported for youngsters classified as personality disorders and only slightly less than that in instances of psychoneurotic or psychotic disorder (Rosen et al., 1965, p. 1570).

It thus appears that many clinics diagnose as having transient situational reactions adolescents who are felt to require ongoing psychotherapy and who subsequently receive it. Hence the apparently large percentage of transient disorders occurring in the sample of Rosen et al. is not inconsistent with the already noted caution about minimizing adolescent disturbance; the high incidence of treatment in these patients suggests that the frequent impression of "transient situational personality disorder" reflected more a reluctance to apply other diagnostic labels than a conviction that these youngsters had self-limiting disturbances for which they did not require treatment.

Rosen et al. also observed age-related diagnostic patterns consistent with the view that the diagnosis of transient situational disturbance may be too frequently applied to adolescents seen in oupatient clinics. They found for both boys and girls that the frequency of brain syndromes, mental deficiency, and particularly transient situational disorders decreased with age, whereas increasing age was associated with more frequent diagnoses of psychotic, psychoneurotic, and personality disorders. Their impression of these findings merits careful consideration:

"Our data on diagnosis shows that until age 18 the largest proportion of patients were diagnosed with transient situational personality disorders. This may be partially due to the reluctance of the psychiatrist to place a label of a serious disorder on a youngster when his identity may be in flux, especially on the basis of only a few interviews, or this may be due to the lack of adequate technics for such early identification. The increase in the number of older adolescents diagnosed as psychotic or psychoneurotic may indicate, in part, that as the patient grows older the seriousness of his disorder becomes more evident. Further research in the early identification of potentially serious mental disorders in adolescents is needed" (Rosen et al., 1965, p. 1571).

Several other interesting age and sex differences in the diagnoses of clinic patients appear in Table 1. One difference is that the much greater incidence of diagnosed situational reactions in adolescent than in adult patients is balanced primarily by a correspondingly greater incidence of psychotic and psychoneurotic disorders among the adults, whereas most categories of personality disorder are as frequently diagnosed in adolescent as in adult patients. Thus personality disorders constitute about one-fourth of the diagnoses for both the adolescent and the adult females, and for the males the greater frequency of personality disorder among the adults (40.9%) than among the adolescents (30.6%) is in large part accounted for by the 6.2% incidence of alcohol addiction in the adults. The greater overall frequency of diagnosed personality disorder in male than in female patients of all ages derives primarily from the greater likelihood of the males being diagnosed as passive-aggressive or sociopathic personality, whereas emotionally unstable personality emerges as a somewhat more common diagnosis for females.

The categories of psychoneurotic disorder also contain some striking sex differences, especially in regard to the diagnosis of depressive reaction. Depression is by far the most common neurotic diagnosis in adult women, and in adult men it is only slightly less common than anxiety reaction. Yet for adolescents depressive reaction is diagnosed less frequently than anxiety reaction in girls and much less frequently in boys. The lower incidence of diagnoses of psychoneurosis in adolescent than in adult clinic patients is thus due largely to the relative infrequency of diagnosed depressive reaction in the adolescents. It also appears that the generally greater frequency of diagnosed psychoneurotic disorder in females than in males relates to the higher incidence of depressive reaction in the females.

The category of psychotic disorder demonstrates both the far greater incidence of serious diagnoses in adult than in adolescent outpatients and a predominance of schizophrenia among psychoses diagnosed for both age groups. It can be seen for adolescents in particular that a diagnosis of psychotic disorder almost always implies schizophrenia. Other data drawn from a variety of settings over a number of years demonstrate that such a predominance of schizophrenia among diagnosed psychotic disorders of adolescence has transcended any variations in diagnostic practice that are associated with time and place (see Carter, 1942; Curran, 1940; Malzberg, 1931; Masterson, 1956). Other studies of psychotic adolescents by Sands (1956) and Toolan (1962) confirm that schizophrenia is by far their most common disorder, with manic-depressive disturbance rarely occurring.

CLINICAL CONTRIBUTIONS TO CLASSIFICATION

Behavioral scientists have long recognized that epidemiologic data are as likely to reflect diagnostic practices as the clinical status of the patients: "Such figures are a function (among others) of the conditions of admission and the reliability of the anamneses" (Bleuler, 1911, p. 341). A number of writers have accordingly attempted to delineate the major categories of adolescent psychopathology primarily from clinical rather than epidemiological data. In one such study Serrano et al. (1962), who interpret psychopathology as the failure to complete various developmental tasks, utilized developmental histories, clinical observations, and psychological testing to assign a series of disturbed adolescents to the following four diagnostic categories:

1. Preadolescent maladjustment reaction.
2. Juvenile maladjustment reaction.
3. Childish maladjustment reaction.
4. Infantile maladjustment reaction.

The preadolescent maladjustment reaction group tended to be youngsters who were in relatively good tune with their peers but, because of problems with autonomy and identity, were contemptuous of the values of their family, school, and community and were inclined to be rebellious or delinquent. These youngsters had typically been free of psychological difficulties until age 16 or later, when they had begun to have difficulty in accepting their peers' normative movement away from the group and toward individual identities.

Juvenile maladjustment reaction was diagnosed by Serrano et al. for youngsters who were anxious and fearful, overly conforming and conscientious, or bothered by such neurotic and somatic complaints as phobias, tics, headaches, and gastrointestinal disturbances. In contrast to the relatively mature youngsters with preadolescent adjustment reactions, the adolescents with juvenile maladjustment reactions were considered to evince persistent oedipal concerns; that is, to behave as if they expected and feared parental retaliation for forbidden acts.

Even less mature than the adolescents with juvenile maladjustment reactions were those whom Serrano et al. regarded as presenting a childish maladjustment reaction. These youngsters had for the most part been referred for apparently uncontrollable aggressive behavior, including temper tantrums, destruction of property, stealing, running away, and a general pattern of arrogance, negativism, and incorrigibility. Unlike the rebellious older adolescents in the preadolescent maladjustment reaction group, these childish youngsters acted out as a way of life and were constantly in trouble because of their impulsive and ill-conceived actions. Manipulation and the accretion of power seemed to be their major aims, and even with their peers they were seldom able to make meaningful affective contact.

The infantile maladjustment reaction outlined by Serrano et al. included adolescents clearly identified as schizophrenic. These youngsters displayed autistic patterns of living typically associated with early infancy: symbiosis with a mothering figure, limited and impersonal relationships with peers, indifference to external events and influences, and illusory concepts of omnipotence based on mastery of a fantasy world.

As Rutter (1965) has pointed out, an adequate classification of be-

havior disorders requires the delineation of syndromes that can be meaningfully differentiated from one another along several dimensions, including symptom clusters, response to treatment, long-term prognosis, etiology,
epidemiology, and age and sex trends. Although Serrano et al. did not
assess all of these dimensions, they were able to demonstrate some differential corollaries among their four diagnostic categories in the nature of
the family-interaction pattern and the approach to treatment associated
with each. The implications of their findings for differential diagnosis and
treatment planning is elaborated in subsequent chapters.

It is also of interest to note that the developmentally oriented categorization scheme successfully applied by Serrano et al. to their patient sample
corresponds closely to traditional diagnostic categories elsewhere suggested
to encompass the common patterns of adolescent psychopathology; for
example, Finch (1960, pp. 299–316) concludes from his experience that
the following five broad categories adequately classify the majority of
psychological disturbances in adolescence:

1. *Adjustment reaction of adolescence,* which pertains to transient situational personality disorders that do not constitute a major disturbance.[1]

2. *Psychoneurosis,* which, with the exception of relatively infrequent
depressive reactions, occurs with similar frequency in adolescents and
in adults.

3. *Psychophysiologic disorder,* among which obesity can be singled out
for its special contribution to psychological difficulties during adolescence.

4. *Personality disorder,* of which delinquency is stressed as being of
particular importance among disturbed teenagers.

5. *Psychotic disorder,* with schizophrenia being by far the most
common.

Finch's particular emphases within these traditional categories neatly
parallel the developmental diagnoses applied by Serrano et al. to their
patient sample. Preadolescent maladjustment reaction appears to represent
the traditional adjustment reactions of adolescence, juvenile maladjustment
reaction combines the psychoneurotic and psychophysiologic categories,
childish maladjustment reaction corresponds to personality disorder with
special attention to delinquency, and infantile maladjustment reaction defines psychotic disorder, with schizophrenia being the major manifestation
of both.

[1] As already noted, however, such reaction patterns are neither normal nor normative in adolescents (see pp. 55–62) and, if sufficiently pronounced to bring
the adolescent to professional attention, are likely to warrant such attention (see
p. 83).

This demonstrated congruence between broad traditional categories of psychopathology and the differential reaction patterns observed in disturbed adolescents by Serrano et al. additionally challenges the arguments that such classification is impossible and/or meaningless (see pp. 77–79). On the other hand, inasmuch as Serrano et al. devised a conceptual diagnostic scheme into which they subsequently fitted their patients, it is reasonable to question the extent to which conventional nosological assumptions influenced their integration of their clinical data.

Relevant in this regard is the work of investigators who have attempted to avoid preconceived diagnostic categories by inferring the primary patterns of adolescent disturbance directly from symptom clusters observed in adolescent patients. One such study is reported by Masterson, Tucker, and Berk (1963, 1966), who based their conclusions on the principal and secondary symptom patterns presented by the 101 adolescent patients in the already described Payne Whitney study. Masterson et al. were able to adduce five clusters of these symptoms, which accounted for 85% of their patient sample and which they consider to be the major psychological syndromes of adolescence. These five syndromes, listed below with their associated symptom clusters, correspond fairly well to traditional broad diagnostic categories:

1. *Thought disorder syndrome*—thought disorder, inappropriate affect, delusions, hallucinations, bizarre ideation, bizarre motor behavior, mutism, ideas of reference, gross confusion of thinking, and disorganization of habits.

2. *Psychoneurotic syndrome*—subjective anxiety, increased psychomotor activity, somatic complaints or symptoms, object or situational fear, and body overconcern.

3. *Acting-out syndrome*—stealing, school rebellion, temper outbursts, general negativism, hostility and physical aggression against others, delinquency, pathological lying, and lack of impulse control.

4. *Depression syndrome*—depressive affect, recurrent crying, suicidal preoccupation or attempt, and pathological guilt or self-depreciation.

5. *Hysterical personality disorder syndrome*—erotic or overdramatic behavior, dramatic attention seeking, marked sexual consciousness or provocativeness, and histrionic behavior.

In a similar approach to classification Jenkins (1964, 1966) and Jenkins, NurErddin, and Shapiro (1966) utilized computer methods to derive clusters of behavioral symptoms observed in 500 children studied in a child-guidance clinic. Although Jenkins focuses primarily on the classification of childhood disturbance, the primary symptom clusters emerging from his analysis typically involve youngsters between 9 and 15 years old and are thus relevant to at least the earlier portion of the adolescent age range. Jenkins identified five groups of children who shared sufficiently distinctive symptoms or traits to justify grouping them according to syndrome. These five groups of children, with the primary shared traits that identified their syndrome, were the following:

1. *Shy-seclusive*—seclusiveness, shyness, absence of close friendships, overimaginativeness, marked inferiority feelings, and nervousness.

2. *Overanxious-neurotic*—sleep disturbances, fearfulness, tearfulness, overimaginativeness, marked inferiority feelings, and nervousness.

3. *Hyperactive-distractible*—hyperactivity, lack of concentration, mischievousness, inability to get along with peers, overdependency, and bashfulness.

4. *Undomesticated*—defiance of authority, malicious mischief, cruelty, vengefulness, sullenness, initiation of fighting, and inadequate guilt feelings.

5. *Socialized delinquent*—bad companions, furtive and coooperative stealing, habitual truancy, and running or staying away from home.

To the extent that the shy-seclusive children in Jenkins' population represent tendencies toward schizophrenic disturbance; the overanxious-neurotic toward psychoneurosis; and the undomesticated and socialized delinquent toward personality disorder, his inferred categorization additionally confirms the applicability of traditional broad diagnostic categories to young adolescent patients. Jenkins views the hyperactive-distractible group of children as most commonly presenting with brain injury, a category of adolescent disturbance not covered by the contributions of Finch, of Serrano et al., and of Masterson et al. However, the hyperactive-distractible group, with its typical member in the 9 to 11 age range, was the youngest of Jenkins' five groups, and the data of Rosen et al. reveal a relatively low incidence of diagnosed brain damage among 11- to 19-year-old psychiatric clinic patients.

DIAGNOSTIC CLASSIFICATION IN CLINICAL PRACTICE

The studies reviewed in the preceding section attest the appropriateness of efforts to classify psychological disturbances in adolescents. These epidemiologic and clinical investigations consistently demonstrate that disturbed adolescents can be differentiated according to the traditional broad diagnostic categories of psychosis, psychoneurosis, and personality disorder. Each of these studies has in addition emphasized the particular prominence of certain subcategories of psychotic, psychoneurotic, and personality disorder among disturbed adolescents. As previously noted, for example, diagnosed psychotic disorders in adolescents are almost exclusively schizophrenic disturbances, more so than in adults, whereas the depressive reaction accounts for fewer adolescent than adult psychoneurotic disorders.

For clinical purposes it is furthermore important to recognize that certain presenting problems are typically associated with the various prominent subcategories of adolescent disturbance and heavily influence their indicated treatment; for example, the experienced clinician is aware that the large majority of passive-aggressive adolescents he sees present with a chief complaint of academic underachievement. Although a passive-aggressive personality style will have maladaptive ramifications in broad segments of a young person's behavior, it is characteristically an unexpectedly poor school performance that influences the parents—or the passive-aggressive adolescent himself in the case of older youngsters—to seek professional counsel. The literature clearly reflects this clinical phenomenon: contributions addressed directly to the passive-aggressive personality in adolescence are sparse, whereas there is a fairly extensive literature on academic underachievement in which the psychodynamics of passive-aggressive behavior are vividly depicted (see Chapter 6).

The important relationship of diagnostic subcategories to presenting behavior problems in adolescents has also been noted by Beckett (1966), who concludes from his experience at the Lafayette Clinic that no more than a third of referred adolescents demonstrate a clear-cut syndrome; the rest, he indicates, present primarily with such disturbed behavior as underachieving in school or getting into repeated fights. It is with these considerations in mind that the topics for Chapters 4 through 8 of this book have been chosen. They represent a practical distillate of the already reviewed diagnostic studies, the author's clinical experience, and the emphases to be found in the literature concerning adolescent psychopathology.

Psychotic reactions in adolescence, as has been noted, appear almost exclusively as schizophrenic disturbance. Adolescent schizophrenia may present in a variety of forms that are initially suggestive of psychoneurotic or personality disorders, and the devastating long-term effects of this disturbance require the clinician to be constantly alert to the possibility that the behavior problems of an adolescent patient might represent the initial phase of a schizophrenic decompensation. The nature of adolescent schizophrenia and its differential diagnosis and treatment are the subjects of Chapter 4.

Depressive reaction, although infrequently diagnosed in adolescents, was identified as a major syndrome in the Masterson study and deserves careful attention because of its relationship to suicidal behavior. As reviewed in Chapter 5, suicide in adolescents is noteworthy not so much for its incidence, which is lower than that in adults, but for the frequency with which it is attempted and its fifth rank among causes of death in this age group (see p. 158). Because of the relatively common occurrence of suicidal gestures among adolescents and the catastrophic consequences of attempts that inadvertently succeed, the clinician must often exercise judgments about the likelihood and probable seriousness of suicidal behavior in his adolescent patients. Although not necessarily tied to a pronounced depressive reaction, suicidal behavior in adolescents usually represents an attempt to communicate feelings of discouragement and frustration that have much in common with depressive reaction.

Neurotic manifestations of anxiety, as defined by Masterson's psychoneurotic syndrome and the overanxious-neurotic pattern identified by Jenkins, consist primarily of symptom clusters involving anxiety and fearfulness, somatic complaints, and feelings of inadequacy. At the clinical level this combination of symptoms in an adolescent is most typically encountered in the setting of school phobia. The school refusal in such cases may represent just one of many phobic patterns, and the somatic complaints may reflect pervasive propensities for conversion reaction, but it is most frequently the refusal or inability to attend school that brings these adolescents to the clinician and remains the basis of their treatment in the eyes of the patient and his family. Hence Chapter 6 is concerned with problems of anxiety, phobia, and conversion in adolescents but is specifically focused on school phobia.

The two most common personality disorders observed in the survey of Rosen et al. were passive-aggressive personality and varieties of sociopathic personality disturbance. As already noted, the dynamics of passive-aggressive personality functioning in adolescents emerge most clearly in the evaluation and treatment of youngsters with academic underachievement, the topic to which Chapter 7 is devoted. The term "sociopathic personality" in standard nomenclature has major implications for the acting-out and delinquent patterns noted by Masterson and Jenkins, respectively, and these patterns of disturbance are the subjects of Chapter 8.

REFERENCES

Ackerman, N. W., *The Psychodynamics of Family Life.* New York: Basic Books, 1958.

Ames, L. B., Metraux, R. W., and Walker, R. N. *Adolescent Rorschach Responses.* New York: Hoeber-Harper, 1959.

Annesley, P. T. Psychiatric illness in adolescence: Presentation and prognosis. *Journal of Mental Science,* **107**:268–278, 1961.

Beck, A. T. Reliability of psychiatric diagnoses: I. A critique of systematic studies. *American Journal of Psychiatry,* **119**:210–216, 1962.

Beckett, P. G. S. Psychiatric symptoms in adolescents: A challenge of the 1960's. *Journal of the American Medical Association,* **198**:359–363, 1966.

Bleuler, E. (1911). *Dementia Praecox or the Group of Schizophrenias.* Translated by J. Zinkin. New York: International Universities Press, 1950.

Carter, A. B. Prognostic factors of adolescent psychoses. *Journal of Mental Science,* **88**:31–81, 1942.

Curran, F. J. Psychotherapeutic problems of puberty. *American Journal of Orthopsychiatry,* **10**:510–522, 1940.

Douvan, E., and Adelson, J. *The Adolescent Experience.* New York: Wiley, 1966.

Edwalds, R., and Dimitri, K. Treatment of the adolescent patient in a state hospital. *Psychiatric Quarterly,* **33**:615–622, 1959.

Eisenberg, L. The role of classification in child psychiatry. *International Journal of Psychiatry,* **3**:179–181, (1967).

Finch, S. M. *Fundamentals of Child Psychiatry.* New York: Norton, 1960.

Hamilton, G. *Psychotherapy in Child Guidance.* New York: Columbia University Press, 1947.

Hathaway, S. R., and Monachesi, E. D. *Adolescent Personality and Behavior.* Minneapolis, Minn.: University of Minnesota Press, 1963.

Havighurst, R. J., and Taba, H. *Adolescent Character and Personality.* New York: Wiley, 1949.

Hollingshead, A. B., and Redlich, F. C. *Social Class and Mental Illness.* New York: Wiley, 1958.

Jenkins, R. L. Diagnoses, dynamics, and treatment in child psychiatry. *Psychiatric Research Report, American Psychiatric Association,* **18**:91–120, 1964.

Jenkins, R. L. Psychiatric syndromes in children and their relation to family background. *American Journal of Orthopsychiatry,* **36**:450–457, 1966.

Jenkins, R. L., NurEddin, E., and Shapiro, I. Children's behavior syndromes and parental responses. *Genetic Psychology Monographs,* **74**:261–329, 1966.

Jones, H. E. *Motor Performance and Growth.* Berkeley, Cal.: University of California Press, 1949.

Larsen, V. L. Physical characteristics of disturbed adolescents. *Archives of General Psychiatry,* **10**:55–64, 1964.

Laufer, M. Assessment of adolescent disturbances. *Psychoanalytic Study of the Child,* **20**:99–123, 1965.

Lehmann, H. E. Empathy and perspective or consensus and automation: Implications of the new deal in psychiatric diagnosis. *Comprehensive Psychiatry,* **8**:265–276, 1967.

Malzberg, G. A statistical study of the prevalence and types of mental disease among children and adolescents. *Psychiatric Quarterly,* **5**:511–537, 1931.

Masterson, J. F. Prognosis in adolescent disorders—schizophrenia. *Journal of Nervous and Mental Disease,* **124**:219–232, 1956.

Masterson, J. F. *The Psychiatric Dilemma of Adolescence.* Boston: Little, Brown, 1967a.

Masterson, J. F. The symptomatic adolescent five years later: He didn't grow out of it. *American Journal of Psychiatry,* **123**:1338–1345, 1967b.

Masterson, J. F., Tucker, K., and Berk, G. Psychopathology in adolescence: IV. Clinical and dynamic characteristics. *American Journal of Psychiatry,* **120**:357–366, 1963.

Masterson, J. F., Tucker, K., and Berk, G. The symptomatic adolescent: Delineation of psychiatric syndromes. *Comprehensive Psychiatry,* **7**:166–174, 1966.

Menninger, K., Mayman, M., and Pruyser, P. *The Vital Balance.* New York: Viking, 1963.

Miller, E. Individual and social approach to the study of adolescence. *British Journal of Medical Psychology,* **35**:211–224, 1962.

Nathan, P. E. *Cues, Decisions, and Diagnoses: A Systems-Analytic Approach to the Diagnosis of Psychopathology.* New York: Academic Press, 1967.

Nicklin, G., and Toolan, J. M. 20-year follow-up of an adolescent service in a psychiatric hospital. *Psychiatric Quarterly Supplement,* **33**:301–316, 1959.

Outpatient Psychiatric Clinics: Special Statistical Report, 1961. Bethesda, Md.: National Institute of Mental Health, 1963.

Patients in Mental Institutions. Part II: State and County Mental Hospitals. Part III: Private Mental Hospitals and General Hospitals with Psychiatric Care. Chevy Chase, Md.: U.S. Department of Health, Education, and Welfare, Public Service Publication No. 1818, 1966.

Reiss, I. L. *The Social Context of Premarital Sexual Permissiveness.* New York: Holt, Rinehart, and Winston, 1967.

Rosen, B. M., Bahn, A. K., Shellow, R., and Bower, E. M. Adolescent patients served in outpatient psychiatric clinics. *American Journal of Public Health,* **55**:1563–1577, 1965.

Rutter, M. Classification and categorization in child psychiatry. *Journal of Child Psychology and Psychiatry,* **6**:71–83, 1965.

Sands, D. E. The psychoses of adolescence. *Journal of Mental Science,* **102**: 308–316, 1956.

Schofield, M. *The Sexual Behavior of Young People.* Boston: Little, Brown, 1965.

Selzer, M. L. The happy college student myth. *Archives of General Psychiatry,* **2**:131–136, 1960.

Serrano, A. C., McDonald, E. C., Goolishian, H. A., MacGregor, R., and Ritchie, A. M. Adolescent maladjustment and family dynamics. *American Journal of Psychiatry,* **118**:897–901, 1962.

Shakow, D. The role of classification in the development of the science of psychopathology with particular reference to research. *Bulletin of the Menninger Clinic,* **30**:150–161, 1966.

Spivack, G., Haimes, P. E., and Spotts, J. Adolescent symptomatology and its measurement. *American Journal of Mental Deficiency,* **72**:74–95, 1967.

Tanner, J. M. *Growth at Adolescence,* 2nd edition. Springfield, Ill.: Thomas, 1962.

Toolan, J. M. Suicide and suicidal attempts in children and adolescents. *American Journal of Psychiatry,* **118**:719–724, 1962.

Ward, C. H., Beck, A. T., Mendelson, M., Mock, J. E., and Erbaugh, J. K. The psychiatric nomenclature: Reasons for diagnostic disagreement. *Archives of General Psychiatry,* **7**:198–205, 1962.

Warren, W. A study of adolescent psychiatric inpatients and the outcome six or more years later: I. Clinical histories and hospital findings. *Journal of Child Psychology and Psychiatry,* **6**:1–17, 1965.

Weiner, I. B. *Psychodiagnosis in Schizophrenia.* New York: Wiley, 1966.

Zubin, J. Classification of the behavior disorders. *Annual Review of Psychology,* **18**:373–406, 1967.

CHAPTER 4

Schizophrenia

Schizophrenia has traditionally been viewed as a disturbance that begins primarily in the adolescent years. In applying the label *dementia praecox* to the variety of conditions currently designated as the schizophrenias, Kraepelin (1899) had specifically in mind that these mental aberrations most typically appear in adolescence or early adulthood. Bleuler (1911) notes in his classic monograph that almost 40% of Kraepelin's large patient sample had experienced onset of their disturbance before age 20 and over 60% before age 25, and he agrees that "the adolescent age period seems to offer a particular predisposition to this disease" (p. 340).

Subsequent studies have established that the onset of schizophrenic disturbance encompasses a broader age range than was postulated in these early contributions. Some forms of schizophrenia begin in childhood (Bender, 1953), whereas paranoid schizophrenia most frequently has its initial onset beyond age 30 (Noyes and Kolb, 1963, p. 347). Nevertheless the average ages of onset for various subcategories of schizophrenic disturbance demonstrate that schizophrenia does often first appear during the adolescent years (see Weiner, 1958, pp. 135–153).

Although the frankly schizophrenic adolescent usually poses little diagnostic difficulty, most young people in the initial stages of a schizophrenic breakdown present a mixed clinical picture in which schizophrenic features are secondary, subtle, or submerged. Because accurate early diagnosis is often essential to the prompt institution of appropriate therapeutic measures, the clinician must be alert to mild and nascent schizophrenic conditions in youngsters who do not present a definitive clinical picture. To overlook schizophrenia in a disturbed adolescent until an advanced or readily apparent stage of the disorder has been reached may delay incisive therapeutic intervention beyond the time of its maximum effectiveness.

This chapter is addressed to the psychopathology, differential diagnosis, prognosis, and treatment of schizophrenia in adolescence.[1] The discussion first reviews the distinctive patterns of personality impairment, diagnostic subcategory, and age of onset commonly observed in adolescent schizophrenia and then considers the clinical aspects of assessing and treating the schizophrenic adolescent.

PERSONALITY IMPAIRMENT IN ADOLESCENT SCHIZOPHRENIA

Schizophrenia may be usefully conceptualized as an impairment of certain major ego or personality functions. The normal individual is generally able to think coherently, logically, and at appropriate levels of abstraction; to assess his experience and his behavior realistically; to establish and maintain rewarding relationships with other people; and to exert adaptive control over his thoughts, feelings, and impulses. Schizophrenic disturbance, on the other hand, is characterized primarily by disordered thinking, poor relation to reality, limited capacity for object relationships, and inadequate control of affects, ideation, and behavior. The clinical phenomena of schizophrenia derive in large part from these four impairments of personality functioning (see Beres, 1956; Weiner, 1968).

Although adolescent schizophrenia corresponds closely to the general psychopathology of schizophrenic disturbance, schizophrenia in the adolescent youngster comprises certain distinctive patterns of personality impairment and presenting symtomatology that provide important guidelines for its differential diagnosis. A number of clinical and research studies have elaborated these general and distinctive patterns of ego impairment in adolescent schizophrenia.

General Psychopathology of Adolescent Schizophrenia

Each of the four major personality impairments associated with schizophrenic disturbance—disordered thinking, poor relation to reality, limited capacity for object relationships, and weakened controls—has been observed in schizophrenic adolescents. This correspondence of adolescent schizophrenia to adult schizophrenia has recently been demonstrated by Spivack, Haimes, and Spotts (1967) in an extensive factor-analytic study of adolescent symptomatology. Spivack et al. collected ratings on 172 problem behaviors for 640 thirteen- to eighteen-year-old boys and girls, including youngsters with diagnosed brain damage as well as schizo-

---

[1] For a broader review of basic concepts in the understanding, diagnosis, and treatment of schizophrenic disturbance than can be included in this chapter the reader is referred to Arieti (1955), Bellak (1958), Bleuler (1911), Broen (1968), Burton (1961), Bychowski (1952), Jackson (1960), Romano (1967), Rosenthal and Kety (1968), and Weiner (1966).

phrenic, psychoneurotic, schizoid, passive-aggressive, and antisocial individuals; a group with adjustment reaction; and a sample of normal youngsters. Analysis of these data yielded 18 behavioral factors on which the diagnostic groups were subsequently compared.

The 93 schizophrenic adolescents in the study of Spivack et al. received the highest score of any diagnostic group on 5 of the 18 factors. These five factors, with the behavior-rating items loading highest on them, were the following:

1. *Bizarre cognition.* The adolescent in this group substitutes, confuses, or misuses pronouns in conversation; uses his name rather than "I" when referring to himself in conversation; his speech is disconnected, incoherent, or not sensible; he reports hearing voices or other hallucinations.

2. *Bizarre action.* This group displays odd facial grimaces, postures, or movements; puts inedible, unhealthy, or even dangerous things into the mouth; shuts out sounds by lifting shoulders or putting fingers in ears; rocks while sitting or standing.

3. *Schizoid withdrawal.* The patient has a blank stare or faraway look in eyes; day dreams; walks around oblivious as if wrapped up in own thoughts; looks puzzled or confused by things happening around him; talks to himself.

4. *Emotional detachment.* The patient keeps his distance or reserve with adults; has a fixed facial expression that lacks feeling; is unemotional, rarely shows feelings; is unaware of how adults feel toward him.

5. *Poor emotional control.* The youngster in this group gets very upset or overemotional if things do not go his way; often expresses anger; is easily upset by peers; expresses anger in poorly controlled fashion; reacts with anger if having difficulty in mastering or learning something.

These observed characteristics of schizophrenic adolescents either directly state or are readily translatable into the defining ego impairments of schizophrenic disturbance delineated by Weiner (1966, 1968). Other studies have confirmed the relevance to adolescent schizophrenia of one or another of the general features of schizophrenic disturbance. With regard to disordered thinking, for example, Masterson, Tucker, and Berk (1963) identified in their Payne Whitney study (see p. 88) an adolescent thought disorder syndrome consisting of looseness of association, concreteness, delusions, ideas of reference, and gross confusion of thinking; Neubauer and Steinert (1952) observed a uniform display of ideas of reference, arbitrary reasoning, and inability to maintain a productive focus of attention in a group of schizophrenic adolescents; and Kates and Kates (1964), using a picture-sorting test to study concept formation in psychotic and in normal adolescent boys, found the psychotic boys to be significantly less able to operate at appropriate levels of abstraction. The psychotic youngsters studied by Kates and Kates tended in particular to pay inordinate attention to trivial differences among the stimuli they were asked to categorize and to base their sorting decisions on strikingly vague and idiosyncratic criteria.

Concerning the relation to reality, Podolsky (1963) found schizophrenic college students typically to exhibit the types of poor judgment that derive from loose reality contact. These students frequently displayed career aspirations beyond their capabilities; bizarre study methods, such as copious note taking far in excess of what was useful; and poorly conceived actions by which they repeatedly drew unsympathetic attention to themselves— such as entering a class discussion despite being unprepared, handing in overelaborate assignments, and performing unrequested favors for classmates or instructors. Kiersch and Nikelly (1966) similarly observed poor relation to reality and consequently impaired judgment in schizophrenic college students, manifested in such behavior as frequent sweeping changes in curricula and unnecessary school transfers.

Work by Colbert and Koegler (1961) confirms that the implications of poor relation to reality for impaired body perception are also characteristic of adolescent schizophrenia. In comparing the psychological test performances of adolescents who had been childhood schizophrenics, of youngsters who became schizophrenic in adolescence, and of nonschizophrenic adolescents with behavior problems, they found that the two schizophrenic groups demonstrated marked distortions of body image that were not evident among youngsters with behavior problems. Particularly in their drawings of the human figure the schizophrenic youngsters exhibited maladaptive concerns over body periphery and inadequate attention to various body parts.

Limited capacity for object relationships is posited as a primary characteristic of adolescent schizophrenia by Burns (1952) and Sands (1956), among others. In Burns' experience the most important early signs of a developing schizophrenic disturbance in adolescents are withdrawal from people and a corresponding increase in sensitivity that impairs tolerance for the give and take of social interactions. Sands (1956, p. 309) draws a similar conclusion from his studies of schizophrenic adolescents:

"The most common denominator in over a hundred such patients was a difficulty in relating themselves to people and situations from early life. This social failure in adaptation was associated with an anxiety which seemed to be intolerable, and they might even be said to be constitutionally allergic to anxiety, and to avoid it by any sacrifice."

Weakened controls have been identified in schizophrenic adolescents in regard both to inadequate affective integration and to limited control over thoughts. The adolescent thought disorder syndrome observed by Masterson et al. (see p. 88) was defined in part by the presence of inappropriate affect and bizarre ideation. From his clinical experience Burns (1952) suggests that blunted affect or apathy is often among the precursors of schizophrenia in adolescence, and Edelston (1949) points out that adolescent schizophrenia may first appear as an incapacity to integrate emotional drives.

It should be noted that the adolescents' display of schizophrenic personality impairments in these clinical and research studies could have derived entirely from their having been diagnosed as schizophrenic on the basis of these same impairments. In other words, the investigator who wishes to assess a generally accepted parameter of schizophrenic disturbance in a designated schizophrenic population must recognize that the parameter itself has probably figured prominently in establishing the diagnosis of schizophrenia. His observations may otherwise involve an unavoidable contamination of the dependent and independent variables. On the other hand, congruence between a clinical impression of schizophrenic disturbance and a subsequent experimental or independent clinical confirmation that the persons designated schizophrenic do indeed display personality impairments that are thoeretically associated with schizophrenia lends convincing construct validity both to the diagnostic process and to the postulated characteristics of schizophrenia.

Distinctive Patterns of Impairment

Although schizophrenic adolescents have been observed to display the full range of ego impairments that generally define schizophrenic disturbance, additional data demonstrate some distinctive profiles of impairment in the clinical picture of adolescent schizophrenia. Rorschach studies of schizophrenic and nonschizophrenic adolescents in particular reveal that certain indices of impaired ego functioning tend to occur more often in nonschizophrenic adolescents than in nonschizophrenic adults, whereas certain other pathological indicators are as significant for schizophrenia in adolescents as they are in older persons.

The already cited contribution of Ames, Metraux, and Walker (1959) summarizes 700 Rorschach protocols of nonpatient 10- to 16-year-old boys and girls. These young people were found at all ages to formulate many of their Rorschach responses in a vague, fluid, overgeneralized, and circumstantial fashion (p. 287). The 16-year-old subjects were particularly likely to give symbolic, overly abstract, and free-associative response elaborations (pp. 241–246). Thus these nonpatient adolescents evinced patterns of arbitrary reasoning and abstract preoccupation that in an adult would suggest thought disorder.

Silverman, Lapkin, and Rosenbaum (1962) substantiated this finding in Rorschach assessments of 11- to 18-year-old schizophrenic and nonschizophrenic patients in a residential treatment center. The mean incidence of formal primary process scores (see Holt and Havel, 1960) among their neurotic and character disorder adolescents, expressed as a percentage of total response frequency, was 43.30; in other words, these disturbed but nonschizophrenic adolescents averaged roughly 9 formal primary process scores for every 20 Rorschach responses they gave. This notable frequency of indices of thought disorder in the nonschizophrenic adolescents was nevertheless significantly surpassed by the schizophrenic subjects, in whom the mean primary process score was 74.15. The data of Silverman et al. therefore confirm the relevance of disordered thinking to the diagnosis of schizophrenia in adolescents, but they also suggest that neurotic and characterologically disturbed adolescents are more likely to display arbitrary reasoning and inappropriate abstraction than are nonschizophrenic adults.

This possibility is supported in a Rorschach study of adult neurotic and schizophrenic subjects by Watkins and Stauffacher (1952). Utilizing types of deviant verbalization originally specified by Rapaport, Gill, and Schafer (1946, pp. 331–336), these investigators derived a Rorschach index of pathological thinking that significantly differentiated schizophrenic from neurotic adults. Interestingly, the incidence of pathological thinking in the Rorschach records of the neurotic adults did not begin to approach the frequency of primary process scores in the neurotic and characterologically disturbed adolescents assessed by Silverman et al., whereas there was a close similarity between the schizophrenic adults and the nonschizophrenically disturbed adolescents in the extent of primary process thinking.

Rorschach studies furthermore suggest that weakened ideational control may be less significant for schizophrenic ego impairment in adolescents than in adults. Ames et al. (1959) report numerous violently aggressive response specifications—explosions, fighting and blood, figures cut or split open, or with parts chopped off or being torn apart—in the Rorschachs of their nonpatient adolescents. Rychlak and O'Leary (1965) similarly found the Rorschachs of 562 eleven- to eighteen-year-old nonpatient boys and girls to embrace a significant number of contents generally considered "unhealthy" in adults. Such "unhealthy" content themes as blood, guts, death, decay, destruction, and sex constituted 15 to 20% of their subjects' Rorschachs, and 75% of their nonpatient adolescents gave one or more "unhealthy" responses for every 10 responses in his Rorschach.

Data reported by Silverman et al. (1962) further confirm that weakened ideational control may have relatively little significance for schizophrenia in adolescents. Specifically, they found virtually no difference in the extent of blatant sexual and aggressive content expressed by their schizophrenic and nonschizophrenic subjects. The schizophrenic adolescents had an average incidence of 20.45% of primary process content scores among their total Rorschach responses, and the comparable figure for the neurotic and character disorder adolescents was 19.50%.

Thus there is evidence to suggest that both disordered thinking and weakened controls have different diagnostic significance in adolescents than they do in adults. Whereas the extent of disordered thinking differentiates schizophrenic adolescents from those with neurotic or characterological disturbances, the latter may display as great an extent of circumstantial and overly abstract thinking as many schizophrenic adults. Evidence for these indicators of ego impairment must accordingly be considerably greater in adolescent patients than in adult patients to suggest schizophrenic disturbance. Weakened ideational control is also prominent in both nonschizophrenic and schizophrenic adolescents, and the extent of manifest sexual and aggressive imagery apparently does not distinguish schizophrenic from nonschizophrenic patients.

However, it is important to recognize that these age-related differences do not extend to other patterns of personality impairment associated with schizophrenia. In the first place, disordered thinking and weakened controls are not unitary phenomena. Although the arbitrary reasoning and abstract preoccupation aspects of disordered thinking should be interpreted more conservatively in adolescents than in adults, there is no convincing evidence to suggest that dissociation or blocking are any more likely to occur in nonschizophrenic adolescents than they are in nonschizophrenic adults. Similarly, whereas conscious awareness of blatant aggressive and sexual imagery may occur in nonschizophrenic adolescents, impaired affective integration has not been demonstrated to be any more common in nonschizophrenic adolescents than it is in nonschizophrenic adults.

Hence, although certain peculiarities in reasoning and concept formation and some lack of ideational control are more likely to appear in nonschizophrenic adolescents than in nonschizophrenic adults, disordered thinking as reflected in dissociation and blocking, and weakened controls as reflected in inadequate emotional integration have equal significance as clues to schizophrenic disturbance in both adolescents and adults.

Secondly, psychodiagnostic studies of nonpatient adolescents reveal few indications of the impaired relation to reality or the limited capacity for object relations that is observed in schizophrenic youngsters. Regarding relation to reality, the average Rorschach scores obtained by Ames et al.

(1959, pp. 26–28) demonstrate a high level of perceptual accuracy and an excellent capacity to recognize and endorse conventional modes of response. Hertz (1960) and McFate and Orr (1949) also found nonpatient adolescents to endorse significant numbers of conventional Rorschach responses. Gravitz (1966) examined the human-figure drawings of several hundred 17- to 19-year-old subjects and found little evidence that nonpatient adolescents have difficulty in maintaining a sexually differentiated body percept. Only 5% of the boys and 5% of the girls in his study produced drawings that lacked clearly differentiating sexual characteristics.

With respect to capacity for object relatedness, the Ames et al., McFate and Orr, and Hertz subjects at all ages rarely excluded human content or impressions of human activities from their Rorschach responses. To the extent that such exclusions reflect withdrawal, disinterest, or incapacity for social relationships, these findings indicate that such withdrawal, disinterest, or incapacity are not consonant with normative adolescent patterns. The interpretative significance of these psychodiagnostic test indices of impaired relation to reality and limited capacity for object relationships is elaborated by Weiner (1966, pp. 104–120, 156–164, and 463–464), who also notes their equivalent implications for adult and adolescent schizophrenia.

In summary, then, schizophrenia in adolescence embraces a range of personality impairments comparable to those that define adult schizophrenia but, particularly in its mild or incipient forms, is likely to present some distinctive profiles of impairment. Circumstantial thinking, abstract preoccupation, and conscious awareness of blatant sexual and aggressive imagery tend to be less conclusive as signs of schizophrenic disturbance in adolescents than they are in adults, whereas poor relation to reality limited capacity for object relationships, and the specific phenomena of blocking, dissociation, and inappropriate affective integration are equally suggestive of schizophrenic disturbance in adolescents and adults.

Presenting Symptoms

Although defined by patterns of personality impairment similar to those characteristic of adult schizophrenia, adolescent schizophrenia frequently presents as a mixed disturbance in which identifying features of schizophrenia are not clinically dominant. For example, Masteron's sample included 24 adolescent patients who initially demonstrated some features of schizophrenic disturbance, of whom 18 were eventually diagnosed as schizophrenic. Of these 18 schizophrenic youngsters, only 7 had exhibited unequivocally disordered thinking, poor reality testing, and inappropriate affect during their first interview. The remaining 11 schizophrenic adolescents had initially presented a mixed and equivocal clinical picture: 5 had displayed many features of personality disorder, 5 had demonstrated prominent depressive phenomena, and 1 had originally appeared to have a psychotic reaction without schizophrenia (Masterson, 1967, pp. 49–58).

More specifically, the five subsequently diagnosed schizophrenic adolescents who initially presented primarily as personality disorder included four with prominent sociopathic traits and one with schizoid tendencies. The apparently sociopathic youngsters presented with complaints of restlessness, concentration difficulty, and insomnia, together with a history of antisocial behavior, academic failure, truancy, and intrafamilial conflict. Although these patients did not initially display disordered thinking or inappropriate affect, their long-standing history of poor social relationships and such interview behaviors as blunted affect, denial, guardedness, evasiveness, and suspiciousness suggested the possibility that they were basically or incipiently schizophrenic. The apparently schizoid youngster who was subsequently diagnosed as schizophrenic similarly presented without disordered thinking or inappropriate affect but manifested sufficient concentration difficulty, scholastic impairment, and social withdrawal to raise the question of schizophrenia.

The five schizophrenic adolescents with prominent depressive features presented primarily with suicidal preoccupation or attempts. For these patients a past history of social difficulty and blunted affect or guardedness on interview, in the absence of thought disorder or inappropriate affect, alerted the initial examiner to possible underlying schizophrenia. The youngster whose initial diagnosis was psychotic reaction presented with some circumscribed delusional preoccupation and social withdrawal but did not manifest pervasive thinking and affective impairments until later in his clinical course.

The frequency with which withdrawal or chronically poor social relationships were the harbinger of schizophrenia in these 11 youngsters, in the absence of initial clinical evidence of thought disorder and inappropriate affect, emphasizes the particular importance of impaired capacity for object relationships in the identification of adolescent schizophrenia. It is further interesting to note Masterson's description of the six patients in his study who initially evoked mixed clinical impressions but were subsequently considered not to be schizophrenic. Two of these youngsters presented with primarily sociopathic features, two demonstrated prominent schizoid patterns, and two were regarded as passive-aggressive personalities.

In other words, among the youngsters in the Masterson sample who initially presented a mixed diagnostic picture with schizophrenic and nonschizophrenic elements, all five for whom the differential diagnosis lay between depressive and schizophrenic reaction were subsequently identified as schizophrenic; of the six with mixed sociopathic and schizophrenic features, four were subsequently diagnosed as schizophrenic and two were not; and just one of the three with schizoid features—and neither of the two with passive-aggressive tendencies—was later considered to be schizophrenic. These findings suggest that depressive phenomena in an adolescent with subtle schizophrenic features, particularly in the case of suicidal preoccupation or attempt, are highly likely to represent a developing schizophrenic disturbance; a mixed picture of sociopathic and schizophrenic disturbance would be somewhat less indicative of developing schizophrenia but still more likely to imply such developments than presenting schizoid and passive-aggressive traits.

Other clinical observations tend to support two of Masterson's major findings:

1. Relatively few schizophrenic adolescents initially present with unequivocally schizophrenic symptomatology.

2. Sociopathic tendencies and symptoms of depression, especially as reflected in suicidal behavior, account for most of the equivocally disturbed adolescents who are subsequently found to be schizophrenic.

For example, Symonds and Herman (1957) report that only 18 of 50 schizophrenic girls seen consecutively in the adolescent ward at Bellevue were admitted because of bizarre or withdrawn behavior that clearly indicated schizophrenic disturbance. This 36% incidence of initially unequivocal schizophrenic symtpoms in subsequently diagnosed schizophrenic adolescents corresponds closely to the 39% rate (7 of 18) observed by Masterson. Of the remaining 32 schizophrenic girls in the Symonds and Herman sample, 12 were admitted because of suicidal attempts or preoccupation with suicide, 10 because of persistent aggressiveness in school or at home, and 4 for running away from home. The other 6 girls were admitted for diverse reasons, many of which involved criminal or antisocial activity.

The particular role of conduct disorder in an underlying or developing schizophrenic disturbance in an adolescent has been noted by several other writers. Sands (1956, p. 309) concludes from his study of 180 psychotic adolescents that such disturbances often evolve from conduct disorders in a manner seldom seen in adults:

"In retrospect it may be found that stealing, truanting, refusal to attend school, screaming attacks, and behaviour sometimes involving court appearances, have marked the onset of disorder that subsequently is diagnosed as schizophrenic."

Djartov (1965) comments that syndromes resembling psychopathy are predominant during the initial period of schizophrenia in adolescents, and in Hamilton's (1947, p. 250) experience, "when marked conduct disturbances or marked personality changes have their onset just before or during puberty, the possibility of schizophrenia must be kept in mind."

DIAGNOSTIC SUBCATEGORIES

In addition to presenting certain distinctive patterns of personality impairment and initial symptomatology, schizophrenia in adolescents also comprises a somewhat different distribution of traditional diagnostic subcategories from that common to adult schizophrenics. Table 2 compares the incidence of major diagnostic subcategories of schizophrenic disturbance among approximately 2550 schizophrenic adolescents and 17,000 schizophrenic adults terminated from outpatient clinics.

Table 2. Subcategories of Schizophrenia in Adolescent and Adult Patients Terminated from Psychiatric Clinics[a]

Subcategory	Adolescents[b]		Adults[c]	
	Males	Females	Males	Females
Paranoid	18.6	14.5	39.2	34.4
Acute undifferentiated	11.6	16.4	5.3	6.7
Chronic undifferentiated	27.9	25.5	32.2	31.3
Childhood	20.9	12.7	—[d]	—[d]
Other	21.0	30.9	23.3	27.6

[a] Expressed as percentage of total.
[b] From Rosen et al. (1965, p. 1566), based on approximately 2550 schizophrenic adolescents.
[c] From *Outpatient Psychiatric Clinics* (1963, pp. 150–151), based on approximately 17,000 schizophrenic adults.
[d] Category not listed.

The table reveals little in the way of sex differences, with the exception of the greater relative incidence of diagnosed childhood schizophrenia in schizophrenic adolescent males than in females. Between adolescents and adults, however, a number of clear differences in diagnostic pattern emerge. Paranoid schizophrenia is a much more common designation for adult schizophrenics (39.2% for men and 34.4% for women) than it is for adolescent schizophrenics (18.6 and 14.5%, respectively). This difference, together with the somewhat greater frequency of chronic undifferentiated schizophrenia in adults, is balanced partly by childhood schizophrenia, which is diagnosed for a significant proportion of schizophrenic adolescents (20.9 and 12.7% for boys and girls, respectively) but is not listed as a separate category in the adult epidemiologic data, and partly by acute undifferentiated schizophrenia, which is more commonly diagnosed in adolescent than in adult schizophrenics.

As already mentioned (see p. 83), it is difficult to know to what extent such diagnostic labeling is determined by the patients' actual clinical status and to what extent by nonpersonality factors. Such considerations aside, however, Sands (1956) presents a cogent rationale for the greater frequency of prominent paranoid features in schizophrenic adults than in schizophrenic adolescents. He suggests that the particular phenomena manifested by a person who becomes psychotic will be partly determined by the degree of his personality development and integration: if a person is immature, so will be the nature of the psychosis he develops. Hence adolescents, because of their relative immaturity, are less likely than adults to develop paranoid psychoses, which, especially in respect to systematized delusional formations, reflect a considerable extent of personality integration and crystallization.

Noteworthy in addition to the traditional subcategories of schizophrenic disturbance is a pattern of *pseudopsychopathic* adolescent schizophrenia described by Lauretta Bender (1959). She notes that some schizophrenic children are able to utilize the developmental processes of puberty to reorganize their defenses in such a way that they compensate for their underlying schizophrenic disturbance and function in a nearly normal fashion, only to reexperience personality disorganization under the increasing demands of later adolescence. A number of such youngsters she observed manifested as the first stage in their adolescent decompensation a number of psychopathic personality characteristics, including inability to identify with or relate to their peers, refractoriness to social standards, diminished tolerance for anxiety, and impulsive behavior. Bender's description of pseudopsychopathic schizophrenia in adolescence has much in common with the already mentioned observations that sociopathic personality features may herald the onset of schizophrenia in disturbed adolescents.

The distinction between acute and chronic disturbance in schizophrenic adolescents has been elaborated in a number of important contributions. For the most part these reports agree with Masterson's (1967, pp. 29–30) delineation of three major patterns of schizophrenia in disturbed adolescents: (a) a childhood schizophrenic condition exacerbated by the stress of puberty; (b) a chronic, insidiously developing schizophrenic disturbance in which the specific biological and psychological events of adolescence play little part; and (c) an acute onset of schizophrenic disturbance at or during adolescence in the absence of a previous history of psychological difficulty. For example, Neubauer and Steinert (1952) divided their group of schizophrenic adolescents into (a) those whose disorder had an original onset in childhood, (b) those whose disturbance apparently first occurred in adolescence but whose history revealed earlier neurotic or schizoid difficulties, and (c) those who demonstrated a clear initial onset of psychological difficulty in adolescence.

These three patterns of adolescent schizophrenia are also described by Symonds and Herman (1957) in their study of 50 schizophrenic girls hospitalized at Bellevue. Eleven of the girls demonstrated a long history, starting in infancy or early childhood, of bizarre behavior and developmental deviations suggestive of childhood schizophrenia; although only three of these youngsters had previously been diagnosed as schizophrenic, all had been regarded by parents and teachers as "strange" girls who were "never like other children."

For 18 of the girls there had been a gradual development of schizophrenic psychosis out of a childhood pattern of serious personality and behavior problems, including truancy, fighting, stealing, running away, temper tantrums, and numerous neurotic complaints. In another 15 girls no serious disturbance had been in evidence prior to the onset of schizophrenia in adolescence. These girls had developed in apparently normal fashion, and their behavior in school and at home had been free from signs of personality deviation. In each case there was a sharp demarcation in time and behavior between the schizophrenic and preschizophrenic states. The remaining six girls in the Symonds and Herman sample presented both an acutely developing psychotic state and a childhood history of behavior disturbance.

Childhood and Chronic Schizophrenia

Other studies have affirmed the distinctive nature of one or more of these three patterns of adolescent schizophrenia. Colbert and Koegler (1961), in their already mentioned study of adolescents who had been diagnosed as schizophrenic in childhood, found that these youngsters had been regarded as pervasively immature by their parents and teachers; had in most cases presented early severe disturbances in eating, sleeping, and toilet training; and in several instances had displayed persistent turning in circles or toe walking. As adolescents they were strikingly immature, both physically and psychologically, demonstrated marked poverty of thought, and were frequently preoccupied with matters of space, time, and motion—drawing rocket ships, studying train schedules, collecting watches and clocks, and so forth (see also Ekstein, 1966). In contrast, the Colbert and Koegler control group of youngsters who became schizophrenic in adolescence presented significantly less evidence of childhood developmental difficulty, appeared their appropriate age, and were free of impoverished thought and space-time-motion preoccupations.

Spivack et al. (1967) also report some significant differences between schizophrenic adolescents who had been diagnosed as schizophrenic in childhood and those who had not. Although all of their 93 schizophrenic adolescents demonstrated the disturbed behaviors summarized on page 97, the 53 childhood schizophrenics in their sample exhibited in addition an extent of emotional, social, and intellectual incompetence that was not observed among the 40 youngsters who became schizophrenic at or during adolescence. As adolescents the childhood schizophrenics were much more likely than the other schizophrenic youngsters to be defiant and resistive in some instances and clinging and dependent in others, to lack heterosexual interest, to display physical weakness and poor coordination, to be hyperactive and expansive, and to demonstrate such poor personal habits as uncleanliness, sloppiness in dress and grooming, and incontinence.

The relatively deteriorated condition at adolescence of youngsters who have been schizophrenic from early childhood is also noted by Eisenberg (1956), who reassessed 63 autistic children at an average age of 15. On follow-up 46 of these youngsters had not emerged from their autism to any extent and were functioning in a markedly maladaptive fashion characterized by apparent feeble-mindedness and/or grossly disturbed behavior. The remaining 17 had had a somewhat more favorable outcome and resembled the picture of chronically developing adolescent schizophrenia. These 17 youngsters had painfully acquired some ability to simulate normal adolescent behavior but were still markedly lacking in social skills. Their inability to empathize with others, their lack of tact, and their incapacity for diplomacy had typically caused them such painful interpersonal experiences that they had withdrawn into a solitary existence. Rutter, Greenfeld, and Lockyer (1967, p. 1195) observed a similar adolescent outcome of infantile psychosis:

"Only a minority of psychotic children reach a good level of social adjustment by the time of adolescence, and very few enter paid employment. About half remain incapable of any kind of independent existence and most of these are cared for in mental subnormality hospitalis."

The adolescent with insidiously developing chronic schizophrenic disturbance often lingers unrecognized on the fringes of teenage groups while a slow deterioration takes place, with declining school performance, diminishing interest in peers and in personal appearance, increased pursuit of solitary or meaningless activities, development of strange, pseudophilosophical attitudes, and affective blunting. In describing this pattern Finch

(1960, p. 313) notes that in many cases these aspects of deterioration go unnoticed in their early stages because parents and others tend to protect the youngster and to attribute his deviant behavior to normal adolescent variability. Sands (1956) similarly observed a progression in chronic schizophrenic adolescents from a prolonged phase of behavior disorder, with temper outbursts, stealing, and the like, through neurotic defensive maneuvers subtly suggestive of schizophrenia, such as obsessional ideas bordering on the delusions, to gradual lapse into an overt psychosis.

Acute Schizophrenia

Detailed attention to acute schizophrenic reactions in adolescents dates back at least to the work of Kasanin and Kaufman (1929), who carefully reexamined the diagnostic status of 21 primarily 13- to 15-year-old youngsters hospitalized with presenting symptoms of schizophrenic psychosis. They concluded that 10 of these patients were not schizophrenic at all but rather demonstrated hysterical, psychopathic, or other personality disorders. Of the remaining 11 cases, they diagnosed 6 as "schizophrenic" and 5 as "reactive psychosis of adolescence." The six schizophrenic youngsters displayed such symptoms as diminished interest in the world, prominent autistic fantasy, hallucinations, peculiar behavior, and irrelevant speech. The youngsters with "reactive psychosis" demonstrated many of these same symptom patterns but differed from those designated schizophrenic in two major respects: (a) their markedly deviant behavior had emerged suddenly after some emotional trauma, in relation to which it could be understood, and (b) their disturbance did not run a malignant course.

Whereas Kasanin and Kaufman reserved the designation "schizophrenia" for apparently chronic and progressive disturbance, their distinctions by contemporary standards serve primarily to distinguish acute schizophrenia from chronic schizophrenia. The seriousness of disturbance in their "reactive psychosis" youngsters was evident not only in the schizophrenic nature of their symptoms but also in the fact that they required extended hospital care, ranging from 1 to 18 months in duration, to achieve remission.

Warren and Cameron (1950) have more recently attempted to distinguish between "schizophrenia" and "reactive psychosis" in adolescents. As in the Kasanin and Kaufman study, the disordered thinking and self-referential, delusional, and hallucinatory symptoms displayed by Warren and Cameron's "reactive psychosis" youngsters suggest that they were by most standards schizophrenic, although in this group the onset of disturbance was more closely tied to specific life events than was the case for the chronically disturbed adolescents whom Warren and Cameron labeled schizophrenic. They differentiate acute from chronic disturbance in psychotic adolescents partly in terms of the clarity of such precipitating events and partly according to the patients' retention of personality integration and capacity for affective rapport:

"The content of the acute phase constituted an emergence into consciousness of hitherto unconscious material of so dominating a character that it led to delusions or hallucinatory experience. It was uniformly found, however, in these cases that affective contact was not lost and that personality disintegration did not occur, so that they remained susceptible to psychotherapy. In retrospect, the situation and emergent material were found to explain the illogical content and to demonstrate the mechanisms at work. The well retained personality and affective rapport after the acute phase, and the relative simplicity of the connection between the situation and the content, are regarded as characteristic of this group of cases." (Warren and Cameron, 1950, p. 456).

To summarize these last two sections, then, many schizophrenic youngsters will present an initially mixed or equivocal clinical picture in which features of psychopathic or depressive disturbances are combined with evidence of social withdrawal and affective blunting. Furthermore, with regard to traditional subcategories of schizophrenia, adolescents are much less likely than adults to present markedly paranoid forms of the disturbance, and the major significant distinctions in schizophrenic adolescents are among the childhood, chronic, and acute forms of the disorder.

AGE OF ONSET AND PRODROMAL INDICES

Aside from recognizing that adolescent schizophrenia may represent a continuing childhood schizophrenic disorder, an insidiously developing chronic schizophrenic process, or an acute and precipitous schizophrenic breakdown, clinicians view differently the age at which a fully developed schizophrenic condition can be said to exist. Some maintain that all schizophrenia is essentially a childhood disturbance, with onset early in life; others focus on the particular role of adolescent difficulties in precipitating the initial onset of schizophrenia at or following puberty; still others regard deviant phenomena in adolescence as merely prodromal to a schizophrenic disturbance that is not fully manifest until early adulthood or later.

Childhood, Adolescent, and Adult Onset

According to Lauretta Bender (1953, 1959), schizophrenia always begins as a childhood disturbance. Whether their disturbance has been acute or chronic, she maintains, all schizophrenic adolescents share a history of more or less overt childhood schizophrenic disorder. Thus the clinical differences between adolescent schizophrenics pertain only to the history of their defensive operations and not to any differences in the age at which the schizophrenic disturbance sets in: "Schizophrenia has been viewed as a lifelong process but a psychosis occurs only when other more satisfactory defenses fail" (Bender, 1959, p. 491).

Finch (1960, pp. 309–310) agrees that the roots of adolescent disturbances extend far back into childhood, but he stresses the adolescent era as the period in which an actual psychotic reaction is first likely to develop. He suggests that coping behaviors which allow a preschizophrenic youngster to maintain a limited but reasonable adjustment during his relatively dependent childhood years may first prove to be inadequate at adolescence, when the increased psychological pressures of the teenage years begin to disrupt his personality integration.

Hamilton et al. (1961) found in fact that a specific pattern of adolescent stress, imposed on a childhood history of inadequate personality adjustment, had precipitated the initial onset of schizophrenia in a group of 100 hospitalized boys. As children these patients had tended to be shy, isolated, and poorly coordinated, with minimal investment in school work, group activities, or the world about them. Their decompensation at adolescence was associated with such events as a disturbing family move to a new environment, a severe physical illness or operation for themselves or one of their parents, mounting concern about homosexuality, or leaving home to attend college.

The role that difficulties in college play in precipitating the intial onset of a schizophrenic disturbance in late adolescence has received specific attention from Kiersch and Nikelly (1966) and from Lichtenberg (1957). Kiersch and Nikelly report that 62 of 105 schizophrenic college students whom they evaluated had experienced their first decompensation while attending the university, primarily in response to the academic stress of collegiate standards and competition.

Lichtenberg comments on the initial onset of schizophrenia in college students whose past history reflects not marginal adjustment but apparently dazzling success. He hypothesizes that some youngsters may achieve conventional academic, athletic, and social success as high school students without developing the self-confidence, flexibility, and interpersonal skills necessary to deal adequately with the many demands of college life. The high school careers of such boys and girls, he continues, are characteristically dominated by a quest for praise and esteem, both of which are readily forthcoming from parents and peers. These youngsters become addicted to success and develop little tolerance for failure, and in the college setting—faced with increased competition, diminished relative excellence, and a new coterie of peers and teachers who do not automatically extend their praise and admiration—they are particularly prone to psychological collapse.

Such a pattern of hollow academic success has also been observed by Demerath (1943) among consistently superior high school students who subsequently became schizophrenic. These youngsters had apparently sought scholarly superiority to compensate for social inadequacies. However, although their good grades had earned them the approval of their teachers and some measure of security in the classroom, academic success had assumed such inordinate importance in their lives that it too had become fraught with fears and anxieties, particularly of failing to maintain their intellectual superiority. These able youngsters accordingly had little tolerance for the academic rigors and competition they encountered in the college setting.

As for the impression that schizophrenic features in adolescents are for the most part prodromal to what is essentially an adult disturbance, Wertheimer (1962, p. 788) suggests that schizophrenia "does not reach its maximum rate until at least some ten years after puberty." She proposes, however, that certain pubertal conditions may influence the pattern of schizophrenic breakdown subsequently experienced by a prepsychotic adolescent; for example, in a study of over 1000 adult schizophrenic women she found that those who had experienced the menarche after age 13 were significantly more likely to have "chronic" diagnoses, whereas those who had begun menstruation before age 13 were more likely to present an acutely schizophrenic picture.

Prodromal Indices

Without necessarily endorsing Wetheimer's view that schizophrenia develops fully only in adults, a number of researchers have attempted to identify prodromal indices in the adolescence of patients who became schizophrenic as adults. The most detailed study of this kind is reported by Bower, Shellhamer, and Daily (1960), who interviewed the high school staffs and reviewed the school records of 44 nineteen- to twenty-six-year-old hospitalized schizophrenic men and 44 nonpatient controls. As high school students these preschizophrenic and control subjects had differed significantly in the frequency with which they displayed each of five broad behavior patterns (see Table 3). On the basis of these and additional data, Bower et al. (1960, p. 278) draw the following general conclusions about the prodomal indices of subsequent schizophrenia in high school boys:

"High school students who later become schizophrenic were found to be significantly different from a randomly selected control group of their peers in the manner in which they are perceived by their school staffs and in certain phases of their school records. . . . The developing schizophrenic boys tended to have less interest in girls, group activities, and athletics. They showed less leadership skills and were more submissive, anxious, dependent, and careless than the average boy. Although they were less liked by their peers and teachers and did less well in school, they were not usually perceived as major problems or as being emotionally disturbed. However, in almost all cases their over-all mental health and school adjustment was rated significantly poorer than the control group. With a few exceptions most of the preschizophrenics could be characterized as tending toward the shut-in, withdrawing kind of personality."

This suggestion that schizoid behavior patterns in adolescence are an important predictor of schizophrenia in adulthood is supported by Demerath (1943) and Kohn and Clausen (1955), who observed social

Table 3. Personality Descriptions of 44 Preschizophrenic High School Students and Their Controls[a]

Personality Description	Incidence in	
	Preschizophrenic Group	Control Group
Unusually striking personality, noted by others to be odd, peculiar, queer, or at times crazy	9	2
Slight personality problems, different but not markedly so; shy, dreamy, lacked concentration, temperamental, and stubborn	19	3
Apparently well-adjusted and well-integrated; moderately popular, sociable, no apparent school difficulty	9	31
Qualities of leadership in athletics or scholarship, "pride of school," eager or overeager for success	3	9
No problem, seldom noticed, seclusive, and quiet; often hazily remembered by teachers; sensitive, shy, passive, and colorless	4	0

$\chi^2 = 38.49$, df $= 4$, $p < .001$.
[a] From Bower, Shellhamer, and Daily (1960).

isolation in many adolescents who subsequently became schizophrenic. Pertinent is this comment by Demerath (1943, p. 516):

"No feature of our subjects' histories stood out any more clearly than their inability to engage in the intimate, informal group life of their peers either in childhood or adolescence."

In the Kohn and Clausen study 20 of 45 first-admission schizophrenic patients reported that at age 13 to 14 they had played alone or primarily alone rather than with friends or siblings, whereas only 2 of 45 control subjects reported such solitary patterns of play.

Yet extensive longitudinal data collected by O'Neal and Robins (1958) and Robins (1966) fail to confirm any predictive significance of schizoid personality traits for subsequent schizophrenia. These investigators conducted a 30-year follow-up study of 382 boys and 142 girls initially seen at a median age of 13 in the St. Louis Municipal Psychiatric Clinic between 1924 and 1929. In their follow-up work they were able to locate and interview 436 of these patients and 90 of 100 originally selected nonpatient controls.

Robins (1966, p. 151) reports that symptoms of withdrawal, reticence, and seclusiveness in the boys and girls they studied were generally not predictive of psychiatric disturbance in adulthood; neither these symptoms nor odd ideas, "nervousness," irritability, and oversensitiveness occurred significantly more frequently among youngsters who were disturbed as adults than among those who subsequently displayed no diagnosable psychopathology. Furthermore, of Robins' 23 male patients who became schizophrenic as adults, none had been described as a shy or withdrawn child (p. 258). On the other hand, the preschizophrenic youngsters displayed more nail biting, depression, worrying, and excessive dependency than patients with nonschizophrenic outcomes, and they additionally demonstrated frequent antisocial symptomatology. Stealing, running away, truancy, and incorrigibility were each noted in more than half the preschizophrenic youngsters. These findings are consistent with the predominance of psychopathic over schizoid features in the presenting symptoms of the schizophrenic adolescents studied by Masterson and Symonds and Herman (see p. 104).

To the extent that the various contradictory data concerning preschizophrenic personality are reliable, they appear to support Arieti's (1955, pp. 61–79) view that *both* schizoid and "stormy" personality patterns in young people may be precursors of psychotic breakdown. The emphasis on social isolation in some investigations of preschizophrenic youngsters and on sociopathic behavior in others may accordingly derive from variations in sampling. This possibility is supported in some contradictory findings that have emerged from the Schizophrenia Research Project at the Judge Baker Guidance Center, in which various records have been utilized to examine the childhood patterns of youngsters seen at the Guidance Center who were subsequently hospitalized with a schizophrenic disturbance.

In one such study Gardner (1967) compared the Guidance Center records of youngsters who were initially seen primarily between the ages of 13 and 17 and had subsequently been hospitalized for schizophrenia, mostly when they were in their early twenties, and those of teenage patients whose subequent history indicated no such hospitalization. Gardner found no relationship in either sex between aggressive acting-out behavior as a presenting symptom and later schizophrenia (p. 99).

Yet Nameche, Waring, and Ricks (1964, p. 236) in a study of patients who had been seen at the Judge Baker Guidance Center at a median age of 14 and subsequently hospitalized for schizophrenia at a median age of 21 report the following:

"A substantial portion of the children who later became schizophrenic had been referred to the clinic by parents, school, and courts because of acting-out behavior superficially not unlike that of delinquents. Most of these adolescents resemble Arieti's 'stormy' personalities, and were far from the passive, withdrawn, quiet, 'shut-in' image of the prechizophrenic child."

The observed frequency of acting-out behavior among preschizophrenic youngsters does not of course demonstrate that such behavior is any more predictive of subsequent schizophrenia than of other clinical developments. In fact in the Robins study antisocial behaviors were considerably more extensive in the youngsters who as adults demonstrated sociopathic personalities than in those who became schizophrenic, and stealing and incorrigibility were as common in patients who displayed no psychological disturbance as adults as in the preschizophrenics (Robins, 1966, p. 290). Robins also discovered some interesting differences in the objects of the antisocial behaviors of her preschizophrenic and presociopathic youngsters. Whereas the presociopaths were relatively more likely to display antisocial behavior in relationships external to their family and friends—that is, in aggressive acts toward strangers, authority figures, and organizations—the preschizophrenics' aggressive acting out was directed primarily toward people they knew rather than strangers, and toward their peers rather than adults (Robins, 1966, p. 153).

Nameche et al. similarly found that most of the acting out in their sample of preschizophrenic youngsters occurred in the family and home environments rather than in the community. These investigators present the intriguing hypothesis that community-directed acting out in a pre-schizophrenic adolescent may have potential developmental value to the extent that it serves successfully to break the bonds of isolation within which his pathogenic family has controlled him.

In summary, these observations indicate that a disturbed adolescent may be suffering the long-term effects of childhood schizophrenia, may be experiencing the initial onset of schizophrenia, or may be just beginning to display some prodromal indices that, if unchecked, will blossom into overt schizophrenia during his adult life. These prodromal indices usually take the form of either a withdrawn, schizoid adolescent adjustment or a stormy youth characterized by antisocial behavior.

GUIDELINES IN DIFFERENTIAL DIAGNOSIS

As already noted, relatively few schizophrenic adolescents initially present unequivocal evidence of thought disorder, detachment from reality, and inappropriate affect. Most exhibit a mixed symptom picture, and the clinician's diagnostic acumen is frequently tested by sociopathic adolescents who manifest poor impulse control and shallow object relationships, by depressed adolescents who are apathetic and emotionally unresponsive, and by schizoid youngsters who demonstrate seclusiveness and social withdrawal.

In such ambiguous instances the diagnosis of schizophrenia must often be tentative and perhaps specified as "incipient" or "mild." Yet it is in the incipient or mild stage of a developing schizophrenic disturbance that the clinician's expert judgment is most needed. The relatively inexperienced observer can identify the disorder when it has reached advanced proportions, and by then the most opportune time for therapeutic intervention may have passed. Hence, at the expense of relying on less than conclusive clinical data, the clinician must attune himself to early and subtle signs of schizophrenia in his adolescent patients and label them as such when they appear. This and the following section focus on differential guidelines and sources of data that contribute to such diagnostic inferences.

Three differential guidelines for the assessment of possible schizophrenia in adolescents presenting a mixed or equivocal clinical picture are the following:

1. The persistence of the symptomatology.
2. The extent of normative adolescent concerns.
3. The prominence of formal, as opposed to content, manifestations of disturbance.

Each of these guidelines, as elaborated below, has specific implications for the types of clinical data that should be elicited in pursuing this diagnostic question.

Persistence of the Symptomatology

Persistence of the symptomatology pertains to the length of time that the apparently schizophrenic features in an otherwise mixed clinical picture persist unabated. The longer such symptoms persist, especially in the face of successful efforts to alleviate situational distress, the more probably the adolescent is experiencing a schizophrenic disorder.

The actual point in time at which the persistence of schizophrenic features in a mixed clinical picture becomes conclusively diagnostic of schizophrenia is difficult to specify. Katz (1967) points out that the significance of persistence may vary considerably with the individual patient and with the particular symptomatology under investigation. The adolescent who manifests disordered thinking, inappropriate affect, or detachment from reality can usually be identified as schizophrenically disturbed after a relatively brief persistence of these symptoms; on the other hand, in the case of such phenomena as poor judgment, limited empathic capacity, inability to experience enjoyment, seclusiveness, and sexual or philosophical preoccupations a considerably longer persistence is typically necessary to rule out a nonschizophrenic basis.

Masterson's (1967) longitudinal study illustrates clearly the role of continued observation in the differential diagnosis of adolescents with initially equivocal symptomatology. Of six adolescents in his sample who presented mixed schizophrenic and sociopathic features, two displayed increasing antisocial behavior with no further development of schizophrenic symptomatology over a five-year follow-up period and hence were considered sociopathic. Three others were hospitalized within a year of their initial interview, two with a clear psychotic breakdown and one with auditory hallucinations, and were accordingly adjudged schizophrenic. The remaining youngster had not appreciably decompensated but had demonstrated five years' persistence of flat affect, suspiciousness, social withdrawal, and pervasive ambivalence and dependency, and on this basis was diagnosed as schizophrenic (Masterson, 1967, pp. 51–53).

Masterson emphasizes the particular difficulty of differentiating between schizophrenia and sociopathy in symptomatic adolescents:

"Since sociopaths frequently are isolated and without friends and have blunted affect and psychotic episodes, while schizophrenics often have poor impulse control and acting-out, the combination of the two elements in a guarded, uncooperative adolescent presents the most intricate of riddles to solve" (p. 52).

In the event of a mixed schizophrenic-sociopathic picture in a disturbed adolescent, he concludes, it is extremely difficult to predict which direction the future clinical course will take, and the point at which persistence of schizophrenic features becomes conclusive for schizophrenia may lie several years in the future (see Chapter 8, pp. 314–322).

For adolescents with mixed features of schizophrenia and depression Masterson's data indicate that the point in time at which schizophrenia can be definitively inferred is highly variable. Although all five of his mixed schizophrenia-depression patients were eventually diagnosed as schizophrenic, one demonstrated clear schizophrenic disturbance during the course of a year's treatment; three others who were initially seen at age 17 had developed a full schizophrenic picture by age 20, but for two of these patients no definitive diagnosis had become apparent during the entire course of their first year's treatment following the initial evaluation; and the fifth youngster responded to treatment with a lifting of her depression but was found on follow-up five years later to manifest a persistence of the blunted affect and vague thinking that had originally suggested schizophrenia (pp. 55–57) (see Chapter 5, pp. 175–176).

The importance of persistent symptomatology in the clinical differentiation of schizophrenia from other adolescent disturbances has also been noted by Spotnitz (1961, pp. 224 and 236):

"There is virtually complete agreement that the persistence of a symptom picture is one of the most reliable differentiating criteria. Periods of seclusiveness, despondency, and sexual or philosophical preoccupations do not last long or lead to a break with reality if the ego is an essentially healthy one which is undergoing one of the transient states of fragmentation normally associated with adolescence. If such behavior is prolonged, however, one must investigate the possibility of a schizophrenic reaction. . . . If such states persist over a period of weeks or months, there is justification for the impression that one is dealing not with an adolescent state, but with an adolescent schizophrenic reaction. . . ."

Extent of Normative Adolescent Concerns

Although the persistence of schizophrenic symptomatology is probably the most reliable guideline in the differential diagnosis of adolescent schizophrenia, it may defer indefinitely the formulation of a definitive treatment plan. The other two guidelines, extent of normative adolescent concerns and prominence of formal manifestations of disturbance, contribute significantly to early diagnosis. In the case of the former, the more a disturbed youngster's current concerns resemble those normatively displayed by adolescents, the less likely he is to be schizophrenic; conversely, the disturbed adolescent who is invested primarily in childish or adult interests and activities is more often schizophrenic than the youngster who demonstrates numerous age-appropriate attitudes and pursuits.

Warren (1949) has documented this diagnostic criterion in a study of 50 thirteen- to eighteen-year-old patients seen at the Maudsley Hospital, 19 of whom were considered psychotic. He found that the symptoms of the nonpsychotic youngsters were frequently colored by such common adolescent concerns as achieving independence, attaining confidence and skill in heterosexual relationships, and mastering anxiety about homosexuality or menstruation, whereas such concerns were much less evident in the psychotically disturbed youngsters. These data imply that, although the presence of normative adolescent concerns cannot rule out schizophrenia in a disturbed adolescent, the absence of such concerns increases the likelihood that a schizophrenic disturbance is present.

The schizophrenic adolescent, in other words, will usually demonstrate marked inability to come to grips with normative adolescent concerns. In some youngsters this inability is reflected in striking immaturity and a general failure of social development; in others the normative concerns and activities of adolescence are skirted in favor of a frequently deceptive pseudomaturity. Both possibilities must be carefully assessed in the clinical evaluation of disturbed adolescents.

Immaturity. The immature adolescent typically seeks to maintain the exclusive chumships that characterize the preadolescent years (see Sullivan, 1953, pp. 245–262). As his peers become increasingly interested in dating and broad circles of friends, he gravitates over the years to younger and younger playmates. The failure to develop any normative heterosexual interest is characteristically accompanied in such youngsters by persistently immature fantasies and activities, and a generally childish demeanor.

> A 15-year-old boy, an urbanite who had never ridden a horse, indicated that his future plans were "to go to college and become a rodeo rider." A 15-year-old girl, asked what she liked to do after school, replied, "I go out and play." Both statements resemble what one would expect to hear from an 8- or 9-year-old and in these teenagers suggested marked immaturity.

Although immaturity by itself does not demonstrate schizophrenia in a disturbed teenager, such evidence of nonparticipation in adolescent frames of reference enhances the possibility of schizophrenia in an otherwise mixed diagnostic picture. To judge such patterns adequately the clinician must have a good grasp of normative adolescent behavior in respect both to age and sociocultural considerations. The 13-year-old boy who likes to play cowboys and Indians is more likely to be psychologically immature than his agemate who collects pictures of baseball players; at age 15 a boy who is concerned with collecting and swapping pictures of athletes should raise more clinical eyebrows than one who builds and races midget auto models; yet at 17 a youth who is still devoted to racing model cars is not displaying normally mature interests.

As for sociocultural considerations, it may, for example, have little pathological significance that a 16-year-old upper-middle-class girl whose family and friends expect her to complete college before contemplating marriage is not particularly interested or involved in dating. If she additionally happens to come from a conservative ethnic or religious background in which youngsters are brought to maturity slowly, her minimal heterosexual activity at age 16 is even less significant. On the other hand, in a lower-class girl of 16 whose peers normatively begin active dating at puberty and expect to marry upon graduation from high school disinterest in dating may imply a maladaptive extent of nonengagement in age-appropriate activities.

Pseudomaturity. Adolescents who respond to the psychological challenges of adolescence by short-circuiting them tend to present a facade of calm, serious, and mannerly behavior that is very appealing to adults and seldom suggests psychological distress to the unsophisticated observer. Such pseudomature boys and girls are responsible and conscientious, discuss world events and the behavior of their peers from their parents' or teachers' viewpoint, and generally begin as early as age 12 or 13 to identify themselves as adults.

> A 15-year-old boy, an only child, attributed his being viciously teased by his classmates to "how unruly young people are today." He referred to his parents' social engagements as, "We had some of our friends over yesterday." Although his measured IQ was 90 and he had virtually never engaged in any activity other than in the company of his parents, except for attending school, a number of people who had discussed his peer-group difficulties with him—principal, guidance counselor, minister—had consistently introduced their initial impressions of him with such statements as, "This bright, alert, clean-cut young man discussed the situation with me in a very open, sensible, and mature manner."

The basic developmental failure in such pseudomature adolescents is usually apparent in their total lack of appropriate and rewarding peer relationships. The clue to their psychological disturbance lies not in their apparently mature interests and excellent relationships with adults, but in their adult investments at the total expense of engagement in age-appropriate activities, interests, and fads. The 16-year-old boy who dresses like a banker, is neither homosexual nor has any interest in girls, and has never heard of the Rolling Stones, the Red Sox, or the "jerk" is in all likelihood reacting to his inadequate psychological preparation for the adolescent years by a maladaptive effort not to live them.

At times the immaturity and basic social inadequacy underlying the pseudomature pattern comes suddenly to the fore in episodes of poor judgment or psychological collapse that come as a total surprise to the parents and teachers. The apparently mature and sophisticated young lady of 16 goes into a frenzied panic when a boy tries to kiss her, because she has never progressed beyond the childhood fantasy that kissing causes pregnancy; or the seemingly self-reliant 14-year-old boy goes off to camp for the first time and must be rescued by his parents after a week in which he has made no friends, clung to his counselor's side, and cried himself to sleep at night.

Some youngsters who mask an underlying schizophrenic disturbance with a facade of adequacy may avoid overt breakdown until late in their adolescence and then decompensate in the face of increasing demands for independent and self-assured behavior and decreasing availability of parental support and protection. As mentioned on page 111, such young-sters may achieve apparent social and academic successes during most of their teenage years, only to have the emptiness of these achievements exposed near the close of their adolescence when they are unable to muster the necessary self-confidence and object-relationship capacity to attain an adequate adult adjustment.

It is important to reemphasize that the relationship between normative adolescent concerns and schizophrenic disturbance is not mutually exclusive. Although a well-developed pattern of peer engagement and age-apppropriate activities greatly diminishes the likelihood of schizophrenia in a disturbed adolescent, it does not entirely contradict such a possibility. Similarly the failure to present adolescent concerns, whether manifest in blatant immaturity or in clinically transparent pseudomaturity, may be associated with such phenomena as intellectual limitation, delayed physical development, and minimal brain dysfunction as well as schizophrenia. Hence it is the nonretarded, nondelayed, non-brain-injured adolescent with difficulties in peer engagement who should be closely evaluated for possible schizophrenic tendencies; the psychoneurotic and personality disorders of adolescence, whatever the problems they pose for interpersonal rela-tionships, seldom interfere with the development of age-appropriate inter-ests and activities.

Prominence of Formal Manifestations of Disturbance

Available data, much of it derived from psychodiagnostic research, indi-cate a direct relationship between the prominence of formal manifestations of disturbance and the likelihood of schizophrenia in adolescent youngsters. As already noted, for example, schizophrenic adolescents and nonschizophrenic controls may produce similar amounts of "unhealthy" content on the Rorschach but will differ significantly in their frequency of formal Rorschach indices of disordered thinking (see p. 100).

Several writers have emphasized the diagnostic importance of such distinctions between formal and content aspects of psychological test data. Piotrowski (1962) stresses that inferences based solely on the verbal content of adolescents' test protocols usually exaggerate the degree of psychopathology present, whereas the formal aspects of an adolescent's thought yield a more accurate estimate of his personality strengths and weaknesses. Symonds (1949, p. 320) draws a similar conclusion from extensive TAT studies in which the content of adolescent subjects' stories proved to have little diagnostic significance. Machover (1961, p. 322) places the following emphasis on formal psychodiagnostic variables in the assessment of possible adolescent schizophrenia:

"The more severe the disturbance of the basic structure of thought, that is, of the cognitive processes, the greater is the likelihood of pathological process. Peculiar thought content . . . may alert us to possible deviations in process, but it is essentially the nature of the process by which the content was arrived at that I feel is significant for the question of pathology in the sense of ego disorganization."

The distinction between formal and content manifestation of disturbance is applicable to interview as well as psychological test data. For example, the adolescent who describes bizarre fantasies, strange dreams, or unusual preoccupations may be experiencing a schizophrenic disturbance; yet this likelihood rests primarily with the extent to which such material is recounted in a blocked, dissociated, or circumstantial manner that demonstrates formal thought disorder.

An additional formal index to the likelihood of schizophrenia is the adolescent's inability to take realistic distance from deviant aspects of his thinking or behavior. Easson (1968, p. 157) describes a group of essentially nonpsychotic adolescent patients with some apparent features of psychosis who could be distinguished from psychotic youngsters by this reality-testing capacity:

"These patients are not at such a distance from reality that they are unable to see the unreality of what they say and do. They may have to deny or project in an active effort to deal with such anxiety-provoking reality, but, unlike the psychotic patient, they cannot comfortably live the unreality."

Wilson (1951) has elaborated the diagnostic significance of a disturbed adolescent's reaction to the content of his thoughts in relation to obsessive-compulsive phenomena, which frequently overlap neurotic and schizophrenic disturbances. He observes that in the nonpsychotic person obsessional anxiety is accompanied by some awareness of the symptom's abnormality, as reflected in such comments as, "I know it's ridiculous to have this idea, but I just can't get it out of my head," or "I can't think of one good reason for doing this over and over again, but I somehow just feel I must." In the adolescent with a developing schizophrenic disturbance, however, obsessional concerns tend to be speculative rather than anxiety provoking, are manifest in odd and detached ruminations that have little personal meaning to the individual, and are seldom accompanied by reflective and self-critical statements. In general, then, the less critically a disturbed adolescent can judge his unusual thought content, the more probably he is experiencing a formal thought disorder that is indicative of schizophrenia.

SOURCES OF DIAGNOSTIC DATA

The psychopathology of adolescent schizophrenia and the differential guidelines in its diagnosis define to a large extent the clinical data necessary to evaluate possible schizophrenia in the individual case. This section specifies further certain aspects of the clinical history, interview behavior, and psychological test findings that contribute significantly to differential diagnosis of the adolescent who presents a mixed clinical picture. It should be emphasized that none of the considerations reviewed is conclusive for, or exclusively related to, schizophrenic disturbance. Schizophrenia is defined by the coexistence of certain personality impairments, each of which may appear in some nonschizophrenic conditions. Furthermore, the diagnosis of schizophrenia in initially equivocal cases of all types is at best a probability statement determined by the extent and number of the schizophrenia-related ego impairments that can be demonstrated.

Clinical History

The clinical history, as collected from the adolescent patient and his parents, school records, family doctor, and various other sources, contributes significantly both to the identification of schizophrenia and to the differentiation between acute, chronic, and childhood schizophrenic conditions. The clinician concerned that a disturbed adolescent may have an underlying or incipient schizophrenic disorder should attend carefully in his clinical history to (a) the nature of the youngster's friendship patterns and engagement in peer-group activities; (b) possible indications of bizarre or unusual behavior or judgment; (c) any family history of schizophrenia; and (d) reports of previous behavior disturbance or developmental deviations.

Peer-Group Engagement. The importance of peer-group relationships in evaluating possible schizophrenia in a disturbed adolescent cannot be overemphasized. For a schizophrenic youngster whose quiet, retiring, over-controlled behavior conceals even from those close to him that he has difficulty thinking clearly and testing reality accurately, an inability to engage in meaningful relationships with his agemates may be the primary or sole manifest clue to the severity of his disturbance. Such youngsters may avoid doing anything "crazy" by avoiding doing anything at all, and the clinician must learn to identify the failure to engage in age-appropriate activities as a potential index of underlying schizophrenia.

As noted on page 103, evidence of an active and rewarding engagement in interpersonal relationships with peers is at times sufficient to rule out schizophrenia in a youngster whose occasionally peculiar ideas or behavior may have raised this possibility. In making such judgments, however, it is necessary to determine that the adolescent's engagements are as real as they are apparent; that is, that they do not represent an empty or superficial facade in which the youngster goes through the motions of socially expected adolescent behaviors without developing any personal involvement in them.

In the case, for example, of a boy in the Boy Scouts or on the football team or a girl who belongs to the dramatics club or is a cheerleader, it is significant whether these activities are pursued because the youngster really enjoys them or because his parents or teachers press them on him. It is additionally relevant whether the activities are large group functions—such as the school band, where the youngster is unlikely to be singled out for any demanding individual contribution—or small group pursuits—such as a combo, in which no member can participate without truly pulling his own oar. The more an adolescent's activities represent others' motives and interests rather than his own and the less they require of him a measure of individual investment and competence, the more likely it is that they are apparent rather than real peer-group engagements.

An adolescent's social relationships should be similarly assessed to distinguish apparent from real peer engagement. As described by Pitt, Kornfeld, and Kolb (1963), a young person's social patterns are defined by the number and duration of his friendships, the frequency with which he interacts with his friends, and the variety of activities he shares with them. The adolescent who has one friend at a time, who sees his friend only occasionally and in connection with a single shared activity, and who moves frequently from one friend to the next demonstrates much less capacity for object relatedness than a youngster who maintains a number of friendships over an extended period of time with peers he sees fairly often around a variety of shared activities.

Also of importance is the mutuality of a youngster's friendships. The less his relationships are characterized by mutual respect, mutual decision-making, mutual exchange of favors, and mutual activity in maintaining the relationship, the less likely they are to represent adaptive capacity for social engagement. The exploited youngster who complies with his "friend's" every wish, waits at his beck and call, and plies him with money and gifts demonstrates little more capacity for rewarding interpersonal relationships than the youngster who claims no friends at all. Such a non-mutual friendship pattern is poignantly illustrated in the following exchange with a lonely 13-year-old boy who elsewhere presented evidence of disordered thinking:

THERAPIST: What are you planning to do during your Christmas vacation?
PATIENT: I don't know. Maybe I'll call up a friend and offer to take him bowling so he'll come over to my house.
THERAPIST: He wouldn't come over to your house if you didn't take him bowling?
PATIENT: No.
THERAPIST: What if you just asked him if he wanted to go bowling, with both of you paying your own way?
PATIENT: Oh, I couldn't get anyone to go with me if I did it that way. The last time I tried it the kid hung up on me before I even got a chance to offer to pay for him.

Behavior and Judgment. Evidence of unusual or bizarre behavior and judgment often dominates the clinical history reported by the parents and teachers of a frankly schizophrenic youngster. In the case of a mildly disturbed adolescent with a mixed clinical picture, however, the pathological import of his actions and opinions may be ambiguous, and the family and school may report diagnostically significant events without being aware of their deviance. The following three examples of peculiar orientations were among the initial indices of subsequently demonstrated schizophrenic disorder in youngsters who presented in an otherwise undramatic fashion:

The parents of a 13-year-old boy, who were concerned that he was "emotionally immature" and argumentative, described almost in passing that he was fascinated with timepieces and could spend hours absorbed in watching a clock tick. From their point of view his preoccupation with watches and clocks was merely a nonproductive hobby.

A 17-year-old high school senior indicated he planned to play football when he entered college the following year. Asked about his high school football career, he reported that he had never played football, because he wanted to avoid the risk of injury and save himself for "the big time."

A 16-year-old boy being evaluated in connection with a variety of obsessive-compulsive symptoms was found to be heavily involved in writing a musical version of *The Hound of the Baskervilles.*

Such instances of apparently unusual ideation and activity must always be carefully considered in light of normative adolescent behavior and in respect to the seriousness with which they are pursued. The more extremely the behavior or judgment deviates from normative patterns and the less able the adolescent is to take some critical distance from it (as in such comments as, "I guess I know that's really not a sensible expectation" or "I'm just doing it for the fun of it, not to be taken seriously"), the more likely becomes the possibility of schizophrenic disturbance.

Family History. A family history of schizophrenia is always important in alerting the clinician to the possibility that a disturbed adolescent may be moving toward an overt schizophrenic condition. This diagnostic criterion does not presume any commitment to a genetic interpretation of schizophrenic etiology. Familial incidence of schizophrenia can be interpreted along psychogenic as well as biological lines (see Laing and Esterson, 1964; Mishler and Waxler, 1965, 1968). Either way it appears empirically to be the case that the greater the incidence of schizophrenia in a patient's family and the more closely his schizophrenic relatives are related to him, the more likely he is to develop a schizophrenic disturbance. This point is neatly made by Meehl (1962, p. 827), who notes that the single fact contributing most reliably to a diagnosis of schizophrenia is the knowledge that the patient has an identical twin who is schizophrenic.

Developmental History. Indications of prior disturbance or developmental deviation are helpful in determining whether an apparently schizophrenic adolescent is experiencing an acute, chronic, or childhood form of the disorder. The youngster who develops fairly rapid onset of schizophrenic symptoms in adolescence, following a childhood free from behavioral disturbances that include identifying features of schizophrenia, is likely to be acutely schizophrenic, whereas the adolescent whose presenting schizophrenic picture is only the end result of a long and gradual development of his symptomatology is probably chronically disturbed. This seemingly simple distinction is at times complicated by the parents' difficulty in reporting accurately their child's preadolescent development, and the clinician may have to rely heavily on his own initial impressions in determining chronicity.

The identification of childhood schizophrenia through history is usually less of a problem, primarily because the childhood schizophrenic usually demonstrates blatantly deviant phenomena that his parents have seldom been able to overlook or deny. The adolescent with childhood schizophrenia typically has had an early history of developmental lags, mutism, bizarre play habits, and withdrawn or autistic behavior (see p. 107), and most parents can reliably report whether or not such phenomena occurred.

Interview Behavior

A number of aspects of an adolescent's interview behavior can assist the clinician in assessing the possibility of schizophrenic disturbance. These behaviors need not be frankly schizophrenic or necessarily indicative of schizophrenia if taken out of context. Rather, they comprise subtle indices of disturbance that, given the set of a mixed clinical picture, increase the probability of a schizophrenic disorder. Of particular diagnostic significance in the adolescent's interview behavior are his speech patterns, his style of relating, his appearance, and the quality of his affect and judgment.

Speech Patterns. An individual's speech patterns are highly likely to reflect any disorder in his thinking (see Kasanin, 1944; Laffal, 1965), particularly with respect to dissociation and blocking, the two major clues to pathologically disordered thinking in disturbed adolescents (see p. 101). In the mildly or incipiently schizophrenic adolescent dissociation may emerge only as subtle discontinuities in the interview, many of which can be overlooked or erroneously attributed to simple misunderstandings if the clinician does not attend closely to the direction and flow of the conversation. The following two interchanges with a 14-year-old boy illustrate subtle discontinuities that initially raised the question of an eventually confirmed schizophrenic disturbance:

THERAPIST: What kinds of things do you like to do?
PATIENT: I like to play basketball; I'm a good aimer.
THERAPIST: You're a good shot?
PATIENT: Yes, last summer at camp we shot at targets with real bullets.

PATIENT: The kids at school tease me and call me all kinds of names.
THERAPIST: Like what?
PATIENT: Oh, like "stupid" and "mental" and "retarded" and like that.
THERAPIST: Do they call your brother those names [reference to patient's younger brother in same school]?
PATIENT: No, no one calls me "brother."

Blocking as a clue to disordered thinking is illustrated in the following excerpt from the psychological testing report on a 19-year-old girl, whose behavior also suggested impaired affective integration:

"Although Mary was cooperative and quite submissive to directions, her obvious and severe blocking considerably hampered her response process. Her reaction times were extremely slow, and her verbal communications were offered in short phrases separated by long pauses during which she seemed constantly on the verge of saying something, but not quite able to sound the words. Additionally of note in her behavior was her inappropriate affect. She maintained a fixed smile during much of the session, a smile punctuated only by occasional laughs for which no appropriate stimuli were apparent."

DeHirsch (1967) has elaborated several other features of language and speech that suggest schizophrenic disorder in young people, including idiosyncratic word usage and unusual variations in pitch, stress, and inflection. The youngster who uses words peculiarly, who displays a monotonous, repetitive, or singsong delivery unrelated to the content of his speech, or whose pronunciation and inflection suggest a speech impediment or that the language he is speaking is not his native tongue, when neither is the case, is more likely to be experiencing a schizophrenic disorder of thinking and affect than the youngster whose conversation has none of these qualities.

Style of Relating. The manner in which the adolescent relates on interview also provides valuable information in the differential diagnosis of schizophrenia, particularly in regard to the patient's capacity for object relatedness. The clinician must judge as best he can the extent to which he feels mutually engaged with the adolescent in an ongoing interpersonal relationship. The adolescent who stares vacantly at the interviewer or is unable to maintain any eye contact with him at all, for example, is often severely deficient in his capacity to relate to others. This inference would of course assume that hostility and defiance were not determining the staring or disinterest, and that situational anxiety, embarrassment, or shyness was not involved in the youngster's inability to look the interviewer in the eye.

Such distinctions usually rest with the general appropriateness of the patient's behavior patterns. Nonengagement with the interviewer may well represent refusal to do so in the resistive youngster who is brought for treatment against his wishes. In the adolescent who comes willingly or submissively and appears eager to return, however, such nonengagement usually reflects basic difficulties in reaching out to people.

Similarly, the youngster who sits huddled in his coat, his body turned away from the examiner and his glance averted, but who nevertheless exhibits an occasional appropriate smile or argumentative retort is much less likely to be schizophrenically disturbed than the youngster who cannot inject such responsiveness into a general posture of withdrawal. For many seriously troubled but not schizophrenic adolescents who come for an initial interview frightened and virtually mute, it may be only through such glimpses of warmth and appropriate affect that a nonschizophrenic diagnosis can be correctly made. In contrast, the pattern of withdrawal described in the following excerpt from the psychological examination of a 16-year-old girl points strongly toward schizophrenia:

"Vera was quite blocked throughout the examination and was frequently out of contact with me. It was quite typical for her abruptly to cease her response process and either look vacantly into space or sit with her eyes tightly closed. At such times she would frown, bite her lips as in fear or embarrassment, or smile inappropriately. These behaviors bore no relationship to the reality situation as I perceived it and seemed rather a function of complete withdrawal on her part into her fantasy."

Appearance. The adolescent's appearance often reflects his level of personality organization. Given the teenager's normative attention to physical appearance, the youngster who appears for an interview unkempt and bedraggled is more likely to be experiencing personality disorganization than one whose dress and grooming reveal a socially oriented attention to his person. As for the sloppy sandals or shaggy locks affected by the self-styled "hippie" or "swinger," it is seldom difficult to differentiate the youngster whose sloppiness is dictated by careful conformity to an "in" style of dress from the one whose disarray derives from apathy or obliviousness.

In this regard Easson (1966) points out that an adolescent's appearance yields diagnostic clues not only in relation to personality organization but also by its congruence with reigning adolescent standards. It is important that the clinician be sufficiently current with these standards to determine accurately whether his patient's dress reflects adequate peer-group engagement. As of this writing, teenage youngsters endorse a wide variety of styles in dress. However, the adolescent whose attire is immediately reminiscent of a much younger child or a stodgy adult is probably not maintaining satisfactory social relationships with his peers. Obviously not every such youngster is likely to be schizophrenic. Yet, given other evidence of schizophrenic ego impairments, failure to exhibit an age-appropriate appearance may be an important piece of evidence contributing to a diagnosis of schizophrenia.

Affect and Judgment. Finally of note is the general appropriateness of the adolescent's interview behavior, particularly in relation to his affect and judgment. The importance of inappropriate affect in suggesting schizophrenic disturbance has been mentioned at several points in this chapter. Such inappropriateness in the interview setting may arise either as acts of commission or omission. The adolescent who is childishly silly, giggles out of context, or responds with extreme reactions—shock, surprise, disbelief, embarrassment, etc.—to relatively insignificant statements demonstrates inappropriate affect; similarly the youngster whose affective tone is so blunted that neither joking, sarcasm, sympathy, nor even browbeating elicit an emotional reaction also exhibits an impaired capacity for affective integration.

Mild displays of inappropriate affect sometimes arise in connection with a disturbed adolescent's inability to judge accurately the nature of the interview situation, as in the following example:

> A 15-year-old obviously anxious and frightened boy was asked some routine, simple questions in order to engage him and reduce his anxiety—how old he was, where he went to school, what grade he was in, and so forth. Although apparently in good contact and not experiencing any blocking, he made a major production of each question. As if he were being cross-examined and enormous consequences were riding on each answer, he furrowed his brow, reflected at great length, and then either gave a vague, noncommittal answer ("I guess I'm 15"; "I think maybe it's Northeast High") or declined to respond at all. That for him the experience of these few questions may indeed have been that of cross-examination is not the issue here; by interpreting the situation disparately from its objective reality, he allowed his poor judgment to produce an inappropriate affective tone.

Unusual interview behavior is often a major index of poor or idiosyncratic judgment, and schizophrenic potential in a mildly disturbed adolescent may first become apparent through minimal and scattered hints of social inappropriateness. The pathological implications of subtly unusual behavior, interpreted in relation to normative adolescent patterns, is illustrated in the following excerpt from the summary of an initial diagnostic interview with a 13-year-old boy:

> "From the beginning of the interview and at several times during it, Jack's behavior left me concerned about the level of his judgment and the appropriateness of his affective responses. He initially exhibited none of the nervousness, guardedness, wariness, or obvious defenses against such

feelings that might be normatively expected of an adolescent brought for his first visit with a psychologist. Rather, as I began to ask him what his understanding of coming to see me was, he broke in with a harangue about his father's always yelling at him, and he talked throughout the interview without hesitation and with no questions about why he was here or what we would be doing. At several points he abruptly interrupted his own sentences with, 'Is there anything else you want to ask me?', which was usually far removed from the context of our interaction. Similarly his affect, though appropriate for the most part, sometimes involved a very unusual, singsong presentation of what he was saying and at times a demonstrative emotional style that in my view was neither appropriate to the content nor within the normal range for an adolescent boy in an interview situation."

Psychological Test Findings

The assessment of possible schizophrenic features in disturbed adolescents constitutes a significant portion of the psychological examiner's consultative work. The frequency of this question among requests for psychodiagnostic consultation derives from (a) the already discussed difficulty in differentiating schizophrenia from certain other maladaptive tendencies in disturbed adolescents on the basis of initial case history and interview data, and (b) the particular sensitivity of psychodiagnostic tests to many of the personality impairments that define schizophrenic disturbance.

In this latter regard the psychological test battery permits relatively clear distinctions between the formal and the content aspects of disorder (see pp. 121–123). On both structured and projective techniques the clinician can usually clarify more readily than he can on interview the extent to which any peculiar content in an adolescent's fantasy is accompanied by peculiarities in the formal thought processes by which the unusual content is arrived at. Furthermore, to the extent that a youngster's thought content reflects his level of maturity, an adolescent's fantasy productions on projective examination provide diagnostically relevant clues to the age appropriateness of his interests and pursuits (see pp. 118–121). The teenager whose Rorschach is dominated, for example, by teddy bears and fairy queens probably does not share normative adolescent frames of reference.

Psychodiagnostic tests additionally allow some quantitative assessment of aspects of ego functioning that are significant for the differential diagnosis of schizophrenia in equivocally disturbed adolescents; for example, in respect to a subject's relation to reality the test battery yields numerical indices of his ability to perceive his environment accurately, to recognize conventional modes of response, and to comprehend social experiences at a level commensurate with his demonstrated intelligence.

Finally, the test battery provides several clues to the distinction between acute and chronic disturbance that otherwise might emerge only in the course of an extended follow-up; for example, the pervasiveness of deviant test responses and the extent to which they appear ego-syntonic to the subject have major implications for the chronicity of a schizophrenic disturbance. The specific application of psychological test findings to the differential diagnosis of schizophrenia is beyond the scope of this discussion but has been treated elsewhere in detail (see Weiner, 1966).

CASE ILLUSTRATIONS

The following three cases illustrate common patterns of initially mild, mixed, or equivocal disturbance in adolescents whose clinical history, interview behavior, and psychological test performance subsequently pointed to schizophrenia. The first two patients, both originally seen at age 16, are a boy who demonstrated a drastic personality change with acute onset of aggressive acting-out behavior and a girl who presented with a gradual development of depression and withdrawal during adolescence. The third youngster is a 13-year-old girl with a long history of apathy and social isolation whose slowly and insidiously developing symptomatology antedated her adolescence and was only peripherally affected by it.

Case 1

Donald is a 16-year-old boy who until six months prior to his admission to the hospital had been considered a bright, creative, quiet, and retiring youngster. He reportedly had many friends, was well liked in school, and had never been in disciplinary difficulty. Shortly before the beginning of his sophomore year in high school he was slightly injured in an unusual accident. Standing in his driveway, he was accidentally struck by a car whose teenage driver had veered off the road purportedly just to scare him. Donald suffered no head injury or lingering physical distress as a consequence of this accident. Yet—in sharp contrast to his previously characteristic restraint, self-control, and even temper—he began shortly after the incident to demonstrate marked hyperactivity and frequent angry outbursts. He shouted obscenities at his mother at the slightest provocation and responded to minor domestic disagreements by stamping around the house and slamming doors. He also began to sleep poorly, to have frequent nightmares, and to thrash so violently in bed that he repeatedly bruised himself against the wall and his bedframe.

Upon returning to school shortly after the sudden onset of his aggressive, poorly controlled behavior he displayed a precipitous decline in his grades, from the "B" and "C" work of his freshman year to "D" and "F" grades. He also became a school discipline problem for the first time, and on one occasion he was apprehended by the police while attempting with some other boys to force entry into the school building at night. His difficulties continued unabated until February of the school year, when he responded to his principal's request that he cut his extremely long hair by storming out of school and refusing to return. The parents at this point sought professional help.

During an initial interview Donald fidgeted, displayed flat affect, tended to stare at the wall with a silly grin on his face, and expressed little concern about his problem behavior and failing grades at school. There was, however, no gross evidence of thought disorder. Because of the extent of his loss of control, his refusal to return to school, and his strained relationship with his mother, it was decided to admit him to the hospital for further evaluation and treatment planning. His admission diagnosis was "adolescent turmoil."

During a subsequent 1-month hospital stay Donald proved refractory to efforts to assist him in controlling his aggressive, antisocial behavior; if anything his hostile, obtrusive, and recalcitrant behavior increased. He repetitively cursed out the staff, particularly his therapist ("You're a shitty doctor"), broke up furniture, threw his shoes and other handy objects at fellow patients, and twice ran away from the hospital. Midway in his hospitalization his continued inability to control himself, poor judgment, and occasional display of dissociation and blocking suggested the possibility of underlying schizophrenia, and psychological consultation was requested.

Donald's performance on psychological examination clearly identified features of schizophrenic disturbance. Particularly notable were poor reality testing and an impaired capacity for social judgments. Almost half of his Rorschach responses were perceptually inaccurate, an extent of perceptual inaccuracy far beyond normal adolescent limits, and he failed to report most of the common and conventional Rorschach responses. He responded to items of social comphrehension on the Wechsler Adult Intelligence Scale in a spotty and inconsistent fashion, at times misinterpreting or suggesting impulsive reactions to fairly clearly defined situations and at other times offering sophisticated, clearly reasoned analyses of complex problems.

Donald's hospitalization at a university medical center ended abruptly with the expiration of his insurance coverage. He was discharged with a diagnosis of acute undifferentiated schizophrenia, and further hospitalization at a nearby state hospital was recommended. His family declined this recommendation, however, and he returned home to continue his treatment on an outpatient basis. Relative to his stormy hospital course and guarded prognosis at discharge, Donald did surprisingly well after leaving the hospital. It was almost as if the hospital regime had somehow perpetuated his misbehavior and that only upon returning to his natural environment could he consolidate and implement psychotherapeutic gains he had made during his hospitalization. At any rate, follow-up over two years indicated that for the most part he had resumed the quiet, controlled personality style that had characterized him before his acute decompensation. He continued to manifest some strange behavior, but he had returned to school without incident, was performing well in his studies, and had presented no behavioral difficulty.

Donald's case illustrates the sudden and acute onset of personality decompensation during adolescence, with a mixture of schizophrenic and sociopathic features. The psychological testing pointed the differential diagnosis toward schizophrenia, and his subsequent course, with continuing personality peculiarities but no further antisocial behavior, bore out this impression. His rapid and reasonably successful remission, together with the preciptious nature of his breakdown, demonstrates the acute nature of his schizophrenic reaction.

Case 2

Karen was first seen at age 16 at the request of her family doctor, to whom she had expressed some suicidal ideas during a routine physical examination. She was an attractive, stylishly dressed, somewhat heavily made up girl who complained initially of having felt depressed for the past two to three years, primarily in relation to the deaths of two horses she had owned. Her apparently erroneous impression that she had in some way been responsible for these deaths had led her to give up riding, which had been her major interest. She reported poor appetite, difficulty in sleeping, preoccupation with the meaning of life, and a generally bleak view of her future. She also described herself as a "loner" who had little interest in being with people and no desire for heterosexual relationships. Although her mood was clearly depressed, she talked freely and without apparent incoherence or irrelevance. In view of the unclear suicidal risk and the fact that her home was some distance from the city, it was decided to admit her to the hospital. Her diagnosis at admission was "adolescent adjustment crisis, with depressive, phobic, and hysterical features."

Karen's behavior during her first week in the hospital, however, together with some emerging details of her history, began to suggest possible schizophrenic disturbance. On the ward she was alternately seductive and markedly withdrawn. As if to shut out the world as much as possible, she at times curled up in a corner of her room, with the blinds pulled and the lights out, wearing sunglasses. She frequently complained that "life is only pain and emptiness" and began to ask if she could remain in the hospital indefinitely. She said that she felt close to no one, particularly her parents—"I love them but I don't care about them." She also admitted that there were times, mostly when she was alone, when she felt that eyes were watching her.

When asked about her disinterest in dating, Karen stated that, since all boys expect heavy petting on the first date and she did not want either to be touched or to have to "put men down," she had always declined dating invitations. It was also learned, however, that between the ages of 13 and 14 she had regularly been embraced and kissed by an older brother whenever the two of them were alone in the house. Her stated reason for neither resisting her brother's advances nor complaining of them to her mother was, "I don't want to put anybody down."

Additional information from Karen's mother revealed that she had generally been a shy, introverted girl with little self-confidence. When asked about her shyness, Karen confirmed that she had always felt uncomfortable around youngsters of her own age and from age seven or eight had preferred associating with older people. The only two organized peer-group activities she had ever pursued were the 4-H Club and a horse club, both of which she had given up during the previous two years. Finally of note was that several months prior to her hospitalization she had become increasingly compulsive in her school work and begun to stay up far into the night pondering over the details of her studies.

Karen's physical and emotional isolation from others, her unusual behavior, and her unrealistic ideas about dating and being watched—viewed in relation to her depressive complaints, uncharacteristic seductiveness, and preocccupation with detail—suggested the presence of an underlying schizophrenic disturbance that was emerging in the form of apparent depression and a last-ditch intensification of hysterical and obsessive-compulsive defenses. Subsequent psychological examination yielded the following confirmatory impressions:

"In general, the data reveal that Karen is a highly intelligent girl with many areas of ego resource who does not seem as seriously disturbed as some aspects of her clinical history and behavior might suggest. On the other hand, she is a very troubled girl, with major problems in the area of sexual identification, and there are times when the nature of her concerns is reflected in circumstantial reasoning and poor reality testing. The pattern of her strengths and weaknesses might be consistent either with an early stage of an incipient schizophrenic reaction or with a mild borderline state."

After 3½ weeks in the hospital, during which she remained depressed and withdrawn but no longer appeared to present a suicidal risk, Karen was discharged to office treatment. Three months later she was back in the hospital, complaining, "I'm not myself, they changed me in the hospital; I started out thinking someone was going to kill me, and now I think everyone wants to kill me." During her outpatient treatment her condition had continued to decline, and by her own report she had done nothing but "sit around and lose all hope." Two weeks before her second admission she had developed the specific delusional idea that a tall man with a knife was after her to kill her. On readmission she appeared sullen and withdrawn, demonstrated flat affect and an inclination to stare blankly ahead of her, and was preoccupied with delusions of impending victimization. Over the next eight months her depressive affect lifted somewhat and her paranoid ideation diminished, and she was again discharged, now with a diagnosis of "schizophrenic reaction, schizo-affective type."

After several months' subsequent outpatient treatment, during which she maintained reasonable ideational control and adequate affective integration, a second psychological consultation was obtained to aid in evaluating her readiness to return to school. On this occasion the examination revealed considerably less anxiety and many fewer ruminations and fears about relationships with other people than had been apparent on her previous testing. However, her decreased interpersonal anxiety appeared to have been achieved at the cost of increased distance and withdrawal from other people, with diminished interest in thinking about others or reaching out for them emotionally.

These developments, together with continued evidence of illogical reasoning and impaired reality testing, suggested that Karen was moving toward a basically chronic schizophrenic adjustment. Although her withdrawal was interpreted as a maladaptive concomitant of her schizophrenic disturbance, it was also seen as a successful means of reducing her anxiety level and allowing her to achieve a more stable course than she had previously been able to realize. Karen's history illustrates the gradual development of a chronic schizophrenic disturbance, apparently beginning in adolescence, with prominent depressive features initially dominating the presenting symptomatology.

Case 3

Alice was first brought by her parents for evaluation at age 13 after several years of borderline academic performance that had recently culminated in her being assigned to a modified class program. During her first two months in this program she had performed very well and now wished to return to her regular class. Her parents were uncertain whether she was too bright for the modified program and should be removed from it or whether it was important for her to continue the unprecedented success experience she was having in this relatively undemanding program.

Although their interest in evaluating Alice's school potential had prompted her parents' request for professional guidance, they readily reported many years' concern about her pervasive apathy and poorly developed social relationships. Alice had never been interested in her school work or in anything else, they indicated, and her only current source of enjoyment was watching television. They had kept her active in the Girl Scouts for a few years, primarily by conducting her to and from all the scouting events, but they felt she had never developed any intrinsic interest in Girl Scouts and had never gained anything from her "participation."

Concerning Alice's social relationships, the parents stated that she had never had many friends and that her few girlfriends of past years had been growing distant from her. In their view her persistent childishness and failure to develop typical teenage interests and attitudes were responsible for her increasing isolation from her peers. Alice's only current companions were younger children in the neighborhood, and her parents had observed with distress her proclivity, at age 13, to engage in hide-and-seek type games with 9- and 10-year olds. They also described Alice as a very quiet girl who kept her feelings to herself and had never presented them with any behavior or disciplinary difficulties. Her growth through infancy and childhood was reported as normal, and she had never had any major health problems.

Alice was a tall, physically developed girl who appeared for her first interview somewhat sedately but appropriately dressed. She sat primly in her chair and responded to questions in a forthright but rather formal and stilted manner. Although her behavior initially suggested merely that she was an anxious and rigid girl, her persistent stiffness and monotonous response style as the interview progressed became increasingly reminiscent of the flat, automatic, repetitive behavior patterns seen in catatonic patients.

Alice additionally displayed a number of peculiarities in the content and form of her conversation. Asked to indicate some things she wished for, she listed a motorcycle, a skindiving outfit, an eagle, and a hawk. The uselessness of a motorcycle to a 13-year-old, who could not be licensed to drive it, and the fact that Alice had never done any skindiving attest the unusual quality of her first two wishes. Regarding the eagle and the hawk, she gave the following strange, clearly childish explanations: the eagle could be used to stop the school bus if she ever wanted to get someone off it, and the hawk could be used for delivering messages. When asked what she liked to do, she listed horseback riding as her favorite activity; yet it turned out she had ridden only once and that had been two years ago. At many points she responded in such subtly discontinuous ways as the following:

THERAPIST: What did you do the past weekend?
PATIENT: Our father took us to visit the museum on Sunday.
THERAPIST: Do you go out together like that very often?
PATIENT: No, my father is too busy, and usually on Sunday he's writing checks.
THERAPIST: What does your father do?
PATIENT: Oh, he took us to the museum and he stayed there with us to hear a man give a talk.
THERAPIST: I said what does he do.
PATIENT: Oh, you mean his business.

Subsequent psychological examination revealed Alice to have clear impairments of reality testing, with a pathological frequency of inaccurate percepts on the Rorschach and pronounced incapacity for adaptive social relationships. The testing also demonstrated below average intelligence, with an IQ in the 85 to 90 range. This intellectual performance indicated that Alice might be expected to achieve no better than borderline performance in a regular class in her particular school but that mental retardation could not be adduced to account for her striking immaturity, peculiar thought content, and poor reality testing. The combined history, interview, and test data strongly suggested an underlying schizophrenic disturbance that, in the absence of any blatant symptomatology or major behavior difficulties, had been slowly and quietly developing for a number of years prior to the advent of her puberty.

PROGNOSIS

Neither the general outcome nor the differential prognosis of schizophrenia has been conclusively explored to date, and the extensive literature in this area is difficult to integrate (see Huston and Pepernik, 1958, pp. 331–333). Variations across studies in the diagnostic criteria for schizophrenia, the nature and extent of treatment received, the length and methodology of the follow-up investigations, and the nature of the control groups, if any, severely limit comparisons across published research studies.

The general notion of prognosis, furthermore, is meaningful only in relation to its criteria. For example, remission of symptoms, discharge from hospital, and successful academic and social readjustment, each of which can be achieved without the other two, have all been used to define favorable outcome. In spite of these difficulties, the available research literature does provide some indications as to the general outcome of adolescent schizophrenia and certain indices that may aid the assessment of prognosis in the individual case.

General Outcome

Follow-up studies of schizophrenic adolescents by Carter (1942), Masterson (1956), and Warren (1965) have employed comparable criteria of patient status and may accordingly be integrated to yield some picture of general outcome in adolescent schizophrenia. Carter's study was based on 78 fourteen- to eighteen-year-old psychotic youngsters consecutively admitted to the Shenley Hospital in England. Follow-up data were collected over a three-year period on 55 of these patients who were diagnosed as schizophrenic or as having an "acute confusional state" with many schizophrenic features. Masterson followed up 83 patients 5 to 19 years after they had first been diagnosed as schizophrenic at the Payne Whitney Clinic when they were age 12 to 18. Warren followed for six years or more 23 schizophrenic patients seen in the adolescent unit of The Bethlem Royal Hospital in England.

Each of these investigators utilized interview and accessory data to assign his patients to four similar adjustment categories on follow-up. Category A was applied by Carter to patients who had been out of the hospital for at least three years, were earning a living, and were completely free of symptoms; Masterson designated as category A patients who were functioning without impairment from symptoms at work or in the home; and Warren used category A to indicate patients who were not in need of psychiatric treatment. Category B was defined by Carter, Masterson, and Warren respectively as remission of psychosis and discharge from hospital but with incomplete recovery and residual symptoms; as functioning with minimum impairment from symptoms (up to 50%) at work or at home; and as requiring ongoing treatment though not necessarily by a psychiatrist. The respective criteria for category C were apparent periods of recovery followed by relapses requiring rehospitalization from time to time; functioning with marked impairment from symptoms (greater than 50%) at work or home; and requirement for psychiatric outpatient treatment. Category D consisted of acute or chronic deterioration requiring permanent hospitalization; inability to function and hospitalization; and requirement for continued hospitalization.

Of the 161 schizophrenic adolescents studied by Carter, Masterson, and Warren, 37 were assigned on follow-up to category A, 18 to category B, 24 to category C, and 82 to category D. It is interesting to note the bimodal nature of this distribution: 84% of the youngsters were eventually either more or less completely recovered (category A), or were continuously hospitalized (category D). Of course many factors other than a patient's state of disturbance influence the likelihood of his being continuously hospitalized or resuming an adequate community adjustment—including the nature of the treatment he receives, the attitudes and economic resources of his family, and the social, academic, and vocational demands he must face (see Cheek, 1965; Freeman and Simmons, 1963; Orr et al., 1955). It is nevertheless tempting to interpret the bimodal follow-up distribution in these studies as being consistent with the distinction between acute or reactive schizophrenic disturbance on the one hand and chronic or process schizophrenia on the other (see Kantor and Herron, 1966).

In other words, these longitudinal studies imply that the large majority of adolescent schizophrenics either achieve fairly complete recovery from their disturbance or progress toward continued incapacitation and institutionalization. The youngsters who fall into intermediate categories of outcome may well represent environmental influences on future course: namely (a) fortunate circumstances that avert continued incapacitation and hospitalization in the chronically disturbed schizophrenic adolescent and (b) unfortunate circumstances that interfere with what might otherwise have been a complete recovery in the acutely disturbed youngster.

These data can also be meaningfully compared with certain other follow-up studies of schizophrenic adolescents and adults. If the Carter-Masterson-Warren category A is interpreted to represent recovery, the B and C categories to indicate some improvement, and the D category as an index of no change or decline, the following conclusion emerges: in general 23% of adolescent schizophrenics will recover, 49% will either recover or realize some improvement, and 51% will fail to improve or become worse. Longitudinal studies by Annesley (1961) and Errara (1957), utilizing these three categories to designate outcome, have yielded similar results. Annesley followed 78 schizophrenic adolescents over a two- to five-year period after their admission to St. Ebba's Hospital in England, and Errara reevaluated 54 patients 8 to 24 years after they had been diagnosed as schizophrenic in an outpatient clinic.

Annesley reports that 19% of his patient sample recovered during the follow-up period, 42% either recovered or improved, and 58% demonstrated no change. For Errara the percentages of good, mediocre, and poor clinical status on follow-up were 26, 52, and 48%, respectively. Together with the work of Carter, Masterson, and Warren, these data suggest that, other things being equal, about one-fourth of adolescent schizophrenics will recover, another one-fourth will demonstrate some improvement, and the remaining one-half will fail to improve. It should be noted, however, that these figures derive in the main from hospital samples; that is, from adolescent patients who were sufficiently disturbed when they were first seen to require hospital admission. Even in Errara's clinic-based study, 83% of the patients were hospitalized at one time or another following their initial clinic contact. The question therefore remains open as to what more favorable outcome statistics might derive from samples of youngsters who, though schizophrenically disturbed, did not require hospital admission.

In regard to similar follow-up studies of adults Huston and Pepernik (1958, p. 533) report that the extensive literature concerning outcome in adult schizophrenics who have received hospital care indicates a range from 22 to 54% who demonstrate improvement or recovery, with most such reports clustering around 40%. From these data it would appear that the expected outcomes for hospitalized schizophrenic adolescents is roughly comparable to that observed among patients who are first hospitalized for schizophrenia as adults.

However, Pollack, Levenstein, and Klein (1968) present some evidence that both adolescent and young adult schizophrenics may have a poorer prognosis than patients with later onset. In a three-year follow-up study of schizophrenic patients first hospitalized as adolescents (age 16–19), young adults (20–29), or older adults (30–57), they found no significant differences between the adolescent and young adult groups on a variety of outcome measures. Yet the adolescent and young adult groups combined rated significantly less well than the older adult group on most of the follow-up indices.

Prognostic Indices

A number of specific prognostic indices of adolescent schizophrenia have been suggested in these various longitudinal studies. Carter found that a favorable outcome was most likely in youngsters who demonstrated an acute, stormy onset of schizophrenic disturbance after an obvious precipitating event, were disoriented and confused on initial interview, and had for the most part been amiable and adaptable prior to their decompensation. On the other hand, the earlier the onset of personality change or psychotic behavior in a shut-in and sensitive type of youngster, without evidence of confusion, acute decompensation, and obvious precipitating factors, the graver the prognosis for recovery. Carter also reported that, whereas sporadic instances of psychosis in the family of a schizophrenic adolescent had little implication for his prognosis, multiple psychotic disturbance in the family history was associated with a poor prognosis.

Masterson confirmed some of Carter's findings, challenged others, and added some additional prognostic criteria. In agreement with Carter he found that confusion in the symptomatology and a predisturbance history of good social adjustment were related to a favorable outcome, whereas seclusiveness and a period of onset (defined as the time between the first evidence of difficulty and subsequent inability to function) of greater than 12 months' duration indicated a poor prognosis. Unlike Carter, however, he found no association between either the presence of obvious precipitating events or a family history of psychosis and outcome.

Masterson also reports that favorable outcome was most common among schizophrenic adolescents who were age 15 or older at admission, presented affective features in their symptomatology, had had a good predisturbance school adjustment, demonstrated rapid improvement without relapse in the hospital, and were assigned a good prognosis at discharge. Those who were 14 or younger at admission, who presented features of hebephrenic or simple schizophrenia and a history of poor school adjustment, and who remained in the hospital four months or longer unimproved and unresponsive to somatic treatment tended to have unfavorable outcomes.

Other studies by Annesley (1961) and Pollack (1960) suggest that schizophrenic adolescents with relatively high IQs and normal electroencephalogram (EEG) tracings are likely to have a more favorable outcome than less intelligent schizophrenic adolescents with abnormal EEGs. Pollack notes that his schizophrenic subjects with relatively low IQs and EEG abnormalities tended also to be the ones with earlier onset of schizophrenia, and he hypothesizes that the earlier a youngster experiences the onset of schizophrenia, the more severe his disturbance and the greater the likelihood of his being a damaged person, with limited intelligence, abnormal brain functioning, and a poor prognosis.

These various prognostic indices of adolescent schizophrenia closely resemble the most commonly reported predictors of outcome among schizophrenic adults. Vaillant (1962, 1964) has extracted from the literature and to some extent validated a prognostic scale comprising the following seven indices, each of which has been found to correlate fairly consistently with remission in adult schizophrenia:

1. Acute onset, with less than six months elapsing between the onset of difficulty and full-blown psychosis.
2. Absence of a premorbid schizoid adjustment.
3. Confusion or disorientation.
4. Clear affective components in the symptomatology.
5. Clear precipitating factors.
6. A family history of psychotic depressive disturbance.
7. A preoccupation with death.

The first five of these indices have also figured prominently in highly successful predictions of outcome in adult schizophrenia reported by Stephens, Astrup, and Mangrum (1967), who additionally found a favorable prognosis for recovery or improvement associated in both American and Norwegian schizophrenics with being married, expressing guilt feelings, presenting no marked emotional blunting during hospitalization, and having no schizophrenia among blood relatives.

Although the clinician will find it useful to have such indices in mind as he estimates the possible future course of a schizophrenic youngster, he must heed Vaillant's (1964, p. 508), caution that "there is no well-documented method for predicting on admission the long-term clinical course of schizophrenics." As already noted, the limited power of available admission predictors of outcome in schizophrenia derives partly from the inconsistency of research design in this area and partly from the fact that many nonpersonality factors affect the subsequent adjustment of the person who experiences a schizophrenic disturbance.

Regarding this latter point, even the most widely validated personality indices cannot transcend the subsequent impact on a schizophrenic adolescent of his family's reaction to his disturbance, the opportunities available to him for continued treatment as indicated, and the academic and vocational horizons open to him. The exeperienced clinician will readily recall instances in which the long-range outlook for a schizophrenic youngster hinged on his parents' capacity to "forgive" him for the anxiety and embarrassment he had caused them by becoming disturbed, on the availability of a half-way house or his family's ability to finance long-term outpatient or residential care, or on his school's willingness to allow him to graduate with his class despite a spotty attendance.

Brown (1966) has recently emphasized that efforts to prognosticate schizophrenic disturbance must take increased cognizance of such complexities. It is interesting to note that Henderson sounded a similar plea in 1923 in what is apparently the earliest article on the prognosis of psychotic disorder in adolescence:

"The prognosis should not be based on symptoms, but should depend on the acuteness of the disorder, on its early recognition, on the individuality and intensiveness of the treatment, which in turn must be modified according to a study of the reactions of the personality" (p. 1095).

In general the prediction of outcome in adolescent schizophrenia is at best difficult. Roughly, the older the adolescent when schizophrenic disturbance first appears, the more adequate his academic and social adjustment during his premorbid years, and the more precipitous the onset of his disturbance, the better are his prospects for early remission or complete recovery. Such immediately available data as a pronounced affective component to the disturbance and no family history of schizophrenia may improve the prognosis, but, as illustrated in case 2 (see pp. 134–136), these indices cannot rule out the possibility of prolonged, chronic disturbance.

Some additional prognostic indices emerge in the course of therapeutic intervention. The youngster who is able to become meaningfully engaged with his therapist and who if hospitalized responds quickly to the inpatient milieu with a diminution of his symptoms is probably more likely to sustain a long-range improvement than the youngster who remains distant and aloof and seems unaffected by a variety of inpatient treatment programs. As illustrated in case 1 (see pp. 132–134), however, refractoriness to the hospital regime does not preclude the possibility of rapid remission after discharge.

Finally, given two schizophrenic youngsters with identical presenting histories and a similar initial response to treatment, the one whose family is best able to accept his disturbance and rally to his support and for whom long-term recommendations for therapy, school, work, and living arrangements can be implemented is the one who is most likely to achieve and sustain maximum recovery.

TREATMENT

Treatment of the schizophrenic adolescent combines general procedures for treating schizophrenia with basic principles of psychotherapy for young people. Psychotherapy for the adolescent youngster is discussed at some length in Chapter 9, and there is an extensive literature concerning the treatment of schizophrenic disturbance through individual psychotherapy (Boyer and Giovacchini, 1967; Fromm-Reichmann, 1959, Part III; Hill, 1955), group, milieu, and family therapy (Edelson, 1964; Friedman et al., 1965), somatic therapies (Davis, 1965; Gerz, 1965; Hoch and Pennes, 1958a,b), home care (Pasamanick, Scarpittie, and Dinitz, 1967), and other modalities (see also Redlich and Freedman, 1966, pp. 511–521; Polatin, 1966, pp. 217–226). Without elaborating these topics, the following discussion presents some general guidelines for individual psychotherapy of the schizophrenic adolescent and some considerations in planning his residential care.

Individual Psychotherapy

Relationship and *reality testing* can appropriately be considered the two R's of therapeutic work with the schizophrenic adolescent. The therapist's major effort in the treatment must be to develop an engaged, trusting, mutual relationship in which he can give the youngster a positive experience of interpersonal relatedness and also help him to recognize and revise his inaccurate and distorted impressions of his environment and life events. These primary guidelines for psychotherapy with schizophrenic adolescents follow directly from the impaired capacities for object relatedness and reality testing that centrally define this disturbance.

Above all, the therapist's success in helping the schizophrenic youngster will depend on how fully he can impress him as a warm, genuine, and understanding person who is interested in his welfare, who can be trusted to nurture without exploiting him, and who can invoke special skills on his behalf beyond those of his parents or other adults who have tried to help him. The schizophrenic adolescent has withdrawn from other people because his disturbed cognitive functioning prevents him from understanding them or because his limited social skills cripple his interpersonal coping capacity. In either case he has usually suffered repetitive frustrations, humiliations, and rejections in his approaches to other people that have rendered him interpersonally aversive. The therapist's task is therefore to demonstrate to the youngster that he is at least one person who can understand and make himself understood and who can be relied on not to ridicule, scold, or reject him for his behavior.

To achieve this goal the therapist needs to employ various procedures generally helpful in initiating treatment and building a psychotherapeutic relationship with disturbed adolescents (see pp. 361–370). For those schizophrenic adolescents who display prominent psychopathic personality features, aspects of the treatment approach to characterologically delinquent youngsters may also be applicable (see pp. 332–338). Beyond a certain point of specificity, however, it is impossible to formulate treatment prescriptions that are broadly applicable to schizophrenic youngsters. Ekstein (1963) cogently points out that generalizations about treating the psychotic adolescent can be given individual life only through considerable inventiveness and spontaneity on the part of the therapist.

Ekstein adds that the therapist treating a psychotic adolescent must be prepared for uncertainty regarding his patient's commitment to the therapy, its ultimate course, and the extent to which the youngster's fears of interpersonal engagement will intrude on the relationship. Because of the schizophrenic youngster's usually impaired repressive capacity, proximity to a therapist may bombard him with homosexual or heterosexual fantasies that frighten him or make him feel worthless, hopeless, and degraded. The therapist may also become the object of deep hostilities the youngster feels toward a world he perceives as unappreciative, rejecting, or about to annihilate him. Such poorly modulated impulses have been observed by S. L. Green (1964) and others to foster passive resistance or overtly aggressive maneuvers by which the schizophrenic young-ster seeks to fend off the therapist's efforts to establish a close relationship with him.

To overcome the schizophrenic youngster's efforts to insulate himself from intimacy the therapist needs to rely heavily on his understanding of the patient's actions and behavior. The greater the youngster's resistance to treatment, the less the therapist's warmth and genuineness alone will suffice to initiate a therapeutic relationship. The therapist will have to recognize and interpret the concerns underlying his patient's initial fears and guardedness, and to continue to build the treatment relationship he must also be attuned to the frequently metaphorical quality of the schizo-phrenic youngster's speech. Thus to the schizophrenic youngster who says, "I'm a machine" the therapist's necessary response may be, "If you were a machine, you wouldn't have any feelings and you wouldn't have to worry about anyone hurting you." Beulah Parker (1962) in her book *My Language Is Me* vividly describes the role of metaphorical communi-cation in establishing a therapeutic relationship with a schizophrenic ado-lescent boy, and her material provides a rich glimpse into the course and vicissitudes of outpatient psychotherapy with the schizophrenic adolescent.[2]

In regard to reality testing, the therapist needs to provide the schizo-phrenic adolescent with continuous and direct corrections of his distorted perceptions. Whether these distorted perceptions involve blatant delusional and hallucinatory experiences or subtle instances of poor judgment, the therapist's role is to identify reality and attempt to impress on his patient the eventual rewards of embracing it. Yet the therapist must avoid be-coming an apostle of reality at the expense of undercutting his relationship with the youngster. As the treatment proceeds he will be able to challenge the youngster's misperceptions only as rapidly as he can instill sufficient trust for the youngster not to interpret the challenge as hostility or rejection.

At times certain other treatment procedures effectively supplement the primary emphasis on relationship and reality testing in the treatment of the withdrawn, schizophrenic adolescent. For example, Gladstone (1964) has noted that the therapist can increase the youngster's contact with his environment by sharing real experiences with him and by using educa-tional techniques to provide him with basic information about living that his previous withdrawal may have prevented him from acquiring. Katz (1967) recommends environmental manipulations and pharmacotherapy

---

[2] For an excellent fictionalized account of Frieda Fromm-Reichmann's treatment of a schizophrenic adolescent the reader is referred to Hannah Green's (1964) *I Never Promised You a Rosegarden.*

to attenuate the deteriorating effects of anxiety on the youngster's condition and allow him to participate more fully in psychotherapy, and he also notes that encouraging the youngster toward artistic, intellectual, or other constructive pursuits that may give him pleasure will help him to overcome the anhedonia common to schizophrenic disturbance.

Planning Residential Care

Inasmuch as schizophrenia is the psychological disturbance for which the adolescent youngster is most likely to require hospitalization, it is relevant to mention briefly some issues concerning the planning of residential care for disturbed adolescents. Beckett (1965) and Holmes (1964) describe all-adolescent services at the Lafayette Clinic and University of Michigan Neuropsychiatric Institute, respectively, and the inpatient treatment of teenage youngsters in adolescent units has also been endorsed by Toolan and Nicklin (1959) at Bellevue Hospital in New York, Shamsie and Ellick (1965) at the Verdun Protestant Hospital in Montreal, and by Warren (1952) at the Maudsley Hospital in London. The rationale for this approach lies primarily in the recognition that adolescents require treatment programs different from those commonly appropriate to the needs of child and adult patients. For many troubled teenagers engagement with their peers, rather than with adults from whom they feel alienated, is necessary for the type of active, engaged, open milieu in which psychological difficulties become readily accessible to psychotherapeutic intervention. Warren (1952, p. 147) observes that adolescents admitted to adult wards "tend to form an uneasy minority usually resented by the older patients."

Yet other experienced clinicians strongly oppose the idea of an adolescent service for the inpatient treatment of disturbed youngsters. Greaves and Regan (1957) at the Payne Whitney Clinic and Norton (1967) at Presbyterian–St. Luke's Hospital in Chicago, among others, argue that an all-adolescent service deprives youngsters of an opportunity to live in a normal social setting and fosters feelings of having been abandoned, deserted, and cut off from society. In a mixed adolescent-adult service, these writers continue, adolescents can maintain various levels of communication with people of different ages. Furthermore, they point out, the presence of adults restrains youngsters from the destructive epidemics of aggressive acting-out behavior that frequently arise when groups of disturbed youngsters are isolated in a setting in which they can stimulate and encourage each other to misbehavior.

These differences of clinical opinion have not been put to any definitive empirical test. The relative effectiveness of the all-adolescent versus the mixed inpatient treatment service for disturbed youngsters remains an open issue, as does the particular benefit of either setting for schizophrenic as opposed to other disturbed youngsters. Miller (1957) reports that in the mixed treatment service at the Menninger Foundation schizophrenic youngsters improved more rapidly and dramatically than adolescents with character disorders, whereas Schmiedeck (1961) at the nearby Topeka State Hospital reports that the mixed treatment service offered more therapeutic potential for adolescents with personality disorders than for those who were schizophrenic. Studies on all-adolescent services by Annesley (1961) and Warren (1965) similarly suggested greater improvements in characterologically disturbed than in schizophrenic youngsters.

It is difficult to evaluate such data without detailed information on the likely prognosis of the youngsters prior to admission and on the nature of the actual treatment they received. On the other hand, findings summarized by Beavers and Blumberg (1968) strongly suggest that a specific adolescent program for hospitalized youngsters, regardless of whether it is administered on an all-adolescent or a mixed service, enhances the likelihood of improvement. Reviewing a number of follow-up studies of hospitalized adolescents, they compared the improvement rates of youngsters who had been treated as adults on adult wards, on mixed wards with a special adolescent program, and on all-adolescent services. For both schizophrenic and character-disordered youngsters the rates of long-term improvement were similar for the all-adolescent units and the mixed units with special adolescent programs. Both of these types of units achieved more frequent long-term improvement than mixed services without special adolescent programs.

Although recognizing the merits of a specialized adolescent program for schizophrenic youngsters who require hospitalization, the therapist should nevertheless approach a decision to hospitalize a teenage youngster with considerable caution. The therapist's recommendation of hospitalization to the adolescent and his family often elicits feelings of distress and resistance that can seriously impair the treatment effort if they are not recognized and discussed. Nealon (1964), studying the parents of adolescents for whom inpatient treatment had been recommended, observed particularly poignant parental reaction in the face of hospitalization for their youngster. All of the parents she interviewed expressed some degree of anxiety, disbelief, guilt, and anger at the referring person and/or their youngster for having put them in this position. As far as the adolescent himself is concerned, his fears and misunderstanding about the meaning of hospitalization have been observed to lead him to employ many resistive devices that can defeat the treatment program if they are not adequately met (see Rinsley and Inge, 1961).

A final point to mention is the danger of regression during hospital care. Easson (1967) and Kwalwasser and Green (1961) point out that the schizophrenic youngster's possible regression in the hospital milieu must be taken into consideration in the decision to hospitalize and in the treatment programming of the inpatient service. Easson (1967, p. 345) in particular has stressed very conservative use of residential care:

"Residential treatment is a specific treatment modality indicated only in certain very definite therapeutic circumstances where external ego control, support, and direction are needed. The injudicious use of inpatient therapy not only may not benefit the patient, but may produce permanent personality stunting and emotional regression. The growing adolescent may be handicapped emotionally and intellectually by unnecessary or ill-timed hospital placement, possibly more than any other age group."

REFERENCES

Ames, L. B., Metraux, R. W., and Walker, R. N. *Adolescent Rorschach Responses.* New York: Hoeber-Harper, 1959.

Annesley, P. T. Psychiatric illness in adolescence: Presentation and prognosis. *Journal of Mental Science,* **107**:268–278, 1961.

Arieti, S. *Interpretation of Schizophrenia.* New York: Brunner, 1955.

Beavers, W. R., and Blumberg, S. A follow-up study of adolescents treated in an in-patient setting. *Diseases of the Nervous System,* **29**:606-612, 1968.

Beckett, P. G. S. *Adolescents out of Step: Their Treatment in a Psychiatric Hospital.* Detroit: Wayne State University Press, 1965.

Bellak, L., ed. *Schizophrenia: A Review of the Syndrome.* New York: Logos, 1958.

Bender, L. Childhood schizophrenia. *Psychiatric Quarterly,* **27**:663–681, 1953.

Bender, L. The concept of pseudopsychopathic schizophrenia in adolescents. *American Journal of Orthopsychiatry,* **29**:491–512, 1959.

Beres, D. Ego deviation and the concept of schizophrenia. *Psychoanalytic Study of the Child,* **11**:164–235, 1956.

Bleuler, E. (1911). *Dementia Praecox or the Group of Schizophrenias.* Translated by J. Zinkin. New York: International Universities Press, 1950.

Bower, E. M., Shellhamer, T. A., and Daily, J. M. School characteristics of male adolescents who later become schizophrenic. *American Journal of Orthopsychiatry,* **30**:712–729, 1960.

Boyer, L. B., and Giovacchini, P. L. *Psychoanalytic Treatment of Characterological and Schizophrenic Disorders.* New York: Science House, 1967.

Broen, W. E. *Schizophrenia: Research and Theory.* New York: Academic Press, 1968.

Brown, G. W. Working with "unrecovered" patients. *International Journal of Psychiatry,* **2**:627–629, 1966.

Burns, C. Pre-schizophrenic symptoms in pre-adolescents' withdrawal and sensitivity. *Nervous Child,* **10**:120–128, 1952.

Burton, A., ed. *Psychotherapy of the Psychoses.* New York: Basic Books, 1961.

Bychowski, G. *Psychotherapy of Psychosis.* New York: Grune and Stratton, 1952.

Carter, A. B. Prognostic factors of adolescent psychoses. *Journal of Mental Science,* **88**:31–81, 1942.

Cheek, F. E. Family interaction patterns and convalescent adjustment of the schizophrenic. *Archives of General Psychiatry,* **13**:138–147, 1965.

Colbert, E. G., and Koegler, R. R. The childhood schizophrenic in adolescence. *Psychiatric Quarterly,* **35**:693–701, 1961.

Davis, J. M. Efficacy of tranquilizing and anti-depressant drugs. *Archives of General Psychiatry,* **13**:552–572, 1965.

de Hirsch, K. Differential diagnosis between aphasic and schizophrenic language in children. *Journal of Speech and Hearing Disorders,* **32**:3–10, 1967.

Demerath, N. J. Adolescent status demands and the student experiences of twenty schizophrenics. *American Sociological Review,* **8**:513–518, 1943.

Djartov, L. B. Les etats psychopathe-similes dans la periode initiale de la schizophrenie chez les adolescents (States resembling psychopathology in the initial period of schizophrenia of adolescents). *Zhurnal Nervopatologii i Psikhiatrii,* **65**:1045–1047, 1965.

Easson, W. M. The appearance of the adolescent as a diagnostic indicator. *Pediatrics,* **38**:842–844, 1966.

Easson, W. M. The sole admission criterion for residential adolescent treatment: The rights of the adolescent minority. *American Journal of Orthopsychiatry,* **37**:345, 1967.

Easson, W. M. Ego defects in nonpsychotic adolescents. *Psychiatric Quarterly,* **42**:156–168, 1968.

Edelson, M. *Ego Psychology, Group Dynamics and the Therapeutic Community.* New York: Grune and Stratton, 1964.

Edelston, H. Differential diagnosis of some emotional disorders of adolescence. *Journal of Mental Science,* **95**:961–967, 1949.

Eisenberg, L. The autistic child in adolescence. *American Journal of Psychiatry,* **112**:607–612, 1956.

Ekstein, R. The opening gambit in psychotherapeutic work with psychotic adolescents. *American Journal of Orthopsychiatry,* **33**:862–871, 1963.

Ekstein, R. *Children of Time and Space, of Action and Impulse.* New York: Appleton-Century-Crofts, 1966.

Errera, P. A sixteen-year follow-up of schizophrenic patients seen in an out-patient clinic. *Archives of Neurology and Psychiatry,* **78**:84–87, 1957.

Finch, S. M. *Fundamentals of Child Psychiatry.* New York: Norton, 1960.

Freeman, H. E., and Simmons, O. G. *The Mental Patient Comes Home.* New York: Wiley, 1963.

Friedman, A. S., Boszormenyi-Nagy, I., Jungreis, J. E., Lincoln, G. E., Mitchell, H. E., Sonne, J. C., Speck, R. V., and Spivack, G. *Psychotherapy for the Whole Family: Case Histories, Techniques, and Concepts of*

Family Therapy of Schizophrenia in the Home and Clinic. New York: Springer, 1965.

Fromm-Reichmann, F. *Psychoanalysis and Psychotherapy* (collected papers, edited by D. M. Bullard). Chicago: University of Chicago Press, 1959.

Gardner, G. G. The relationship between childhood neurotic symptomatology and later schizophrenia in males and females. *Journal of Nervous and Mental Disease,* 144:97–100, 1967.

Gerz, H. O. Combined psycho and pharmacotherapy of schizophrenia. *International Journal of Neuropsychiatry,* 1:643–655, 1965.

Gladstone, H. P. Psychotherapy with adolescents: Theme and variations. *Psychiatric Quarterly,* 38:304–309, 1964.

Gravitz, M. A. Normal adult differentiation patterns on the figure drawing test. *Journal of Projective Techniques and Personality Assessment,* 30: 471–473, 1966.

Greaves, D. C., and Regan, P. F. Psychotherapy of adolescents at intensive hospital treatment levels. In B. H. Balser, ed., *Psychotherapy of the Adolescent.* New York: International Universities Press, 1957, pp. 130–143.

Green, H. *I Never Promised You a Rosegarden.* New York: Holt, Rinehart, and Winston, 1964.

Green, S. L. Psychotherapy with adolescent girls. *American Journal of Psychotherapy,* 18:393–404, 1964.

Hamilton, D. M., McKinley, R. A., Moorhead, H. H., and Wall, J. H. Results of mental hospital treatment of troubled youth. *American Journal of Psychiatry,* 117:811–816, 1961.

Hamilton, G. *Psychotherapy in Child Guidance.* New York: Columbia University Press, 1947.

Henderson, D. K. Discussion on prognosis of psychoses in adolescence. *British Medical Journal,* 2:1090–1095, 1923.

Hertz, M. R. The Rorschach in adolescence. In A. I. Rabin and M. R. Haworth, eds., *Projective Techniques with Children.* New York: Grune and Stratton, 1960, pp. 29–60.

Hill, L. B. *Psychotherapeutic Intervention in Schizophrenia.* London: Cambridge University Press, 1955.

Hoch, P. H., and Pennes, H. H. Insulin shock treatment. In L. Bellak, ed., *Schizophrenia: A Review of the Syndrome.* New York: Logos, 1958a, pp. 397–422.

Hoch, P. H., and Pennes, H. H. Electric convulsive treatment and its modifications. In L. Bellak, ed., *Schizophrenia: A Review of the Syndrome.* New York: Logos, 1958b, pp. 423–455.

Holmes, D. J. *The Adolescent in Psychotherapy.* Boston: Little, Brown, 1964.

Holt, R. R., and Havel, J. A method for assessing primary and secondary process in the Rorschach. In M. A. Rickers-Ovsiankina, ed., *Rorschach Psychology.* New York: Wiley, 1960, pp. 263–315.

Huston, P. E., and Pepernik, M. C. Prognosis in schizophrenia. In L. Bellak, ed., *Schizophrenia: A Review of the Syndrome.* New York: Logos, 1958, pp. 531–542.

Jackson, D. D., ed. *The Etiology of Schizophrenia*. New York: Basic Books, 1960.

Kantor, R. E., and Herron, W. G. *Reactive and Process Schizophrenia*. Palo Alto, Cal.: Science and Behavior Books, 1966.

Kasanin, J. S., ed. *Language and Thought in Schizophrenia*. Berkeley, Cal.: University of California Press, 1944.

Kasanin, J. S., and Kaufman, M. R. A study of the functional psychoses in childhood. *American Journal of Psychiatry*, **9**:307–384, 1929.

Kates, W. W., and Kates, S. L. Conceptual behavior in psychotic and normal adolescents. *Journal of Abnormal and Social Psychology*, **69**:659–663, 1964.

Katz, P. The diagnosis and treatment of borderline schizophrenia in adolescence. *Canadian Psychiatric Association Journal*, **12**:247–251, 1967.

Kiersch, T. A., and Nikelly, A. G. The schizophrenic in college. *Archives of General Psychiatry*, **15**:54–58, 1966.

Kohn, M. L., and Clausen, J. A. Social isolation and schizophrenia. *American Sociological Review*, **20**:265–273, 1955.

Kraepelin, E. (1899). *Clinical Psychiatry*, 1st edition. Translated by A. R. Diefendorf from the 6th edition of *Lehrbuch der Psychiatrie*. New York: Macmillan, 1902.

Kwalwasser, S., and Green, S. L. Institutional treatment. In S. Lorand and H. I. Schneer, eds., *Adolescents: Psychoanalytic Approach to Problems and Therapy*. New York: Hoeber, 1961, pp. 282–300.

Laffal, J. *Pathological and Normal Language*. New York: Atherton, 1965.

Laing, R. D., and Esterson, A. *Sanity, Madness, and the Family*. Vol. I. *Families of Schizophrenics*. New York: Basic Books, 1964.

Lichtenberg, J. D. Prognostic implications of the inability to tolerate failure in schizophrenic patients. *Psychiatry*, **20**:365–371, 1957.

McFate, M. Q., and Orr, F. G. Through adolescence with the Rorschach. *Rorschach Research Exchange*, **13**:302–319, 1949.

Machover, S. Diagnostic and prognostic considerations in psychological tests. In S. Lorand and H. I. Schneer, eds., *Adolescents: Psychoanalytic Approach to Problems and Therapy*. New York: Hoeber, 1961, pp. 301–345.

Masterson, J. F. Prognosis in adolescent disorders—schizophrenia. *Journal of Nervous and Mental Disease*, **124**:219–232, 1956.

Masterson, J. F. *The Psychiatric Dilemma of Adolescence*. Boston: Little, Brown, 1967.

Materson, J. F., Tucker, K., and Berk, G. Psychopathology in adolescence: IV. Clinical and dynamic characteristics. *American Journal of Psychiatry*, **120**:357–366, 1963.

Meehl, P. E. Schizotaxia, schizotypy, schizophrenia. *American Psychologist*, **17**:827–838, 1962.

Miller, D. H. The treatment of adolescents in an adult hospital. *Bulletin of the Menninger Clinic*, **21**:189–198, 1957.

Mishler, E. G., and Waxler, N. E. Family interaction process and schizophrenia: A review of current theories. *Merrill-Palmer Quarterly,* **11**:269–316, 1965.

Mishler, E. G., and Waxler, N. E. *Interaction in Families: An Experimental Study of Family Processes and Schizophrenia.* New York: Wiley, 1968.

Nameche, G. F., Waring, M., and Ricks, D. F. Early indicators of outcome in schizophrenia. *Journal of Nervous and Mental Disease,* **139**:232–240, 1964.

Nealon, J. The adolescent's hospitalization as a family crisis. *Archives of General Psychiatry,* **11**:302–311, 1964.

Neubauer, P. B., and Steinert, J. Schizophrenia in adolescence. *Nervous Child,* **10**:128–134, 1952.

Norton, A. H. Evaluation of a psychiatric service for children, adolescents, and adults. *American Journal of Psychiatry,* **123**:1418–1424, 1967.

Noyes, A. P., and Kolb, L. C. *Modern Clinical Psychiatry,* 6th edition. Philadelphia: Saunders, 1963.

O'Neal, P., and Robins, L. N. Childhood patterns predictive of adult schizophrenia: A 30-year follow-up study. *American Journal of Psychiatry,* **115**:385–391, 1958.

Orr, W. F., Anderson, R. B., Martin, M. P., and Philpot, D. F. Factors influencing discharge of female patients from a state mental hospital. *American Journal of Psychiatry,* **111**:576–582, 1955.

Outpatient Psychiatric Clinics: Special Statistical Report, 1961. Bethesda, Md.: National Institute of Mental Health, 1963.

Parker, B. *My Language Is Me.* New York: Basic Books, 1962.

Pasamanick, B., Scarpitti, F. R., and Dinitz, S. *Schizophrenics in the Community: An Experimental Study in the Prevention of Hospitalization.* New York: Appleton-Century-Crofts, 1967.

Piotrowski, Z. A. Treatment of the adolescent. 1. The relative pessimism of psychologists. *American Journal of Orthopsychiatry,* **32**:382–389, 1962.

Pitt, R., Kornfeld, D. S., and Kolb, L. C. Adolescent friendship patterns as prognostic indicators for schizophrenic adults. *Psychiatric Quarterly,* **37**:499–508, 1963.

Podolsky, E. A note on the schizophrenic college student. *American Journal of Psychiatry,* **119**:782–783, 1963.

Polatin, P. *A Guide to Treatment in Psychiatry.* Philadelphia: Lippincott, 1966.

Pollack, M. Comparison of childhood, adolescent, and adult schizophrenics. *Archives of General Psychiatry,* **2**:652–660, 1960.

Pollack, M., Levenstein, S., and Klein, D. F. A three-year posthospital follow-up of adolescent and adult schizophrenics. *American Journal of Orthopsychiatry,* **38**:94–109, 1968.

Rapaport, D., Gill, M. and Schafer, R. *Diagnostic Psychological Testing,* Vol. II. Chicago: Year Book, 1946.

Redlich, F. C., and Freedman, D. X. *The Theory and Practice of Psychiatry.* New York: Basic Books, 1966.

Rinsley, D. B., and Inge, G. P. Psychiatric hospital treatment of adolescents:

Verbal and nonverbal resistance to treatment. *Bulletin of the Menninger Clinic,* 25:249–263, 1961.

Robins, L. N. *Deviant Children Grown Up: A Sociological and Psychiatric Study of Sociopathic Personality.* Baltimore: Williams and Wilkins, 1966.

Romano, J., ed. *The Origins of Schizophrenia.* Amsterdam: Excerpta Medica, 1967.

Rosen, B. M., Bahn, A. K., Shellow, R., and Bower, E. M. Adolescent patients served in outpatient psychiatric clinics. *American Journal of Public Health,* 55:1563–1577, 1965.

Rosenthal, D., and Kety, S. S., eds. *The Transmission of Schizophrenia.* New York: Pergamon, 1968.

Rutter, M., Greenfield, D., and Lockyer, L. A five to fifteen year follow-up study of infantile psychosis. II. Social and behavioral outcome. *British Journal of Psychiatry,* 113:1183–1199, 1967.

Rychlak, J. F., and O'Leary, L. R. Unhealthy content in the Rorschach responses of children and adolescents. *Journal of Projective Techniques and Personality Assessment,* 29:354–368, 1965.

Sands, D. E. The psychoses of adolescence. *Journal of Mental Science,* 102: 308–316, 1956.

Schmiedeck, R. A. A treatment program for adolescents on an adult ward. *Bulletin of the Menninger Clinic,* 25:241–248, 1961.

Shamsie, S. J., and Ellick, E. Disturbed adolescents: A suggested community approach to treatment. *Canadian Psychiatric Association Journal,* 10:399–404, 1965.

Silverman, L. N., Lapkin, B., and Rosenbaum, I. S. Manifestations of primary process thinking in schizophrenia. *Journal of Projective Techniques,* 26: 117–127, 1962.

Spivack, G., Haimes, P. E., and Spotts, J. Adolescent symptomatology and its measurement. *American Journal of Mental Deficiency,* 72:74–95, 1967.

Spotnitz, H. Adolescence and schizophrenia: Problems in differentiation. In S. Lorand and H. I. Schneer, eds., *Adolescents: Psychoanalytic Approach to Problems and Therapy.* New York: Hoeber, 1961, pp. 217–237.

Stephens, J. H., Astrup, C., and Mangrum, J. C. Prognosis in schizophrenia: Prognostic scales cross validated in American and Norwegian patients. *Archives of General Psychiatry,* 16:693–698, 1967.

Sullivan, H. S. *The Interpersonal Theory of Psychiatry.* New York: Norton, 1953.

Symonds, A., and Herman, M. The patterns of schizophrenia in adolescence. *Psychiatric Quarterly,* 31:521–530, 1957.

Symonds, P. M. *Adolescent Fantasy.* New York: Columbia University Press, 1949.

Toolan, J. M., and Nicklin, G. Open door policy on an adolescent service in a psychiatric hospital. *American Journal of Psychiatry,* 115:790–792, 1959.

Vaillant, G. E. The prediction of recovery in schizophrenia. *Journal of Nervous and Mental Disease,* 135:534–543, 1962.

Vaillant, G. E. Positive prediction of schizophrenic remissions. *Archives of General Psychiatry,* **11**:509–518, 1964.

Warren, W. Abnormal behavior and mental breakdown in adolescence. *Journal of Mental Science,* **95**:589–624, 1949.

Warren, W. Inpatient treatment of adolescents with psychological illness. *Lancet,* **262**:147–150, 1952.

Warren, W. A study of adolescent psychiatric in-patients and the outcome six or more years later: II. The follow-up study. *Journal of Child Psychology and Psychiatry,* **6**:141–160, 1965.

Warren, W., and Cameron, K. Reactive psychosis in adolescence. *Journal of Mental Science,* **96**:448–457, 1960.

Watkins, J. G., and Stauffacher, J. C. An index of pathological thinking in the Rorschach. *Journal of Projective Techniques,* **16**:276–286, 1952.

Weiner, H. Diagnosis and symptomatology. In L. Bellak, ed., *Schizophrenia: A Review of the Syndrome.* New York: Logos, 1958, pp. 107–173.

Weiner, I. B. *Psychodiagnosis in Schizophrenia.* New York: Wiley, 1966.

Weiner, I. B. Diagnosing schizophrenia. In *Sound Seminars,* No. 75416. New York: McGraw-Hill, 1968.

Wertheimer, N. M. Schizophrenic sub-diagnosis and age at menarche. *Journal of Mental Science,* **108**:786–789, 1962.

Wilson, H. The early diagnosis of schizophrenia. *British Medical Journal,* **1**:1502–1504, 1951.

CHAPTER 5

Depression and Suicide

As noted in Chapter 3, depressive disorders are infrequently diagnosed in adolescent patients and constitute a much smaller part of adolescent than of adult psychopathology. The topic of depression nevertheless merits detailed consideration in any discussion of psychological disturbance in adolescence. In the first place, depressive symptomatology is far more common in disturbed adolescents than the relatively rare diagnosis of a depressive syndrome in this age group would indicate; for example, of the 101 twelve- to eighteen-year-olds studied in the Payne Whitney Symptomatic Adolescent Research Project only 7 were considered to demonstrate a primarily depressive syndrome (Masterson, Tucker, and Berk, 1963), but 41 displayed such depressive symptoms as dysphoric affect, prominent guilt and self-depreciation, and frequent crying spells (Masterson, 1967, pp. 139 and 166). Among the subjects followed longitudinally in this project, 28% of those eventually diagnosed as having personality disorders and 44% of those diagnosed as schizophrenic exhibited depressive symptom patterns during their initial evaluation.

Secondly, depressive phenomena demand careful clinical attention because of their relationship to suicidal behavior. The available literature on suicide and attempted suicide reveals that, of all mental disturbances, depressive disorder—with sadness, pessimism, feelings of futility and worthlessness, and tendencies to excessive guilt feelings and self-reproach—is the one that poses the greatest suicidal risk (Stengel, 1964, p. 51). In reviewing the epidemiology of depression Silverman (1968, pp. 889–890) draws the same conclusion:

"In epidemiologic terms, there . . . appears to be a strong association between depressive illness and suicide. Examination of both the contribution of depressive disorder to the suicide problem and the termination of depressive disorder in suicide leads to a reasonable hypothesis that suicide is the mortality of depressive mental illness."

These data together with the similarity of the dynamic constellations associated with depression and suicidal tendencies (see pp. 181–189) indicate that suicidal potential must be assessed with particular care in the depressed person. The implications of depression for suicidal behavior are particularly important in clinical work with disturbed adolescents, because it is in this age group that suicide reaches its peak relative incidence as a cause of death. In 1965 suicide ranked as the tenth leading cause of death in the United States population at large, whereas for the 15 to 19 age group suicide was the fifth leading cause of death, exceeded only by accidents, malignant neoplasms, major cardiovascular-renal disease, and homicide, in that order (*Vital Statistics of the United States,* 1965).

Furthermore, even though the actual incidence of suicide is far lower in adolescents than it is in adults, adolescents are as likely as adults to make suicide attempts. Faigel (1966) reports that more than 25,000 youngsters attempted suicide in the United States in 1965, which means that somewhat more than one of every 1000 teenagers in this country attempts suicide each year. Data from Stengel and the *Vital Statistics* suggest a similar incidence of approximately one suicide attempt per 1000 persons in the general population.

The first part of this chapter reviews the general psychopathology of depressive disorder and then considers the particular clinical manifestations, personality dynamics, and problems of differential diagnosis that are associated with adolescent depression. The second part reviews the demography and dynamics of suicidal behavior in young people and elaborates the clinical assessment and management of suicidal risk in adolescent patients.

PSYCHOPATHOLOGY OF DEPRESSION

In his 1917 paper "Mourning and Melancholia" Freud provided the following clinical description of depression:

"The distinguishing mental features of melancholia are a profoundly painful dejection, cessation of interest in the outside world, loss of the capacity to love, inhibition of all activity, and a lowering of the self-regarding feelings to a degree that finds utterance in self-reproaches and self-revilings and culminates in a delusional expectation of punishment" (p. 244).

Freud observed that this symptom picture, except for the decline in self-esteem, also characterizes normal grief reactions, or mourning. He accordingly inferred that melancholia, like mourning, originates in the loss of loved objects. However, he added, whereas mourning typically occurs in response to an actual object loss, melancholia derives from fantasied or unconscious losses.

Freud's distinction between mourning and melancholia corresponds to current conceptualizations of *reactive* and *endogenous* depression. Reactive depression is a self-limiting disturbance that is specifically related to an actual, readily apparent object loss or disappointment—a woman mourns the death of her husband, a girl reacts to her fiance's breaking their engagement, a man experiences failure to achieve an expected and desired promotion. Endogenous depression is a more chronic, lingering condition in which neither the patient nor an untrained observer can readily comprehend the origins of the distress, typically because the nature of the loss or disappointment remains unconscious: a woman becomes depressed after giving birth because she unconsciously equates motherhood with loss of her previously enjoyed dependent gratifications; a man becomes depressed on being promoted in his work because he unconsciously fears that his success will attenuate his father's affection for him; or a man becomes depressed on his 50th birthday because, despite being in fact vigorous, virile, and in execllent health, he fantasies 50 as the age at which men begin to lose their potency.

Symptomatology

Although Freud drew his inferences from a small clinical sample, subsequent work has affirmed many aspects of his descriptive and dynamic formulation of depressive disorder; for example, Beck (1967, pp. 14–36) reports that the following four categories of symptoms were each directly related to the rated depth of depression in 966 psychiatric patients he studied:

1. *Emotional manifestations*—dejected mood, negative self-attitudes, reduced experience of satisfaction, decreased involvement with people and activities, crying spells, and loss of sense of humor.

2. *Cognitive manifestations*—low self-esteem, negative expectations for the future, self-punitive attitudes, indecisiveness, and distorted body imagery.

3. *Motivational manifestations*—loss of positive motivation to perform tasks, escapist and withdrawal wishes, suicidal preoccupations, and increased dependency.

4. *Vegetative and physical manifestations*—appetite loss, sleep disturbance, decreased sexual interest, and increased fatigability.

A number of investigators have utilized factor-analytic techniques to identify the symptom patterns that are most commonly associated with depressive disturbance. Raskin et al. (1967), using interview, self-report, and ward-rating data on 124 hospitalized depressed patients, extracted nine major defining characteristics of depression:

1. Decreased interest and involvement in activities.
2. Hostile attitudes toward oneself and others.
3. Feelings of guilt and worthlessness.
4. Prominent anxiety and tension.
5. Sleep disturbance.
6. Somatic complaints.
7. Retarded speech and behavior.
8. Conceptual disorganization.
9. Depressive mood.

A particularly detailed factor-analytic study of depressive disturbance is reported by Grinker et al. (1961), who carefully rated 96 depressed patients on 47 traits describing feelings and concerns and on 84 items of current behavior. Their data yielded 5 factors pertaining to feelings and concerns and 10 factors of current behavior. By combining these factors they were able to derive the following four factor patterns, each of which describes a constellation of feelings and behavior that is likely to characterize some depressed patients (Grinker et al., 1961, p. 233):

Pattern A—hopelessness, low self-esteem, and slight guilt feelings; isolated, withdrawn, apathetic behavior, with slowed speech and some cognitive disturbances.

Pattern B—hopelessness, low self-esteem, considerable guilt feelings, and high anxiety; agitated behavior with clinging demands for attention.

Pattern C—feelings of abandonment and loss of love; agitated, demanding, and hypochondriacal behavior.

Pattern D—gloom, hopelessness, and anxiety; demanding, angry, and provocative behavior.

These empirically demonstrated patterns of depressive behavior correspond closely to Freud's description of melancholia. The work of Grinker et al. additionally demonstrates that depressive disturbance encompasses multiple patterns of clinical phenomena. Of two depressed patients with, for example, hopelessness and low self-esteem, one may manifest withdrawn, apathetic behavior (Pattern A), and the other, agitated and demanding behavior (Pattern B).

In Kolb's (1965) view such differing patterns should not be lumped under the single designation of *depression,* but should rather be regarded as constituting a "depressive complex." Yet Kolb (p. 68) also stresses that certain core symptom patterns define the depressive complex and are common to its multiple clinical manifestations; namely, a more or less intensely felt unpleasant ego affective state, feelings of helplessness, diminution of self-esteem, and the inhibiton of personality function. Lorr, Sonn, and Katz (1967) similarly report that psychotically depressed patients can be distinguished from other psychotic individuals by the extent to which they manifest anxious self-blame; retarded action and thought; impaired ability to work, concentrate, and make decisions; and general dejection, sadness, hopelessness, and apathy.

Dynamics

With regard to the dynamics of depressive disturbance, Beck (1967, pp. 273–274) endorses Freud's designation of fantasied object loss as a central etiologic element in the characteristic sadness of the depressed person. According to Beck, however, fantasied deprivation is only one of three patterns of misinterpretation of experience that participate in endogenous depressions. The other two are (a) unrealistic negative impressions of oneself, which lead to the apathy, feelings of helplessness, increased dependency wishes, and suicidal tendencies associated with depression; and (b) unrealistic negative expectations of the future, which underlie the depressed person's usual pessimism and hopelessness.

In Beck's opinion all three of these patterns of misinterpretation are secondary to idiosyncratic cognitive operations, to which he assigns the primary etiologic responsibility for endogenous depression. In reactively depressed persons who have suffered actual as well as fantasied losses, he concludes, characteristic depressive phenomena derive directly from this same triad of negative attitudes, on a reality basis, without the intervention of cognitive distortions.

Another significant addition to Freud's dynamic formulation of depression is contributed by Bibring (1953), who postulates failure to realize one's aspirations as the essential element in depressive disorders:

"What has been described as the basic mechanism of depression, the ego's shocking awareness of its helplessness in regard to its aspirations, is assumed to represent the core of normal, neurotic and probably psychotic depressions. . . . According to the viewpoint adopted here, *depression represents a basic reaction* to situations of narcissistic frustration which to prevent appears to be beyond the powers of the ego. . . . In general, one may say that everything that lowers or paralyzes the ego's self-esteem without changing the narcissistically important aims represents a condition of depression" (pp. 39–42).

It thus becomes clear that depression, like schizophrenia, is not a unitary phenomenon but rather a multiply determined and variably manifest psychological disorder. Several psychodynamic constellations contribute to its onset, and a number of symptom patterns define its clinical course. Integrative surveys of the literature on depression by Wittenborn (1965), Mendelson (1960), and Gaylin (1968) yield similar conclusions. In a general overview of the symptom patterns, dynamics, and treatment of depressive disorder Wittenborn emphasizes that depressed patients demonstrate appreciable individual variation in their symptomatology. Mendelson (p. 139) likewise stresses that the term "depression" applies to a variety of overtly and subjectively differing affective states, and he additionally notes that within the psychoanalytic framework neither object loss nor collapse of self-esteem is by itself sufficient to account for all depressive reactions. Gaylin recommends a broad definition of *loss* that encompasses disappointment both in object relations and in respect to desired goals:

"What is important to realize is that depression can be precipitated by the loss or removal of *anything* that the individual overvalues in terms of his security. To the extent that one's sense of well-being, safety, or security is dependent on love, money, social position, power, drugs, or obsessional defenses, to that extent one will be threatened by its loss. When the reliance is preponderant the individual despairs of survival and gives up. It is that despair which has been called depression" (p. 390).

CLINICAL MANIFESTATIONS OF ADOLESCENT DEPRESSION

As reviewed in the preceding section, depressive disorder is typically manifest in dysphoric affect, retardation of thought, speech, and action, and pervasive apathy, lethargy, and hopelessness; various patterns of depression may additionally include guilt and self-depreciation, irritability, agitation, hypochondriacal concerns, and suicidal preoccupation or attempts; and depressive disturbance may also affect basic biological and cognitive functioning, as reflected in decreased appetite, weight loss, sleep disruption, bowel irregularity, and impaired conceptual ability.

Among adolescents the clinical manifestations of depression may vary considerably from these typical patterns, particularly in the younger teenager. The traditional symptom picture of depression, with retardation, apathy, dysphoria, suicidal preoccupation, and biological signs, rarely appears prior to age 16 or 17. The epidemiological data of Rosen et al. (1965; see p. 81) included approximately 475 boys and 650 girls age 10 to 19 who were terminated from outpatient psychiatric clinics in the United States with a diagnosis of neurotic depressive reaction. An age breakdown of this sample of youngsters reveals for both sexes a steadily increasing relative incidence of depressive disorder, presumably as diagnosed from traditional symptomatology, over the adolescent years. As noted in Table 4, of all diagnosed 10- and 11-year-old boys and girls in the Rosen et al. study 1.3 and 1.6%, respectively, were considered to be neurotically depressed, whereas for age 18 to 19 these proportions increased to 3.2% for boys and 9.9% for girls.

Table 4. Incidence of Neurotic Depressive Reaction among Adolescents Terminated from Outpatient Clinics[a,b]

	Age					
	10–11	12–13	14–15	16–17	18–19	Total
Boys	1.3	1.6	1.9	2.5	3.2	1.4
Girls	1.6	1.9	3.4	5.2	9.9	3.3
Total	1.4	1.7	2.5	3.5	5.7	2.1

[a] Expressed as percentage of total.
[b] From Rosen et al. (1965, p. 1567), based on approximately 42,000 diagnosed adolescents.

Despite the infrequent emergence of traditional depressive symptomatology before late adolescence, clinical experience indicates that essentially depressive disorders are by no means rare in early adolescence. However, the younger person, more than the older teenager, tends to manifest depression primarily through a number of nontraditional symptomatic expressions, and an adult-oriented diagnostic attitude often overlooks important depressive aspects of early adolescent psychopathology. It is accordingly helpful to consider separately for early and late adolescents the clinical manifestations by which depression can be recognized.

Depression in Early Adolescence

The early adolescent, as a consequence of his usual disinclination to express his feelings openly and his tendency to deny negative and self-critical attitudes, is relatively unlikely to exhibit the gloom, hopelessness, and self-depreciation that commonly keynote adult depression. Furthermore, the relative impulsivity of children and early adolescents typically leads them to express depressive states through behaviors that cloak the depression and disguise the diagnosis (see Gould, 1965).

Nontraditional behavioral manifestations of depression that both reflect the underlying disturbance and serve to camouflage its nature are commonly designated as depressive equivalents. Although depressive equivalents appear in persons of all ages (see Lesse, 1967; Spiegel, 1967), it is particularly in the child and early adolescent that they may constitute the only index to an underlying depression. The major depressive equivalents observed in young people—as elaborated by Glaser (1967), Toolan (1962a), and others—include (a) boredom and restlessness, (b) fatigue and bodily preoccupation, (c) difficulty in concentration, (d) acting out, and (e) flight to or from people.

Boredom and Restlessness. Persistent boredom and restlessness in adolescents frequently reflect underlying depression. The youngster who alternates between total disinterest and intense preoccupation with activities and events, who takes up pursuits with unbounded enthusiasm only to lose interest quickly and search desperately for something new to engage him, who craves constant activity as his only escape from intolerable boredom, and who cannot endure being alone is in most instances defending against underlying feelings of emptiness and isolation that in an older person would produce traditional depressive symptomatology.

Fatigue and Bodily Preoccupation. The adolescent who alternately feels buoyantly energetic and overwhelmingly fatigued, particularly when his fatigue persists after adequate sleep, is very likely to be suffering the inhibiting effect of a depressive disorder on his personality functioning. Pronounced somatic concerns, beyond the body interest that normally characterizes the physically developing pubescent youngster, often have similar implications for underlying depression, as do such psychophysiological reactions as headaches, abdominal pain, and vomiting.

Concentration Difficulty. Difficulty in concentration has specific significance as a depressive equivalent among disturbed adolescents because of the frequency with which it is the chief or sole complaint that brings a youngster for help. The concentration difficulty is typically described in relation to declining school performance, about which the adolescent can usually say only that, no matter how hard he tries or how long he studies, he is just unable to absorb and retain the information. The depressed adult can usually trace such concentration difficulties to general apathy or to dysphoric preoccupations. The depressed early adolescent, however, is seldom able to account for his concentration problem, and underlying depressive disorder can be suspected from the fact of his concentration difficulty alone.

Acting Out. In many instances acting-out behavior—including temper tantrums, running away, and a variety of defiant, rebellious, antisocial, and delinquent acts—serves to defend an early adolescent against coming to grips with underlying concepts of himself as an unloved, inadequate, and unworthy person. Not only does acting preclude thinking—as the common adage prescribes, "Try to keep busy and not think about it"—but the actions themselves, to the extent that they are hazardous or exploitative, may be designed to inflate the youngster's self-image as a tough, brave, and clever person. The particular utilization of aggressive behavior to avoid depression is elaborated by Bonnard (1961) and by Burks and Harrison (1962):

"In our series, we encountered a number of devices utilized by the children, apparently aimed at avoiding recognition of a fundamental state of helplessness or powerlessness of the ego, which was associated with a depressed affect. The children were cocky braggarts who scoffed at ordinary conventions and dangers. They were adamant in denying fears of inadequacies. It is not uncommon for even a casual observer, unaware of the frequency of insomnia and somatic complaints in this group, to recognize the ineffectiveness and futility of these obvious efforts" (Burks and Harrison 1962, p. 419).

It is also not infrequent for delinquent acts to appear directly after the loss of a loved person and thus to represent a manifestation of the mourning process. Keeler (1954) and Shoor and Speed (1963) report a number of cases in which death of a parent or relative was closely followed by conspicuously antisocial behavior in previously conforming youngsters who gave no other evidence of psychological disturbance (see p. 305).

Flight to or from People. A final clue to underlying depression in adolescents who do not otherwise display traditional depressive symptomatology is an exaggerated approach to, or withdrawal from, people. The flight to people has much in common with the already mentioned dread of being alone in that the pervasive sense of isolation felt by many depressed youngsters may create a need for constant companionship. In some instances the urgent necessity to ward off underlying feelings of being unloved and unwanted pushes the adolescent toward promiscuous sexual behavior, in which the close physical contact with another person who expresses interest and affection, for whatever reason, provides the major gratification (see p. 306).

The depressed adolescent's feeling of abandonment and unworthiness often leads him to turn away from, rather than toward, people. Withdrawal as a depressive equivalent is usually unrelated to the traditional depressive apathy that inhibits interpersonal interests and to the limited social skills that participate in schizophrenic withdrawal. Rather, the depressed adolescent often shuns people primarily to avoid being reminded that he feels abandoned and rejected by them.

It is not unusual for a depressed youngster to turn his attention specifically away from people and toward animals. The adolescent who selects animals as his love objects and devotes major attention to their care and feeding may be revealing underlying depressive reactions to feeling rejected by the important people in his life. Not only can he relate to a pet with little risk of rejection, but he often can also vicariously assuage his ungratified dependent needs through identification with the animals for whom he is caring.

Depression in Late Adolescence

As adolescence progresses the clinical manifestations of depressive disorder increasingly resemble the symptom patterns that are characteristic of adult depression; for example, Coon's (1961, p. 125) experience at the Harvard University Health Services indicates that by late adolescence depression commonly comprises much traditional depressive symptomatology—gloomy forebodings, a sense of hopelessness, suicidal preoccupations, insomnia, and reduced interest and appetite—as well as poor concentration, depleted energy, and such somatic complaints as headache and indigestion.

Binger (1961) notes that college girls are particularly prone to traditional depressive reactions marked by apathy and fatigue, considerably lowered self-esteem, and an inability to get work done. Yet he also describes three defensive reactions to underlying depression that often appear as depressive equivalents in this late adolescent group. The first, which he calls "whipping the tired horse," consists of increased drivenness and worry about classroom requirements, frequently to the point of exhaustion or physical collapse. The second is demonstrated by girls who adopt a cynical, supercilious attitude toward the college experience and disregard their work entirely. These girls are apparently defending themselves against the depressive impact of the academic community by withdrawing from it. They are inclined to sleep through or to cut classes and affect a studied disinterest in their declining grades, even though their self-esteem plummets and their underlying depression mounts with each failure to succeed. The third prominent pattern observed by Binger in depressed college girls is a marked change in eating habits, with either bulimia or anorexia developing in reaction to an underlying depressive disturbance.

A particularly common channel for underlying feelings of hopelessness, despair, and inadequacy in late adolescents of both sexes is a pervasive apathy that simultaneously expresses and defends against what is essentially a depressive disorder. As elaborated by Walters (1961), apathetic young people are frequently mired in self-depreciatory expectations of failure in their academic efforts, humiliation in their interpersonal engagements, and defeat in their quest for an independent and mature identity. Their depressive state can usually be recognized from their physical lethargy, decreased interest in people and events, and emptiness of feeling, all of which they fully sense. At the same time, by an apathetic focus on "playing it cool," such youngsters defend themselves against dysphoric moods and avoid any significant pursuits or personal investments in which they might risk failure or disappointment.

This pattern of personality restriction as a manifestation of depression is not limited to the late adolescent who is in college. Shainberg (1966) observed a similar pattern of apathy in a group of late adolescent boys, most of whom were school drop-outs, who had gotten into disciplinary difficulty while in military service. Similarly to apathetic college students, these youngsters were reluctant to think about anything but immediately current circumstances, were persistently hopeless about their situations, and were willing to settle for anything that came their way in life without requiring them to exert themselves. Shainberg saw their apathy as arising from their overall needs to avoid anxiety and challenge by aiming toward "smoothness without friction" in their lives.

DYNAMICS OF ADOLESCENT DEPRESSION

The underlying theme in adolescent as well as in adult depression is the experience of loss: loss of a personal relationship through death, separation, or a broken friendship; loss of self-esteem after failure to attain a desired and anticipated goal or the commission of a regretted act; loss of bodily integrity in connection with illness, incapacitation, or disfigurement. All such losses are common precursors to depressive reaction in adolescents and adults alike. In adolescents as in adults these losses may be actual events that precipitate a reactive, self-limited depression—such as rejection by a boyfriend, failure to make the football team, or an eruption of acne; or they may constitute unconscious or unrealistic fantasies that lead to the more persistent endogenous depressions ("My parents don't love me any more," "I'll never be able to succeed at anything," "My body is weak and unattractive").

Adolescent depression additionally relates to specific developmental tasks that sensitize teenage youngsters to the experience of object loss. It is during the adolescent years that young people are encouraged to loosen their ties to their parents, who have previously been their primary love objects, authority figures, and sources of dependent gratification. The adolescent is increasingly expected to forego dependent gratification, to pursue peer-group activities outside his home, and to rely on teachers and other extrafamilial models for guidance. Even though the normally developing youngster welcomes such changes in his life, both for their own sake and as evidence of his progressive maturity, he typically experiences mixed feelings about relinquishing his childhood prerogatives and about the diminished significance of his parents in his life.

This aspect of adolescent development has been most clearly elaborated in the psychoanalytic literature. Freud (1905, p. 227) in one of his early works described the detachment from parental authority as "one of the most significant, but also one of the most painful, physical achievements of the pubertal period. . . ." Root (1957) asserts that all adolescents must sooner or later renounce and suffer the "loss" of their childhood aims and objects, and Lorand (1967, p. 53) explains the role of such loss in the following way:

"The painful psychic achievement of the adolescent—his detachment from parental authority—is so painful precisely because he experiences it not as a liberation but as an abandonment by those objects on whom he relies for guidance and support. Hence the reluctance sets in, accompanied by feelings of aloneness, emptiness, and helplessness, and a resentment toward the idea of abandoning the past."

Anna Freud (1958) and Jacobson (1961) suggest that such losses frequently induce apparent states of grief or mourning in adolescents that may persist until they have successfully disengaged themselves from their parents and embarked on a quest for new objects. These and other discussions of mourning as a general adolescent phenomenon are reviewed by Laufer (1966, p. 290), who ascribes the impact of actual object loss in adolescence in part to its being imposed on a normal mourning process:

"While not itself pathogenic, object loss can become the nucleus around which earlier conflicts and the latent pathogenic elements are organized. . . . The detachment from the oedipal object is a normal developmental task in adolescence, which may be greatly complicated by the actual loss of the object."

As pointed out in Chapter 2, however, there is little basis for expecting every adolescent to display states of disturbance that resemble adult psychopathology. It would accordingly be misleading to regard depressive states as normal or normative adolescent phenomena. On the other hand, a dynamic understanding of personality development indicates that adolescence, like other transitional periods of life that involve surrender of previous gratifications, does enhance the individual's susceptibility to depressive reaction. What remains from the clinical standpoint is to elucidate those particular circumstances that combine with the adolescent's depressive propensity to produce diagnosable depressive disorder.

It is generally the case that, the less able a youngster is to embrace adolescent development and to give up his infantile attachments, the more prone he will be to experience loss and subsequent depression in the face of parental and environmental expectations that he grow up. Beyond this principle the sufficient conditions for depressive reaction lie for the most part in the nature of definable losses the adolescent happens to experience and the extent of his predisposition to depressive reactivity in the face of stress.

A number of studies suggest that the propensity for depression in the face of loss is directly related to childhood experiences of parental deprivation that sensitize the individual to such losses (see Bowlby, 1961). Brown (1961), for example, found that 41% of a sample of depressed adults had experienced loss of a parent prior to age 16, as against a 16% incidence of such loss in the general adult population from which his depressed sample was drawn. Masterson, Tucker, and Berk (1963) similarly noted a prominent incidence of parental death, separation, or divorce in depressed 16- to 18-year-old youngsters they studied.

Yet there is clearly no one-to-one relationship between parental loss and the likelihood of depressive disorder in adolescents. Jacobs and Teicher (1967) found an equal incidence of parental loss in childhood among suicidal and nonsuicidal teenagers matched for age, sex, race, and family income; on the other hand, 80% of their suicide attempters and only 45% of their control subjects demonstrated depressive affect or withdrawal. In assessing their data Jacobs and Teicher emphasize that it is not the actual loss or presence of a parent that is crucial in the etiology of depressive disorder in adolescents, but rather the entire process by which love objects participate in the youngster's development. If a loved parent is lost, they continue, the impact of the loss is relative to when it occurred; whether through remarriage there is replacement of the object; and whether there are recurrences of the loss through repetitive deaths, separation, or divorce and general family instability. They also call attention to the obvious fact that a youngster can experience a sense of parental alienation and loss of love within a home that by objective standards is unbroken.

Elson (1964) discusses the similarly variable impact of separation on the late adolescent who goes off to college. The nature of the depressive features in the students he sampled was related to the stability and orientation of the family subsequent to the youngster's leaving for school. Where parents denoted the college student's departure as the time for a major shift in their orientation, such as increased attention to younger children or previously dormant commitments, decision to divorce, preparation for an extended trip, or move to a different house, the youngster's reaction to the separation was more likely to have overtones of anger and guilt than if he was voluntarily relinquishing parental ties.

DIFFERENTIAL DIAGNOSIS

Depressive symptoms participate in a wide range of psychopathology, and it is frequently necessary to distinguish primary depressive disorder from depression that is secondary to organic brain dysfunction, sociopathic personality, and schizophrenia. Observed depresssion may be a specific reaction to losses of cognitive functioning associated with organic impairment; sociopathic persons often become markedly depressed in response to even minor frustrations of their immediate, narcissistic needs; and depression commonly appears as an accessory symptom of schizophrenic disturbance.

The relationship of depressed states to organic impairment and schizophrenia may be especially complex. Depression frequently develops after the onset of organic impairments as a secondary reaction to the loss of function that such impairments entail. Even when depressive phenomena arise prior to the appearance of any demonstrable organic impairment, such a pattern of depression secondary to brain dysfunction cannot be ruled out. It is generally recognized that depressive reactivity to subliminally sensed organic changes is not unlikely to precede the actual progression of these changes to a measurable point (Brosin, 1959, p. 1188; Mulder, 1959, p. 1149). When an observed depressive state cannot be traced to any other instance or area of loss, real or fantasied, the patient's symptoms may well be the initial diagnostic index to a developing organic syndrome. Similarly, although mood changes often accompany schizophrenic disturbance, a depressed state may be prodromal to developing schizophrenia and arise prior to the appearance of clearly schizophrenic phenomena (see Chapter 4).

By and large, observed depression can be designated as secondary or accessory to the extent that unequivocal evidence of organic impairment, sociopathy, or schizophrenia emerge in the course of clinical assessment. However, such decisions are complicated in adolescents by the frequency with which they express depression through depressive equivalents of various types. Three of the already noted depressive equivalents are also characteristic symptoms of other major disturbances: concentration difficulty may reflect organic brain dysfunction, acting out is often associated with sociopathic tendencies, and flight from people may indicate a developing schizophrenic disorder. As elaborated below, the differential diagnosis of the youngster who presents such symptoms hinges on an adequate clinical history and appropriate utilization of neurological and psychological consultation.

Organic Brain Dysfunction

The differential diagnosis between depression and brain dysfunction in a youngster with impaired attention and concentration hinges on several phenomenological and dynamic considerations. With regard to clinical phenomena, the more the youngster's attention and concentration difficulties are accompanied by other diagnostic indices of minimal brain dysfunction, the less they are likely to reflect solely an underlying depressive disorder. The major indices of brain dysfunction that contribute to ruling out primary depressive disorder in such instances are hyperactivity, perceptual-motor impairments, emotional lability, general coordination deficits, impulsivity, disorders of memory, specific learning disabilities, disorders of speech and hearing, equivocal neurological signs, and electroencephalographic irregularities (see Clements, 1966, p. 13; see also pp. 248–255). Conversely, the absence of these phenomena enhances the probability that reported difficulties in attention and concentration derive from an essentially depressive disorder, other things being equal.

Concerning dynamics, the more clearly an experience of psychological loss can be demonstrated in the period immediately preceding the onset of attention and concentration difficulty, the greater is the likelihood that a basically depressive, rather than organic, disturbance is present. The following complex case illustrates the differential diagnosis of depressive disturbance in a youngster who had an apparent seizure disorder but whose thinking difficulty could be more clearly attributed to psychological than to organic determinants.

Clara was 15 when her family doctor referred her for a neurological evaluation in connection with reported memory loss, declining school performance, and the apparent onset of mild convulsive seizures. Although electroencephalographic studies revealed abnormalities consistent with a seizure disorder, gross neurological examination was entirely negative. In addition the neurologist learned that Clara had been more or less upset since the death of her mother and subsequent dissolution of her family life four years earlier. An older brother had left home, and she had been sent to live with an aunt and uncle with whom she got along poorly. According to the history she typically moped around the house in a bored and apathetic fashion, complained of being unable to concentrate on things, and expressed the feeling that no one really wanted her, and she had been particularly upset over a recent break-up with a boyfriend.

The neurologist was uncertain whether Clara's memory and concentration difficulty and declining school performance were related to organic dysfunction associated with her apparent seizure disorder, with depression arising in reaction to the organic problem, or whether her thinking and academic problems were purely psychological concomitants of a depressive disorder that antedated and was only peripherally influenced by her abnormal brain functioning. Psychological examination was particularly helpful in clarifying this diagnostic issue and pointing toward appropriate treatment. As measured by the tests, Clara's basic capacity to attend was unimpaired, and her abilities to concentrate and to think in the abstract were commensurate with her overall level of intellectual functioning. Furthermore, she exhibited no decrement of visual organization or perceptual-motor coordination, and her memory both for visual and auditory stimuli was quite good. Significantly, her performance on memory tasks was in no way handicapped either by anxiety or by any indications of actual cognitive deficit.

In addition to thus contraindicating cognitive deficit secondary to brain dysfunction, the psychological test data identified unresolved ambivalent feelings toward her mother. The negative aspects of these feelings seemed to be perpetuating prominent guilt feelings in Clara and a general impression of herself as a worthless person who could not expect to be loved by others. These findings indicated that depressive disorder, developed in response to the loss of her mother and exacerbated by (a) her alienation from her foster parents, (b) the apparent onset of a seizure disorder, and (c) loss of her boyfriend, was the major factor in her concentration and school difficulty. Her treatment was accordingly directed both toward medical management of her possible seizure disorder and a psychotherapeutic focus on her feelings toward herself and her future.

Sociopathic Personality

The differentiation between acting out as a symptomatic depressive equivalent and acting out as a reflection of sociopathy requires a thorough delineation of the adolescent's developmental history and basic personality style. The more a youngster's acting-out behavior contrasts with his prior modes of adaptation, as revealed by the history, and his current defensive style, as inferred from interview or psychological test data, the greater is the likelihood that the behavior is symptomatic rather than characterological in nature (see pp. 321–322).

The sociopathic adolescent has typically been an aggressive, demanding, self-centered child with minimal frustration tolerance and little inclination to subordinate his gratification to the needs of others. In the youngster who begins at adolescence to act out symptomatically as a defense against underlying depression, on the other hand, parental reports are likely to indicate that he had been a quiet, retiring child, obedient and restrained, kind and gentle with his siblings and pets, and well behaved in school, and that the emergence of his rebellious or delinquent behavior has come as a complete surprise. Such a contrast between adolescent acting out and a previous history of exemplary conduct usually identifies symptomatic rather than characterological misbehavior.

Regarding defensive style, it is relatively straightforward in some youngsters to interpret any antisocial behavior they manifest as consistent with their personality orientation. Sociopathy as the basis of acting-out behavior becomes increasingly likely the more an adolescent's interview behavior and performance on psychological examination suggest that he is an unreflective and emotionally labile individual who relates to others in a shallow and superficial manner, seldom exercises self-restraint or an analytic approach to his experience, prefers doing things to talking or thinking about them, and operates in terms of what is concrete and immediate rather than abstract and conceptual (see Blatt, 1965).

On the other hand, there are youngsters in whom acting-out behavior stands in marked contrast to a basically ideational character structure. Rebellious, poorly conceived, antisocial conduct in an adolescent whose demeanor and test protocols suggest that by nature he is a thoughtful, introspective person, disinclined to motor activity or spontaneous expression of his feelings, in all probability represents a depressive equivalent rather than a characterological propensity for acting out. Particularly when indices of dysphoria or self-depreciation are also in evidence, a depressive rather than sociopathic interpretation of the problem behavior is indicated. The following two cases illustrate patterns of acting-out behavior that arose in response to essentially depressive disturbances.

> Martha was brought by her parents for evaluation at age 15 after she had taken $80 from her mother's purse and made off in the family car with her 14-year-old boyfriend. The youngsters had gone as far as a neighboring state before they were apprehended by the police and returned to their homes. Martha was an adopted child whose parents felt they had spoiled her with lavish attention. Martha herself initially presented as a composed, self-assured girl with no real difficulties; she could not explain her behavior, nor did she admit to any interest in attempting to.
>
> Yet Martha's fantasy productions on subsequent psychological examination suggested that she was deeply troubled by a number of specific concerns. Above all she revealed ungratified longings for dependency and nurturance, and an underlying view of her mother as a distant and haughty person who went through the motions of mothering

without ever really giving of herself or communicating feelings of love and devotion. Probably in respect to her difficult relation with her mother, Martha appeared to regard herself as a small, insignificant person, lacking in any intrinsic value or worth, who could expect little else than rejection in her relationships with other people.

Martha's interview behavior and test performance nevertheless demonstrated that, despite such long-standing concerns, she had a basically well-rounded and flexible reservoir of defensive resources. In a fashion consistent with normative expectation in a 15-year-old she displayed a variety of adaptive modes without any premature commitment to one or another. She seemed able both to deal with her experience in a reflective and introspective manner, when she wished to, and also to exercise appropriate and spontaneous affective responses to situations. Her flexible personality style and apparent capacity to control her behavior contraindicated a developing sociopathic personality disorder as the basis for her acting out. Rather, in view of the clear dynamic indications of depressive disorder, her behavioral difficulty could be interpreted as a depressive equivalent and approached accordingly in treatment planning.

Sixteen-year-old Karol was admitted to the hospital as a result of her parents' progressive inability to control her behavior and their fears that she would carry out the threats of suicide with which she had been blatantly manipulating them. Over the previous six months she had become increasingly rebellious at home, refusing to obey any parental orders, using the family car without permission, and on occasion staying out all night. It was learned that several months prior to the onset of her acting-out behavior, in the setting of being assigned major supervisory responsibilities for her younger siblings while the family was vacationing at their summer home, Karol had come to the conclusion that her parents did not love her. At this same time a boyfriend broke off their dating relationship, and her younger brother developed a serious kidney infection that temporarily threatened his life.

Clinical exploration of these real and fantasied losses suggested that Karol was experiencing a basically depressive disorder for which her acting out was an equivalent that diverted her attention from her feelings of loss and powerlessness. Subsequent psychological examination supported this impression. On tests Karol revealed many unresolved concerns about the extent to which she wished to be independent of her parents, with urges for independence competing with ungratified needs for parental nurturance and support. Yet she gave no indications of poor impulse control, nor did she display any particular tendencies toward labile or spontaneous emotional expression. Rather, she seemed fairly interested in imaginative ideational activity. These test findings helped to identify her acting out as a symptomatic reflection of an underlying depression rather than as a characterological commitment to such behavior.

Schizophrenia

Distinction between withdrawal as a depressive equivalent and withdrawal as a manifestation of underlying schizophrenia depends primarily on the extent to which other evidence of a schizophrenic disorder is present. The more the social withdrawal of a disturbed adolescent is accompanied by indices of disordered thinking, detachment from reality, and inadequate affective integration (as reviewed in Chapter 4), the greater the likelihood that he is schizophrenic rather than manifesting the inhibiting effects of a basically depressive disorder. Conversely, the absence of other schizophrenic phenomena enhances the possibility that an observed disinterest in, or avoidance of, people is a symptomatic derivative of an underlying depression.

This explicit formula notwithstanding, differentiation between depressive and schizophrenic withdrawal may prove to be extremely difficult in the individual case. As noted on p. 98, Burns (1952) and Sands (1956) have observed that withdrawal may be the first manifestation of developing schizophrenia in a disturbed adolescent, preceding the appearance of any difficulties in thinking, reality testing, or affective integration. Consequently some period of observation may be required to determine whether social withdrawal in the absence of other schizophrenic phenomena is a depressive equivalent or is rather the earliest manifestation of an incipient schizophrenic disorder. The following case illustrates the sequential development of acting out and then withdrawal as symptomatic equivalents of a depressive disorder in a youngster who caused concern to many observers that he might be basically schizophrenic.

Donald was 16 when a suicide attempt with 20 aspirin tablets led to his hospitalization. The previous several years of his life had been marked by family instability. His mother had had multiple hospital admissions in connection with a chronic schizophrenic condition, and during her periods at home she had been generally disorganized and unable to handle the routine responsibilities of running a household. For his junior high school years his father had sent him to live with his grandparents in another community in order to spare him the distress of their home life, and he had done reasonably well.

Upon returning home to begin his freshman year in high school, however, Donald was distressed to discover that his father was carrying on an intimate relationship with their neighbor, a divorced woman whose children were his schoolmates.

At this point Donald began increasingly to withdraw from activities and to isolate himself from his former friends. He began to frequent bars, where he used false identification papers to be served, and he took to late hours, delinquent companions, and neglect of his studies. This period of acting out, which very probably was a depressive equivalent, culminated in Donald's running away to a distant metropolitan area, where he spent two weeks hanging around bars, living in rooming houses, and developing increasing feelings of isolation.

He then returned home, only to learn that in his absence his father had been to Mexico for a divorce and had married the neighbor. Thus in two short weeks Donald's home as he had known it before had ceased to exist. He declined an invitation to move in with his father and new stepmother and instead rented a room by himself, and in this setting his apparent depressive equivalent, the acting out, rapidly gave way to a full-blown depression. In his own words his life at this point, "seemed like a big pointless nothing; nothing was good for me in the past, and I'll probably end up in a mental hospital or as a bum." After four days of progressive gloom, lethargy, and despair he ingested the aspirins and called his father to ask for help.

Donald's recent history of social withdrawal and his mother's known schizophrenic disturbance initially suggested he might be proceeding toward a schizophrenic decompensation. However, no peculiarities of affect, thinking, or judgment were apparent in his behavior, and he quickly developed appropriate and positive relationships with the hospital staff. Psychological testing further helped to rule out the presence of any impairments of his thought processes, reality testing capacity, or basic ability to establish meaningful social relationships. Donald accordingly was considered to present an adjustment reaction with primary depressive features, and after a brief hospitalization he was discharged to outpatient care. Although he was lost to follow-up soon after, it is significant that he did not require rehospitalization in the subsequent five years.

DEMOGRAPHY OF ADOLESCENT SUICIDAL BEHAVIOR

The extensive literature on the demography, dynamics, and clinical management of suicidal behavior in general has been thoroughly reviewed by

Shneidman (1963), Shneidman and Farberow (1957), Stengel (1964), Stengel and Cook (1958), and Weiss (1966). The remainder of this chapter focuses on these aspects of suicidal behavior as they relate specifically to the adolescent age group.

Regarding demography, the *Vital Statistics of the United States* (pp. 158–159) reports that known deaths by suicide in this country in 1965 included 1 child less than 10 years old, 103 ten- to fourteen-year-olds, and 685 youths aged 15 to 19. These 789 youngsters constituted 3.7% of the 21,507 suicides reported for the entire population during 1965, whereas the age range 20 to 29 accounted for 11.5%, 30 to 39 for 15.5%, 40 to 49 for 20.1%, 50 to 59 for 21.7% and 60 and above for 27.5%. From this age distribution it appears that actual suicide very rarely occurs in children under 10, is infrequent up to age 15, and then rises steadily in incidence during the years 15 to 19 and beyond. There is in fact an almost sevenfold greater frequency of suicide among the 15- to 19-year olds (685) than the 10- to 14-year-olds (103). The *Vital Statistics* furthermore indicates (pp. 20–21) that the suicide rate in 1965 climbed from 0.5 per 100,000 population in 10- to 14-year-olds to 4.0 per 100,000 in the 15 to 19 age range, with a progressively increasing rate up to age 60.

These recent national statistics for adolescent suicide resemble earlier data summarized by Bakwin (1957) and Balser and Masterson (1959), thus indicating a reasonably stable relationship between age and incidence of suicide over the last decade. Balser and Masterson also noted a dramatic increase in suicide attempts during the late adolescent years. In their estimate 10- to 19-year-old youngsters account for 12% of the suicide attempts made each year in the United States, which is considerably larger than the known proportion of adolescent suicide completers (3.7%) in the suicide population.

Studies of selected samples of suicidal adolescents have yielded incidence data that are comparable to these national estimates. Jacobinzer (1960, 1965a) found a steady increase in attempted suicide during the 12 to 20 age range in samples of 299 and 597 youngsters seen consecutively at the Poison Control Center in New York City. Bergstrand and Otto (1962) observed a similar linear increase in the frequency of suicide attempts with age, with progression each year from age 10 to age 19, in over 1500 Swedish youngsters hospitalized after suicide attempts. As for the estimated disproportion of suicide attempts among adolescents, Schrut (1964) reports that in Los Angeles County youngsters under 20 commit 3% of the known suicides each year but make 8% of the reported suicide attempts.

Data from college health services suggest that during the transition from late adolescence to early adulthood the frequency of actual suicide continues to climb, whereas the disproportion of suicide attempts begins to decrease from its adolescent peak; for example, a 10-year study of suicide among Berkeley students by Bruhn and Seiden (1965) demonstrated a positive correlation between completed suicide and chronological age. Furthermore, whereas suicide is the fifth leading cause of death among 10- to 19-year-olds in the United States (see p. 158), Parrish (1957) at Yale and Rook (1959) at Cambridge report that suicide has long been the second leading cause of death among students at their universities. For suicide attempts, on the other hand, Raphael, Power, and Berridge (1937) noted a declining incidence from the freshman to senior years at the University of Michigan, and Braaten and Darling (1962) at Cornell observed a higher incidence among undergraduate than among graduate students.

Other work tends to confirm a much greater ratio of attempted to completed suicides in adolescents than in adults. According to Stengel (1964, p. 75) there are approximately 6 to 10 suicide attempts for every actual suicide among the general population. In contrast, studies of suicidal adolescents have suggested attempt-to-completion ratios of 50:1 (Jacobinzer, 1960), 100:1 (Jacobinzer, 1965b), and even 120:1 (Tuckman and Connon, 1962).

It should also be noted that the known number of completed and attempted suicides in young people probably grossly underestimates the actual frequency of these events. Parental attempts to conceal suicidal actions and the inclination of well-meaning professional persons to disguise them as accidents account for much of this underestimation. The prevailing feeling at the Sucide Prevention Center in Los Angeles is that as many as 50% of the suicidal behavior in young persons is disguised or not reported for such reasons (Schrut, 1964).

Nevertheless various studies of known suicidal adolescents have yielded some consistent demographic findings that are probably representative of the suicidal population from which they are drawn. With regard to sex, all available data point to clear differences between adolescent boys and girls in the frequency with which they attempt and complete suicide. Of the 788 ten- to nineteen-year-old youngsters known to have killed themselves in the United States in 1965, 613 (77.8%) were boys (*Vital Statistics of the United States*). This 3.4:1 ratio of boys to girls in the incidence of completed suicide closely approximates a 3:1 incidence noted by Balser and Masterson (1959) in their earlier report. Among suicide attempters, however, these sex ratios appear to be completely reversed, with a 3.5:1 ratio of girls to boys (Gaultier, Fournier, and Garceix, 1961; Jacobinzer, 1960).

Concerning the means by which adolescents attempt and complete suicide, the *Vital Statistics* reveals that, of the 613 ten- to nineteen-year-old boys who committed suicide in 1965, 52% used firearms or explosives, 26% died by hanging or strangulation, 15% poisoned themselves, and the remaining 7% perished by a variety of other methods. The 175 adolescent girls known to have committed suicide in 1965, on the other hand, died by shooting in 46% of the instances, poisoning in 32%, hanging in only 6%, and by other means in 6%. It therefore appears that boys and girls who kill themselves are both most likely to employ firearms and explosives, but that the second choice is more commonly hanging in boys and poisoning in girls.

An entirely different pattern of preferred method has been observed among adolescents who attempt but do not complete suicide. Clinical experience at Bellevue suggests that the use of poison is not only more common in girls than in boys who attempt suicide but is the most frequent method employed by girls (Toolan, 1962b). Bergstrand and Otto (1962) found ingestion to be by far the most common method among boys (77%) as well as girls (90%) in their large sample of Swedish adolescents who attempted suicide, and a study of all 14- to 17-year-old suicide attempters of both sexes known to the Philadelphia Police Department over a two-year period revealed an 83% incidence of poisoning (Tuckman and Connon, 1962).

Thus both boys and girls prefer hanging and shooting as a means of completing suicide and ingestion as a means of attempting it. One compelling explanation of this difference is the relative lethality of the various methods: ingestion of a poison allows more chance for survival, particularly given the wide range of possible nonlethal doses, than hanging or shooting oneself. Although lethality alone may determine the higher incidence of completed suicide among the hangers and shooters, it can additionally be hypothesized that the individual who means to kill himself selects the more lethal method, whereas the youngster who intends to attempt suicide but not to die chooses a method that gives him reasonable assurance he will not perish in the attempt.

These characteristics of adolescent suicidal behavior are not unique to the young. From data summarized by Stengel (1964, p. 34) it appears that male and female adults complete suicide in approximately the same manner as adolescents: by firearms and explosives in 53% of men and 25% of women, by shooting or hanging in 20% of men and 23% of women, and by poisoning in 17% of men and 35% of women. Adult females thus prefer suicide by hanging somewhat more than adolescent girls and suicide by shooting somewhat less, but in other respects the adult figures closely resemble those reported for adolescents. The shift to less dangerous and fatal methods in attempted suicide is also characteristic of adults, with poisoning accounting for more than 50% of attempts in both men and women (Stengel, 1964, pp. 77–78).

Although a number of investigators have assessed the extent and nature of psychopathology associated with adolescent suicidal behavior, the data have thus far yielded no consistent picture. Gaultier et al. (1961) report that major mental disturbance was rare in their sample of 47 adolescent suicide attempters, with only one instance of psychosis. Yet Schneer and Kay (1961), examining 84 adolescents who had attempted or threatened suicide, considered that more than half were "very disturbed." They specifically noted clearly depressive tendencies in 34 of these youngsters.

Other clinical studies of suicidal adolescents confirm that depression very commonly participates in their personality dynamics (see Gould, 1965). Yet the apparently prominent role of depressive dynamics in suicidal behavior, as elaborated below, does not preclude its being secondary to that of other psychopathological states. Balser and Masterson (1959) in fact report that 19 of 32 adolescents hospitalized at the Payne Whitney Clinic after suicide attempts were diagnosed as schizophrenic, and these authors maintain that schizophrenic rather than depressive psychopathology predominates among adolescents who attempt suicide.

Problems of sampling and definition prevent any meaningful integration of these data. In none of the studies has careful attention been paid to base-rate data, such as the percentage of diagnosed schizophrenics among the total adolescent population admitted to Payne Whitney, and no clear criteria for "major mental disturbance" or "very disturbed" are provided by Gaultier et al. and by Schneer and Kay, respectively. Additionally there is reason to expect that the diagnostic status of adolescent suicide attempters varies with their sex. Otto (1964b) reports that, whereas neurotic depression was generally the most common psychological state in his large Swedish sample, neurotic states were more characteristic of the girls than of the boys who attempted suicide and psychotic states predominated among the boys.

Few diagnostic data are available concerning adolescents who have actually committed suicide. Studies from college campuses by Parrish (1957) and Temby (1961) indicate that students who kill themselves have seldom appeared for evaluation or treatment. At Yale only 11 of 25 students who committed suicide had previously been seen in the student health service, and at Harvard only 3 of 25 had been seen. Other data on students who committed suicide, gathered after the fact by Temby at Harvard and Seiden at Berkeley, suggested that the majority of these young people had given some indications of emotional disturbance prior to their fatal act, but no specific diagnostic conclusions were possible from the information available to the investigators.

DYNAMICS OF SUICIDAL BEHAVIOR IN ADOLESCENTS

Psychodynamic interpretations of suicidal behavior must take into account motivational as well as statistical distinctions between attempted and completed suicide. Suicide attempts are generally defined as self-harmful but nonfatal physical acts committed against themselves by persons who have no conscious wish to die. Yet there are instances in which miscalculation, such as an unintended fatal dose of poison or the failure of an expected rescue, results in a would-be attempter's actually killing himself. Thus a recorded group of suicide completers, though largely comprising persons who wished to kill themselves, may also include some whose death was accidental. Similarly an individual who fully intends to die by his own hand may be saved by some fortuitous circumstances and become for statistical purposes an attempted suicide.

It is of course possible that deeply unconscious wishes lead the "accidental" suicide to miscalculate or the intended "completer" to leave open the possibility of rescue. These complexities of suicidal behavior have led some writers to suggest that, at least from a dynamic standpoint, the distinction between attempted and completed suicide should be drawn on the basis of intent rather than the outcome (e.g., Rubenstein, Moses, and Lidz, 1958). Available clinical and research studies of suicidal behavior, however, have for the most part defined attempted and completed suicide groups according to outcome.

Although there is no single explanation for adolescent suicidal behavior, clinical experience and a wealth of data indicate that the most common denominator in both suicide attempters and suicide completers is a depressive constellation of feelings of deprivation, guilt, helplessness, and rejection. More definitive understanding of the teenager who actually kills himself, beyond the post facto conclusion that he probably wished to die, has been limited by the finality of his act. For the adolescent suicide attempter, however, numerous investigations have elaborated the precipitating circumstances and underlying conflicts that are associated with his behavior.

Precipitating Circumstances

A number of years ago Bender and Schilder (1937), on the basis of their initial studies of suicidal adolescents at Bellevue, reported that escape from an unbearable situation provides an obvious conscious motive in the majority of instances. Subsequent studies of large samples of adolescent suicide attempters have confirmed that these youngsters do readily attribute their actions to specific distressing events, most commonly conflicts within the family (particularly about discipline), problems with the opposite sex, and feelings of anxiety, depression, and impending mental breakdown (Bergstrand and Otto, 1962; Jacobinzer, 1960; Tuckman and Connon, 1962). School problems, pregnancy, and addiction are also mentioned by suicidal adolescents as precipitating circumstances, but with relative infrequency; for example, Otto (1965) noted that fewer than 5% of his large sample of Swedish youngsters related their suicidal behavior to school problems.

Despite the immediate availability of conscious ideation that apparently accounts for an adolescent's suicidal actions, however, the motive mentioned immediately after a suicide attempt typically differs from what the youngster will say about it a few days later. The various precipitating circumstances and underlying conflicts involved in the suicidal behavior are seldom fully apparent from a youngster's immediately conscious or reported motives.

Suicidal behavior in young people has traditionally been viewed as an impulsive act. Jacobinzer (1960, 1965a) regards adolescent suicide attempts as precipitous, impulsive reactions to stressful situations, and he attributes the higher incidence of such behavior in adolescent girls than in adolescent boys to the generally greater impulsiveness of girls. Gould (1965) and Schneer and Kay (1961) concur that the greater impulsiveness and histrionic tendencies of adolescent girls, together with their relatively limited recourse to socially approved outlets for aggression, contribute to their making suicide attempts more frequently than boys. Gould additionally attributes the sharp rise in suicidal behavior during the adolescent years to the general increase in impulsiveness that follows puberty. He further suggests that this adolescent impulsiveness, as manifested in hasty, ill-conceived suicide attempts, decreases the likelihood of death and thus explains the relatively high ratio of attempted to completed suicides in teenagers.

However appealing these formulations may be, they do not stand up well to close examination. Regarding sex differences, first, there is no necessary relationship between the unavailability of socially approved aggressive outlets and the selection of suicidal behavior as a means of aggression against oneself or others. Bosselman (1958, pp. 33–34) in fact suggests that girls are more likely than boys to direct self-destructive urges along such nonsuicidal channels as school failure, sexual delinquency, and neurotic ill health, and she credits this phenomenon with accounting for the greater frequency of completed suicide among young males than among females.

Second, to attribute the high ratio of attempted to completed suicides in adolescents to their impulsiveness is to overlook the possibility that young people who engage in suicidal behavior may simply be less frequently motivated by a wish to die than are suicidal adults. Thirdly, it seems reasonable that a hasty, ill-conceived suicide attempt in a youngster who does not intend to kill himself can present as much or even more risk of death than an attempt he has carefully planned and executed.

Finally, intensive studies of 50 fourteen- to eighteen-year-old suicide attempters and their families by Teicher and Jacobs (1966) and Jacobs and Teicher (1967) seriously challenge the role of impulsiveness in adolescent suicidal behavior. These investigators found little evidence that their youngsters' suicidal behavior was in any way impulsive, temporary, insincere, or irresponsible. Rather, these suicide attempts were for the most part carefully premeditated acts that (a) had been weighed rationally against other alternative solutions to a progressively mounting series of problems and (b) had been chosen only after such other methods as rebelling, withdrawing, running away, and conversion symptom formation had failed to alleviate the situation.

In all of the youngsters studied by Teicher and Jacobs the decision that attempted suicide was the only available solution came as the end result of a long-unfolding process. Characteristic in each case was a long-standing history of such family problems as extreme conflict, instability, mobility, or poverty that had begun to escalate some time within the five years preceding the suicide attempt. During this escalation period the youngsters had felt increasingly alienated from their families. Some had desperately sought an intimate relationship with a boyfriend or girlfriend, often to the exclusion of any other commitments or interpersonal contacts. Then, after a rupture of this relationship or with the prospect of continuing dissolution of meaningful family and social ties, these adolescents had all experienced a pervasive sense of isolation and helplessness that had convinced them suicide was the only road left open.

This combined process of long-standing conflicts, progressive escalation of problems, dissolution of meaningful social relationships, and the failure of nonsuicidal efforts at resolution clearly differentiated Jacobs and Teicher's suicidal adolescents from a group of nonsuicidal controls matched for age, race, sex, and family income. Yet Teicher and Jacobs recognize that not every adolescent faced with such a constellation of difficulties attempts suicide. They suggest that a sufficient condition for suicidal behavior very often resides in suicidal models that lessen social restraints against suicide. For 44% of their suicidal adolescents there had been an actual or attempted suicide by one or more close friends or relatives, and 25% of the youngsters' mothers or fathers had previously attempted suicide.

Other work tends to confirm segments of this unfolding suicidal process formulated by Teicher and Jacobs. Regarding long-standing family problems, a majority of Toolan's (1962b) suicide attempters came from chaotic homes with one or both parents missing; and Bergstrand and Otto (1962) report that, among 927 adolescents in their sample for whom adequate family information was available, there was alcoholism in one or both parents in 15%, prominent mental disturbance in a parent in 28%, and a broken home in 44%. Bigras et al. (1966) observed a 50% incidence of family disorganization—with a history of abandonment, foster parents, and frequent separations—in the families of suicidal adolescents whom they studied intensively; and Sutter, Luccioni, and Scotto (1964) propose from their experience with suicidal youngsters in France that a syndrome of inadequate parental authority is the prime factor in adolescent suicidal behavior.

As these studies suggest, it is not a broken home per se that is implicated in the genesis of suicidal behavior, but rather an accompanying pattern of family disorganization. Bruhn (1962) confirmed a higher incidence of a childhood history of broken homes among adults who attempt suicide than among nonsuicidal psychiatric patients; but, when he next compared suicidal and nonsuicidal patients all of whom had come from broken homes, he found that a broken home became causally significant for suicide only when frequent moves, marital disharmony, and other indications of social disorganization were also in evidence. Jacobs and Teicher (1967) similarly demonstrated with their adolescent subjects that a broken home is meaningful only in relation to the total pattern of social relationships that characterize it. Among their suicidal adolescents such events as divorces, step-parents, and broken romances had *without exception* been unwelcome events that the youngster had viewed with dismay.

Escalating problems, events signaling alienation from significant others, and the failure of nonsuicidal efforts to improve the situation have also been repetitively observed in the period immediately preceding adolescent suicide attempts. Schneer, Kay, and Brozovsky (1961), examining the recent history of 84 twelve- to sixteen-year-old suicide attempters, noted a particular frequency of parental criticism or restriction, defiance of parents or other authorities, actual separations from important objects, and the disclosure of forbidden activities in which the youngster was engaged. These events were typically accompanied by thoughts about punishment, ridicule, deprivation, and being unloved and unwanted by their parents, and also about harming or killing their parents or siblings. Although such events and ideas are neither unusual in adolescence nor specific for suicidal behavior, Schneer et al. (1961, pp. 508–509) remark, "They led to suicidal behavior in the adolescents studied here, because they represented an overwhelming crisis in sexual development and control of aggressive urges, as predetermined by reactions to previous traumatic experiences." The following case excerpt illustrates such a pattern of manifest events preceding suicidal behavior.

> Seventeen-year-old Peggy, athough an attractive and appealing girl, had been plagued throughout her adolescence with feelings of inadequacy and fears of being rejected by others. Over the previous year she had become heavily involved with a group of youngsters whose chief interest was drinking parties that featured promiscuous sex play. Her main pleasure in these parties was not in having intercourse, which she seldom did, but rather in stimulating boys to the point of orgasm where "they were completely in my power and would do anything to have me keep it up."

> These parties came to an abrupt halt after some neighbors alerted the police that Peggy was hosting such a party in her home during her parents' absence. During the week after the discovery she ingested aspirin twice and finally slashed her wrists seriously enough to require hospitalization. Peggy attributed her actions to her terrible guilt over what she had done to her parents by her actions. The clinical data, however, indicated that her suicidal behavior derived mainly from her intense feelings of deprivation at having lost the opportunity for these parties, which had been an important source of gratification to her and had reassured her that her attention could be needed and sought by others.

The development of various psychological symptoms as apparent reactions to mounting difficulties in the months preceding a suicide attempt has been clearly demonstrated among 581 Swedish adolescents carefully studied by Otto (1964a). Otto reports that 38% of these youngsters displayed prominent depressive disturbance during the three-month period preceding their attempt. Another 30% exhibited marked behavior change, with the appearance of such neurotic symptoms as sleep disturbance, psychosomatic complaints, nail biting, and restlessness; and for another 12% the onset of such problem behaviors as drinking, defiance, delinquency, and declining school performance was noted prior to the suicide attempt.

Although there is therefore no specific overt presuicidal syndrome in adolescents, multiple patterns of maladaptive behavior change are likely to appear as the presuicidal youngster attempts to resolve or call attention to his difficulties. The failure of such efforts in the youngster who eventually attempts suicide is emphasized by Powers (1954), who ascribes the theme of aloneness and powerlessness to all suicide attempts. In his view the suicidal young person is attempting by his act to communicate to others his unfulfilled needs and the unbearable circumstances in which he finds himself. He suggests that the suicidal youngster has typically been so unsuccessful in his previous efforts to convey such a message that his self-destructive maneuver may be both the last way he has left of focusing attention on his needs and the only way he can mobilize power of any kind. The following excerpt illustrates the suicidal outcome of longstanding depressive concerns that other means had failed to communicate:

> Polly, at 14, had had depressive concerns for the previous four years. She considered herself "a bad, unworthy daughter" who neither received nor merited attention and affection from her parents. Upon entering puberty she had become additionally alarmed that she was an ugly, unattractive person with little hope of establishing rewarding peer or heterosexual relationships. She had in fact experienced some major frustrations and disappointments in her efforts to make friends with girls she admired and to gain the attention of boys.
>
> At about this time she began to steal money from her parents, purportedly in order to "buy some friends." This sudden and uncharacteristic misbehavior could be understood both as a depressive equivalent and as an attempt to communicate to her previously unaware or indifferent parents that she was in distress and needed their immediate help. After a few months of the stealing, she was caught in the act by her mother. Her mother even at this point made no definite response, but rather said, "I'll have to go and think about what would be an appropriate punishment for this." A few minutes later Polly went upstairs and ingested a nearly fatal dose of barbiturates.

Underlying Conflicts

As noted on page 181, there is considerable evidence to suggest that the essential dynamics of adolescent suicidal behavior is a constellation of feelings of abandonment, guilt, and helplessness that cannot be adequately alleviated or communicated by other methods. The adolescent suicide attempter attributes his actions to a host of frustrating or anxiety-provoking circumstances other than specific depressive complaints, and the manifest events preceding suicide attempts include neurotic symptom formation and acting-out behavior as well as mounting depression; yet the underlying dynamic core of such behavior almost always revolves around depressive themes.

Regarding these depressive themes, the extensive experience of Bender and Schilder (1937), Gould (1965), and Toolan (1962b) with suicidal adolescents has prompted the following formulation of the essential dynamics of suicide attempts in the young: the youngster experiences loss of love, deprivation, and rejection in relation to important persons in his life, primarily his parents; he develops feelings of anger and resentment toward these depriving persons for denying him the affection and nurturance he desires; his aggressive impulses toward these loved objects cause him to experience guilt and a sense of being a bad person; and his need to assuage such guilt feelings leads him to self-destruction attitudes and behavior.

Several authors have additionally suggested that reawakened oedipal conflicts often contribute to guilt formation and consequent self-destructive tendencies in adolescents. More specifically, pubescent youngsters who are troubled by sexual thoughts about their parents may come to regard themselves as bad and worthless for having such thoughts, and their negative self-attitudes are likely to enhance their anticipation of rejection and abandonment and their need for guilt-assuaging punishment (see Mason, 1954; Schneer and Kay, 1961; Zilboorg, 1937). It is interesting in this connection to note that 7 of 21 fourteen- to seventeen-year-old girls examined by Bigras et al. (1966) after suicide attempts reported that sexually seductive behavior by their father was the immediate precipitating event.

Although the dynamic interplay of deprivation, anger, and guilt probably participates in all adolescent suicidal behavior, it must also be kept in mind (a) that attempted or completed suicide is far from being the only outcome of such conflicts and (b) that suicidal behavior is a complex phenomenon that serves important purposes in addition to self-punishment and self-destruction. With respect to outcome, not every youngster who experiences or anticipates rejection from his parents subsequently develops pathological guilt feelings. Schrut (1964) reports from his studies at the Suicide Prevention Center in Los Angeles that in the majority of instances the parents of youthful suicide attempters had sensitized them to guilt reactions by unconsciously conveying to them over the years that they were in some way a "burden." These youngsters accordingly presented a long history of viewing themselves as bad, of being prone to marked guilt feelings, and of engaging in various self-destructive acts prior to the suicide attempt.

Furthermore, not every youngster who is prone to guilt feelings ultimately reaches the point of attempted suicide. Many experience transient suicidal thoughts or develop depressive disturbances marked by suicidal preoccupations, without ever coming close to overt suicidal behavior. Others who experience strong self-punitive needs fulfill them in a variety of nonsuicidal ways. A youngster may punish himself by an ascetic code of life or by undermining his future prospects through failure in his studies; he may provoke external punishment by purposefully irritating, irascible, or antisocial behavior; or he may develop a number of depressive equivalents that defend him against awareness of his depressive ideation while also crippling him with neurotic symptomatology.

Concerning the complexity of suicidal behavior, it is widely acknowledged that self-destructive acts serve extrapunitive as well as self-punitive needs and also bring into dramatic focus the youngster's previously unheeded appeals for attention and help. In many instances a suicidal act is consciously or unconsciously intended to punish the parents as well as the self. Zilboorg (1936) speaks specifically of the "spite reaction" type of suicide, which is a retaliation against those who have withheld their affection from the suicidal person and is accompanied by the thought, "They'll be sorry." The young person typically conceives the retaliatory suicidal act in terms of the distress, humiliation, and regret it will cause his parents.

In the case of youngsters who actually kill themselves it is likely that expectations of reunion with a dead parent or other loved person have also participated at some level in their thoughts. Thoughts about being dead pose a particular risk to life among suicidal adolescents because they have for the most part not yet developed a mature conception of death. The younger adolescent in particular may still view death as a trivial or temporary phenomenon, as it is for a slain actor who later appears for a curtain call or for a deceased relative who, he has been told, "has gone away on a trip." Questionnaire data gathered by Kastenbaum (1959) and Schilder and Wechsler (1934) from high school students confirm that many teenage youngsters still have limited capacity to look far into the future or to understand death as the natural end of life.

Finally, suicide attempts are with few exceptions communications by which the youngster is desperately trying to signal intense distress and to achieve some modification of what have become intolerable life circumstances. There is virtually unanimous agreement among clinicians and researchers who have investigated adolescent suicidal behavior that it is intended to capture the attention of significant people in the youngster's life and to effect some change in their attitudes toward him.

Previously defective communication between suicidal adolescents and their parents has been clearly demonstrated in studies by Teicher and Jacobs (1966) and Tuckman and Connon (1962). Teicher and Jacobs found an average 35% difference between suicidal youngsters and their parents in their estimation of what the youngster's behavioral problems were; these suicidal adolescents felt that their parents were unaware or indifferent to one-third of the problems they actually had and that one-third of the problems their parents attributed to them did not exist. Tuckman and Connon report that one-third of the parents they interviewed could not even venture a guess as to the circumstances that had precipitated their child's suicide attempt.

The relevance of communicative and manipulative intent to adolescent suicidal behavior is further implied by Tuckman and Connon's finding that 87% of their adolescent suicide attempters had made their attempt at home. Jacobinzer (1960) reports that 29% of one of his samples of suicidal youngsters ingested poison at home while their mothers were in the house. As these data indicate, the decision to attempt suicide usually arises in an active interpersonal context. Rubenstein et al. (1958) were able to demonstrate specific desired effects on other people in 36 of 44 adults they studied who had attempted suicide. They emphasize that a suicide attempt is intended by the individual to modify his situation and that it is typically made by a person who is actively engaged in interpersonal struggles with persons important to him. The person who actually intends to die or who kills himself tends in contrast to be an isolated individual with minimal interpersonal engagements.

ASSESSMENT AND MANAGEMENT OF ADOLESCENT SUICIDAL BEHAVIOR

It is seldom possible to predict an adolescent suicide attempt or its consequences. Yet the clinician can be alert to circumstances that enhance the likelihood of suicidal behavior; he can estimate the seriousness of suicide attempts that occur and weigh their implications for further or more destructive suicidal behavior; and he can institute procedures that help to minimize risk of suicide where he feels it is present. The guidelines for such assessments and procedures, as elaborated in this section, follow for the most part from the demography and dynamics of adolescent suicidal behavior that have been already outlined.

Anticipating Suicidal Behavior

As noted in the preceding discussion, the psychological event that is most likely to precede adolescent suicidal behavior, and hence to warn of its imminence, is the onset of depressive symptoms or their equivalents. The possibility of suicide should *always* be considered when a youngster begins to exhibit a depressed mood, eating and sleeping disturbances, withdrawn or rebellious interpersonal behavior, and declining school performance. Such behavior changes have been labeled a "syndrome of adaptive decompensation" by Perlstein (1966), who asserts from his review of the literature that recognition of this syndrome would help to detect impending suicide attempts in 70% or more of instances. Similar prodromal syndromes have been observed among adolescent poison ingesters (Jacobinzer, 1960) and among college students who eventually killed themselves (Seiden, 1966).

Obviously to regard every adolescent who is despondent, agitated, irritable, anorexic, insomniac, withdrawn, or rebellious as a possible candidate for suicidal behavior is to overestimate considerably the occurrence of such behavior. However, it is certainly preferable to institute superfluous preventive measures than to fail to recognize danger of suicide in youngsters who are on the verge of killing themselves. The clinician can nevertheless avoid an excessively inclusive diagnostic attitude by employing several other considerations to sharpen his estimate of the risk of suicide in youngsters who present apparent syndromes of adaptive decompensation.

First, since suicidal behavior characteristically occurs as the culmination of a period of progressive adaptive decompensation—that is, as a final attempt to resolve difficulties after all other efforts have failed—the course and severity of depressive symptoms or their equivalents give many clues to the magnitude of the risk of suicide. The youngster who has recently developed mild symptomatology apparently related to essentially depressive dynamics has usually not begun to exhaust available nonsuicidal avenues for ameliorating his situation. The youngster who already presents an extended history of multiple and increasingly incapacitating symptom formation, on the other hand, particularly when he is no longer able to maintain a realistic appraisal of his situation or of possibilities for improving it, may be rapidly approaching the point of contemplating suicidal behavior as the only remaining solution or mode of communication.

Second, as elaborated by Tabachnik and Farberow (1961), certain aspects of an individual's style of relating to other people have major implications for his inclination to suicidal behavior as a means of communication. The greater the extent and directness of an individual's communication with others, the less is the danger of a suicidal act. Conversely, the less he is able to talk explicitly with significant figures in his life about matters that concern him, and the less these people facilitate or are receptive to such direct communication, the greater is the risk that he will be driven to suicide as a means of conveying his needs.

The risk of suicide is particularly acute when there has been a recent and marked breakdown of previously existing communication channels or when the individual's characteristic mode of expressing his needs to others has been indirect, nonverbal, and manipulative. Thus the youngster who has already resorted to talk, threats, or notes with suicidal overtones should always be considered as having serious potential for acting on such warning signals if improved communication is not forthcoming. Especially when the clinician himself is unsuccessful in establishing lines of communication with a youngster whom he considers to be a suicide risk, the utmost in caution and surveillance is indicated.

On the other hand, the ability to communicate meaningfully with other people and such personal resources as good physical health, emotional stability, and adequate intellect have been observed to decrease the likelihood that a syndrome of adaptive decompensation will result in suicidal behavior (Glaser, 1965). The risk of suicide is further reduced when the parents are aware of the youngster's difficulties, are in good health, and have a stable marital relationship. In general, then, the more a disturbed youngster suffers from physical ailments or emotional disturbance, and the greater the extent of physical or mental illness or discord in his family, the greater is the likelihood that he will be drawn to suicidal behavior.

Third, the potential for suicidal behavior in a troubled adolescent is markedly enhanced by a previous history of suicide attempts or accident proneness. Jacobinzer (1960) noted a 6% incidence of previous suicide attempts and a 15% incidence of previous accidents in one of his large samples of suicidal adolescents. The 6% incidence of previous attempts among adolescent suicide attempters exceeds by many times the estimated 0.1% yearly incidence of suicide attempters among the general adolescent population (Faigel, 1966). Although careful follow-up studies of adolescent suicide attempters have not been reported, Dorpat and Ripley (1967) found in a survey of the literature on suicidal behavior in adults that as many as 22% of adult suicide attempters have been found eventually to die by their own hand.

Estimating the Seriousness of Suicidal Behavior

It follows from the communication aspects of suicidal behavior that many adolescents come to professional attention not before but after they have made a suicide attempt; only with the occurrence of suicidal behavior has the extent of the youngster's disturbance been sufficiently appreciated for the family to take some action. In such instances one of the clinician's first major tasks is to assess the seriousness of the act that has occurred and the likelihood of its being repeated with even more devastating consequences. Many of the following guidelines for such assessment are also noted by Litman and Farberow (1961), Ross (1966), and Tabachnik and Farberow (1961).

In evaluating an adolescent who has made a suicide attempt, the clinician should focus his attention on the onset, the method, and the intent of the suicidal behavior. Concerning onset, the more acute and precipitous the development of the suicidal behavior, the greater is the possibility that some specific efforts to modify the situation, whether through brief psychotherapy or environmental manipulation, will obviate further attempts at suicide. On the other hand, a chronic history of self-destructive behavior patterns, particularly previous suicidal behavior, increases the risk of subsequent attempts and the need for extended treatment or surveillance.

With regard to the method by which a youngster has attempted suicide, it is important to weigh carefully the lethality of the means he employed and the possibilities for rescue, if any, that he left open. Generally a youngster who has survived an attempt to hang or shoot himself has a far greater potential for further and more serious suicidal behavior than one who has ingested a few aspirin tablets or made some superficial scratches on his wrist. In addition it is important to use the adolescent's own appraisal of lethality as well as objective standards. The youngster who has taken a dozen aspirin tablets fully expecting them to kill him is probably a more serious risk for subsequent suicide than one who has become seriously ill after ingesting a dozen barbiturate capsules in the mistaken belief that "only a few pills" would not do anything to him.

In the course of eliciting this kind of information the clinician should also inquire about how the attempt was planned. Generally, the more a youngster has selected in advance a particular time, place, and method for his act by which he maximized both lethality and isolation from potential rescuers, the greater is the subsequent risk that he will kill himself. On the other hand, to the extent that he has acted on the spur of the moment, with whatever means happened to be available, or selected a time and place where other responsible people were either present or certain to come on the scene, the greater is the possibility that further or more serious suicidal acts can be averted.

As for the suicidal adolescent's intent, the clinician should ascertain as best he can the extent to which communicative or manipulative purposes participated in the behavior. Generally, the more clearly a suicide attempt has been meant to impress others and to effect some change in their behavior or attitudes, and the more cognizant the youngster is of such communicative or manipulative intent, the less his behavior implies further, more serious self-destructive acts. On the other hand, when a youngster does not subsequently account for his suicide attempt in interpersonal terms, particularly when not even unconscious interpersonal motives can be identified, the possibility of subsequent and fatal self-destructive acts mounts considerably. Most serious of all is the adolescent whose suicide attempt occurred in total isolation from others and was accompanied by conscious wishes to die. The following case illustrates favorable prognosis after a suicide attempt and the efficacy of a brief clinical contact:

> Noreen, age 13, had consumed eight ounces of straight whiskey and had been brought to the hospital unconscious the evening before she was seen in consultation. She had drunk the alcohol in the bathroom of her home immediately after an argument with her parents. The sound of her falling to the floor had alerted her parents, who

had rushed to her assistance. Significantly, the bathroom door had not been locked or even closed.

When Noreen was seen the following day, she was alert and responsive to questions and seemed quite eager to discuss what had happened. She could not account for her suicide attempt, beyond emphasizing that she considered it a silly and stupid thing to have done and that she most certainly had had no wish to kill herself. It seemed clear that she had not anticipated the full physical consequences of her act and had been very frightened by losing consciousness.

Although Noreen did not spontaneously provide an explanation for her conduct, other readily available information allowed a clear reconstruction of her motives. The argument she had been having with her parents just prior to her suicide attempt concerned her relationship with a particular girlfriend of whom they did not approve. There seemed to be little substantial basis for their disapproval, other than that the girlfriend was a somewhat nonconforming, intellectually oriented youngster who did not fit well with the family's conservative, upper-middle-class, business-oriented approach to the world. Over many months Noreen's parents had become increasingly insistent that she find other companionship. Then, on the day of the suicide attempt, they learned that Noreen had gone with her girlfriend to a nearby shopping center wearing slacks, which violated a family rule against such informal dress. For them this was the last straw, and, during the argument just preceding the attempt, they forbade any further association with the girlfriend.

These data revealed both Noreen's concern about having to give up a valued friendship and her needs to impress on her parents the extent of her distress, in the hope they might change their minds. When these communicative and manipulative aspects of her suicidal behavior were suggested to her, she readily recognized and acknowledged their accuracy. She added that her parents generally did not understand her and that getting through to them when something was troubling her had often proved difficult.

The acute nature and clearly communicative intent of Noreen's suicidal behavior pointed to mild rather than serious suicidal risk, and several additional pieces of information helped to suggest that only minimal professional care might be necessary. Noreen appeared free from any pervasive personality disturbance or decompensation. There were no suggestions in the history or on interview of any schizophrenic tendencies, antisocial behavior, or neurotic symptom formation, and she had maintained consistently excellent achievement in school.

Although there were clear problems of communication within the family and some history of apparent marital disharmony, the parents were sympathetically concerned about Noreen's behavior. They requested and effectively utilized counsel concerning why Noreen had attempted suicide, how they might have contributed to her distress, and what they might do to diminish the danger of such behavior subsequently. The positive treatment response of all family members enhanced the likelihood that the communicative gap between them would be narrowed sufficiently to preclude further suicidal behavior. Eighteen months' follow-up to the time of this writing has confirmed this expectation.

The positive response of the parents in the above case merits further comment. Perhaps equally important as the onset, method, and intent of suicidal behavior in estimating the seriousness of its implications is the impact the behavior has had on the youngster's environment. As elaborated by Sifneos (1966) in relation to adults, there is considerable variation in the environmental manipulation that is achieved by a suicide attempt. The attempt of an adolescent to take his own life may elicit immediate remorse and accession to all of his wishes, or indifference and disbelief, or anger, scorn, and ridicule. Which of these particular reactions the suicidal adolescent has experienced subsequent to his attempt is likely to have considerable prognostic significance.

The more a suicidal adolescent's parents and others have rallied to his cause and been willing to reassess the events and attitudes that led to the attempt, the greater the possibility for some favorable resolution of the adolescent's distress. On the other hand, if there is neither positive parental concern nor any change in family patterns the danger of further suicide attempts is enhanced. Bakwin and Bakwin (1966), Gaultier et al. (1961), Powers (1956), and others who have worked with suicidal adolescents generally agree that it is the youngster who achieves no gratification, whose message remains unheard or unheeded, that requires the greatest clinical surveillance and is most likely to meet with subsequent tragedy. The following case illustrates such near tragedy.

Sara, age 16, had been in more or less constant conflict with her mother since the latter had remarried six years earlier. Sara's father had died when she was four, and she and her mother had been alone together from that time until the advent of her current stepfather, for whom she harbored neither respect nor affection. Sara and her mother fought about anything and everything—dress, friends, table manners, dating privileges, proper attitude toward stepfather, and so forth. When Sara was 15, her mother in desperation sought professional help.

In the course of an evaluation and brief treatment relationship with Sara it seemed clear that both mother and daughter were strong-willed, argumentative, stubborn individuals who regularly magnified minor issues and greatly exaggerated the nature of any differences between them. Sara herself gave no indications of major personality disturbance or symptom formation. In the course of some joint sessions mother and daughter recognized some of the sources of tension between them and agreed to a truce, with compromises on both sides.

Matters improved steadily for over a year after these sessions. Rules of conduct were discussed and compromise agreements reached, and family bickering declined markedly in both frequency and intensity. Then on New Year's Eve, as Sara was dressing for a date that had been arranged long in advance, her mother suddenly and without warning decreed that she could not go out, purportedly because she was not old enough for a New Year's Eve date. Rather, her mother insisted, she should remain at home with the family. Sara stayed at home, crushed by this precipitous and arbitrary reversal, only to have her mother and stepfather subsequently go out and leave her alone in the house. At this point, feeling abandoned and hopeless and convinced that her parents had little appreciation of her needs and feelings, she swallowed some barbiturates. She was careful, however, to limit herself to a small dose that only made her groggy. She went to bed and the next morning told her parents what she had done. At this, fury descended on her head. Her mother became hysterical and called an aunt over to the house to manage the situation. The aunt berated Sara, calling her an actor and a fake and accusing her of trying to drive her mother crazy. At the height of the argument Sara left the room, went upstairs, and severely lacerated both wrists with a razor blade, cutting through several nerves. She then came downstairs, dripping blood, to ask, "Am I acting now?" There seemed little question that the dismal failure of her initial, mild suicide attempt to focus constructive attention on the family issues directly precipitated her second, much more serious self-destructive act.

Treating the Suicidal Adolescent

The demography and dynamics of adolescent suicidal behavior identify the major considerations in treating the youngster who has made a suicide attempt. Above all, *every such attempt must be taken seriously*. Although suicide attempts vary in severity and implications for subsequent suicidal behavior, even the least serious gesture is intended to communicate something significant to the important people in the youngster's life. It is therefore almost inevitable that, as illustrated above, the failure of others to attach significance to his behavior will presage additional and increasingly more dangerous self-destructive actions.

It is to be hoped that family or friends will give an adolescent's suicide attempt sufficient credence to seek professional help, even when the physical consequences do not demand such attention. Then, regardless of whether the youngster has ingested a near fatal dose of barbiturates or merely a few aspirin tablets, the therapist can begin to act on the almost certain knowledge that some otherwise incommunicable distress and some failure in interpersonal relationships have contributed to the youngster's actions.

It is essential first that the therapist take up the communicative slack and convey to the patient that he is interested in, and concerned about, the youngster's welfare and that there are reasons for the suicide attempt that must be identified and understood. It may seem gratuitous to advise a clinician to be interested and concerned. Yet the suicidal adolescent has typically arrived at his self-destructive resolve through a progressively increasing conviction that he is cut off from the affection, nurturance, and support of others. He is thus exceedingly sensitive to indications that his suicidal behavior has earned him even more condemnation and rejection than he was already feeling. Consequently the casual banter that frequently serves to engage adolescents in a therapeutic relationship (see Chapter 9) is ill-advised for the youngster who has attempted suicide. There must be no doubt in his mind that the therapist neither takes the situation lightly nor views it as a culpable act by which he has burned behind him all bridges to self-respect and personal worth.

In the setting of a warm emotional interaction the therapist should seek with the adolescent to identify the motives for his suicidal behavior. If the therapist appears to regard it as "just one of those things" or implies that there is a mystery about such behavior that defies understanding, he simply adds himself to the list of those who have not gotten the youngster's message. Rather, it is necessary to use whatever understanding the patient can provide and whatever relevant information can be assembled from other sources to formulate some dynamic explanations of the patient's actions. When the adolescent himself can volunteer a clear explanation of what has happened, the therapeutic task of resolving the suicidal risk is that much easier. Conversely, further suicidal behavior should be considered an acute and present danger for as long as the patient and the therapist remain unable to identify and discuss directly the communicative or manipulative dynamics involved in his current attempt.

Another mandatory aspect of treating the suicidal adolescent is the inclusion of the parents in the process (see Schechter, 1957). To the extent that an experienced loss of love has participated in the adolescent's suicidal behavior, the therapist should seek to replace such losses not only by making himself available but also by encouraging more positive patterns of family attitudes and interactions. Talking with the parents or with the whole family together is therefore essential to adequate therapeutic intervention. It is vital that the parents too understand the motives for their child's suicide attempt, and that the youngster's covert communication be expressed and shared with them openly. The more the suicidal youngster subsequently encounters warm concern, attempts to understand his behavior, and desired changes in family patterns, the less likely he is to contemplate future suicidal behavior, and these are the considerations that should govern the treatment approach.

This formulation may initially appear to be contrary to reinforcement theory, which would suggest that a rewarding experience subsequent to an act would enhance the likelihood of the act's being repeated. The point, however, is that it is the *communication,* not the suicide attempt, that is reinforced by an adequate treatment approach. The therapist should stress that increased communication is the main key to resolving the intrafamilial difficulty the adolescent has experienced and at the same time should demonstrate and encourage a wide variety of communication techniques that are neither as painful nor as dangerous as a suicide attempt.

REFERENCES

Bakwin, H. Suicide in children and adolescents. *Journal of Pediatrics,* **50**:749–769, 1957.

Bakwin, H., and Bakwin, R. M. *Clinical Management of Behavior Disorders in Children,* 3rd edition. Philadelphia: Saunders, 1966.

Balser, B. H., and Masterson, J. F. Suicide in adolescents. *American Journal of Psychiatry,* **116**:400–404, 1959.

Beck, A. T. *Depression: Clinical, Experimental, and Theoretical Aspects.* New York: Hoeber, 1967.

Bender, L., and Schilder, P. Suicidal preoccupations and attempts in children. *American Journal of Orthopsychiatry,* **7**:225–234, 1937.

Bergstrand, C. G., and Otto, U. Suicidal attempts in adolescence and childhood. *Acta Paediatrica,* **51**:17–26, 1962.

Bibring, E. The mechanism of depression. In P. Greenacre, ed., *Affective disorders.* New York: International Universities Press, 1953, pp. 13–48.

Bigras, J., Gauthier, Y., Bouchard, C., and Tasse, Y. Suicidal attempts in adolescent girls. A preliminary study. *Canadian Psychiatric Association Journal,* **11** (Suppl.):275–282, 1966.

Binger, C. A. L. Emotional disturbances among college women. In G. R. Blaine and C. C. McArthur, eds., *Emotional Problems of the Student*. New York: Appleton-Century-Crofts, 1961, pp. 172–185.

Blatt, S. J. The Wechsler scales and acting out. In L. E. Abt and S. L. Weissman, eds., *Acting Out: Theoretical and Clinical Aspects*. New York: Grune and Stratton, 1965, pp. 242–251.

Bonnard, A. Truancy and pilfering associated with bereavement. In S. Lorand and H. I. Schneer, eds., *Adolescents: Psychoanalytic Approach to Problems and Therapy*. New York: Hoeber, 1961, pp. 152–179.

Bosselman, B. C. *Self-Destruction*. Springfield, Ill.: Thomas, 1958.

Bowlby, J. Childhood mourning and its implications for psychiatry. *American Journal of Psychiatry,* **118**:481–498, 1961.

Braaten, L. J., and Darling, C. D. Suicidal tendencies among college students. *Psychiatric Quarterly,* **36**:665–691, 1962.

Brosin, H. W. Psychiatric conditions following head injury. In S. Arieti, ed., *American Handbook of Psychiatry*, Vol. II. New York: Basic Books, 1959, pp. 1175–1202.

Brown, F. Depression and childhood bereavement. *Journal of Mental Science,* **107**:754–777, 1961.

Bruhn, J. G. Broken homes among attempted suicides and psychiatric outpatients: A comparative study. *Journal of Mental Science,* **108**:772–779, 1962.

Bruhn, J. G., and Seiden, R. H. Student suicide: Fact or fancy? *Journal of the American College Health Association,* **14**:69–77, 1965.

Burks, H. L., and Harrison, S. I. Aggressive behavior as a means of avoiding depression. *American Journal of Orthopsychiatry,* **32**:416–422, 1962.

Burns, C. Pre-schizophrenic symptoms in pre-adolescents' withdrawal and sensitivity. *Nervous Child,* **10**:120–128, 1952.

Clements, S. D. *Minimal Brain Dysfunction in Children*. National Institute of Neurological Diseases and Blindness Monograph No. 3. Washington, D.C.: U.S. Department of Health, Education, and Welfare, 1966.

Coon, G. P. Acute psychosis, depression, and elation. In G. R. Blaine and C. C. McArthur, eds., *Emotional Problems of the Student*. New York: Appleton-Century-Crofts, 1961, pp. 116–132.

Dorpat, T. L., and Ripley, H. S. The relationship between attempted suicide and committed suicide. *Comprehensive Psychiatry,* **8**:74–79, 1967.

Elson, M. The reactive impact of adolescent and family upon each other in separation. *Journal of the American Academy of Child Psychiatry,* **3**:697–708, 1964.

Faigel, H. C. Suicide among young persons: A review of its incidence and causes, and methods for its prevention. *Clinical Pediatrics,* **5**:187–190, 1966.

Freud, A. Adolescence. *Psychoanalytic Study of the Child,* **13**:255–278, 1958.

Freud, S. (1905). Three essays on the theory of sexuality. *Standard Edition,* Vol. VII. London: Hogarth, 1953, pp. 135–243.

Freud, S. (1917). Mourning and melancholia. *Standard Edition,* Vol. XIV. London: Hogarth, 1957, pp. 243–258.

Gaultier, M., Fournier, E., and Gorceix, A. A propos de 47 cas de tentatives de suicides chez des adolescents (A study of 47 cases of attempted suicide in adolescents). *Hygiene Mentale,* 50:363–369, 1961.

Gaylin, W., ed. *The Meaning of Despair: Psychoanalytic Contributions to the Understanding of Depression.* New York: Science House, 1968.

Glaser, K. Attempted suicide in children and adolescents: Psychodynamic observations. *American Journal of Psychotherapy,* 19:220–227, 1965.

Glaser, K. Masked depression in children and adolescents. *American Journal of Psychotherapy,* 21:565–574, 1967.

Gould, R. E. Suicide problems in children and adolescents. *American Journal of Psychotherapy,* 19:228–246, 1965.

Grinker, R. R., Miller, J., Sabshin, M., Nunn, R., and Nunnally, J. C. *The Phenomena of Depressions.* New York: Hoeber-Harper, 1961.

Jacobinzer, H. Attempted suicides in children. *Journal of Pediatrics,* 56:519–525, 1960.

Jacobinzer, H. Attempted suicides in adolescents by poisoning. *American Journal of Psychotherapy,* 19:247–252, 1965a.

Jacobinzer, H. Attempted suicides in adolescence. *Journal of the American Medical Association,* 191:7–11, 1965b.

Jacobs, J., and Teicher, J. D. Broken homes and social isolation in attempted suicides of adolescents. *International Journal of Social Psychiatry,* 13:139–149, 1967.

Jacobson, E. Adolescent moods and the remodeling of psychic structures in adolescence. *Psychoanalytic Study of the Child,* 16:164–183, 1961.

Kastenbaum, R. Time and death in adolescence. In H. Feifel, ed., *The Meaning of Death.* New York: McGraw-Hill, 1959, pp. 99–113.

Keeler, W. R. Children's reactions to the death of a parent. In P. Hoch and J. Zubin, eds., *Depression.* New York: Grune and Stratton, 1954, pp. 109–120.

Kolb, L. C. Psychopathology of depressions. In D. Maddison and G. M. Duncan, eds., *Aspects of Depressive Illness.* London: Livingstone, 1965, pp. 63–84.

Laufer, M. Object loss and mourning during adolescence. *Psychoanalytic Study of the Child,* 21:269–293, 1966.

Lesse, S. Hypochondriasis and psychosomatic disorders masking depression. *American Journal of Psychotherapy,* 21:607–620, 1967.

Litman, R. E., and Farberow, N. L. Emergency evaluation of self-destructive potentiality. In N. L. Farberow and E. S. Shneidman, eds., *The Cry for Help.* New York: McGraw-Hill, 1961, pp. 48–59.

Lorand, S. Adolescent depression. *International Journal of Psycho-Analysis,* 48:53–60, 1967.

Lorr, M., Sonn, T. M., and Katz, M. M. Toward a definition of depression. *Archives of General Psychiatry,* 17:183–186, 1967.

Mason, P. Suicide in adolescents. *Psychoanalytic Review,* 41:48–54, 1954.

Masterson, J. F. *The Psychiatric Dilemma of Adolescence.* Boston: Little, Brown, 1967.

Masterson, J. F., Tucker, K., and Berk, G. Psychopathology in adolescence: IV. Clinical and dynamic characteristics. *American Journal of Psychiatry,* **120**:357–366, 1963.

Mendelson, M. *Psychoanalytic Concepts of Depression.* Springfield, Ill.: Thomas, 1960.

Mulder, D. W. Psychoses with brain tumors and other chronic neurological disorders. In S. Arieti, ed., *American Handbook of Psychiatry,* Vol. II. New York: Basic Books, 1959, pp. 1144–1162.

Otto, U. Changes in the behaviour of children and adolescents preceding suicidal attempts. *Acta Psychiatrica Scandinavica,* **40**:386–400, 1964a.

Otto, U. Suicidal attempts in adolescence and childhood: States of mental illness and personality variables. *Acta Paedopsychiatrica,* **31**:397–411, 1964b.

Otto, U. Suicidal attempts made by children and adolescents because of school problems. *Acta Paediatrica Scandinavica,* **32**:348–356, 1965.

Parrish, H. M. Epidemiology of suicide among college students. *Yale Journal of Biology and Medicine,* **29**:585–595, 1957.

Perlstein, A. P. Suicide in adolescence. *New York State Journal of Medicine,* **66**:3017–3020, 1966.

Powers, D. Youthful suicide attempts. Part 1. *Northwest Medicine,* **53**:1001–1002, 1954.

Powers, D. Suicide threats and attempts in the young. *American Practitioner,* **7**:1140–1143, 1956.

Raphael, T., Power, S. H., and Berridge, W. L. The question of suicide as a problem in college mental hygiene. *American Journal of Orthopsychiatry,* **7**:1–14, 1937.

Raskin, A., Schulterbrandt, J., Reatig, N., and Rice, C. E. Factors of psychopathology in interview, ward behavior, and self-report ratings of hospitalized depressives. *Journal of Consulting Psychology,* **31**:270–278, 1967.

Rook, A. Student suicides. *British Medical Journal,* **1**:599–603, 1959.

Root, N. N. A neurosis in adolescence. *Psychoanalytic Study of the Child,* **12**:320–334, 1957.

Rosen, B. M., Bahn, A. K., Shellow, R., and Bower, E. M. Adolescent patients served in outpatient psychiatric clinics. *American Journal of Public Health,* **55**:1563–1577, 1965.

Ross, M. The practical recognition of depressive and suicidal states. *Annals of Internal Medicine,* **64**:1079–1086, 1966.

Rubenstein, R., Moses, R., and Lidz, T. On attempted suicide. *Archives of Neurology and Psychiatry,* **79**:103–112, 1958.

Sands, D. E. The psychoses of adolescence. *Journal of Mental Science,* **102**:308–316, 1956.

Schechter, M. D. The recognition and treatment of suicide in children. In E. S. Shneidman and N. L. Farberow, eds., *Clues to Suicide.* New York: McGraw-Hill, 1957, pp. 131–142.

Schilder, P., and Wechsler, D. The attitudes of children toward death. *Journal of Genetic Psychology*, **45**:406–451, 1934.

Schneer, H. I., and Kay, P. The suicidal adolescent. In S. Lorand and H. I. Schneer, eds., *Adolescents: Psychoanalytic Approach to Problems and Therapy*. New York: Hoeber, 1961, pp. 180–201.

Schneer, H. I., Kay, P., and Brozovsky, M. Events and conscious ideation leading to suicidal behavior in adolescents. *Psychiatric Quarterly*, **35**:507–515, 1961.

Schrut, A. Suicidal adolescents and children. *Journal of the American Medical Association*, **188**:1103–1107, 1964.

Seiden, R. H. Campus tragedy: A study of student suicide. *Journal of Abnormal Psychology*, **71**:389–399, 1966.

Shainberg, D. Personality restriction in adolescents. *Psychiatric Quarterly*, **40**:258–270, 1966.

Shneidman, E. S. Orientations toward death: A vital aspect of the study of lives. In R. W. White, ed., *The Study of Lives*. New York: Atherton, 1963, pp. 200–227.

Shneidman, E. S., and Farberow, N. L., eds. *Clues to Suicide*. New York: McGraw-Hill, 1957.

Shoor, M., and Speed, M. H. Delinquency as a manifestation of the mourning process. *Psychiatric Quarterly*, **37**:540–558, 1963.

Sifneos, P. E. Manipulative suicide. *Psychiatric Quarterly*, **40**:525–537, 1966.

Silverman, C. The epidemiology of depression: A review. *American Journal of Psychiatry*, **124**:883–891, 1968.

Spiegel, R. Anger and acting out. Masks of depression. *American Journal of Psychotherapy*, **21**:597–606, 1967.

Stengel, E. *Suicide and Attempted Suicide*. Baltimore: Penguin Books, 1964.

Stengel, E., and Cook, N. G. *Attempted Suicide: Its Social Significance and Effects*. New York: Basic Books, 1958.

Sutter, J. M., Luccioni, H., and Scotto, J. C. Suicide et carence d'autorité (Suicide and the lack of authority). *Hygiene Mentale*, **53**:197–204, 1964.

Tabachnik, N. D.. and Farberow, N. L. The assessment of self-destructive potential. In N. L. Farberow and E. S. Shneidman, eds., *The Cry for Help*. New York: McGraw-Hill, 1961, pp. 60–77.

Teicher, J. D., and Jacobs, J. Adolescents who attempt suicide: Preliminary findings. *American Journal of Psychiatry*, **122**:1248–1257, 1966.

Temby, W. D. Suicide. In G. R. Blaine and C. C. McArthur, eds., *Emotional Problems of the Student*. New York: Appleton-Century-Crofts, 1961, pp. 133–152.

Toolan, J. M. Depression in children and adolescents. *American Journal of Orthopsychiatry*, **32**:404–415, 1962a.

Toolan, J. M. Suicide and suicidal attempts in children and adolescents. *American Journal of Psychiatry*, **118**:719–724, 1962b.

Tuckman, J., and Connon, H. E. Attempted suicide in adolescents. *American Journal of Psychiatry*, **119**:228–232, 1962.

Vital Statistics of the United States, 1965. Vol. II, *Mortality.* Washington, D.C.: U.S. Department of Health, Education and Welfare, 1967.

Walters, P. A. Student apathy. In G. R. Blaine and C. C. McArthur, eds., *Emotional Problems of the Student.* New York: Appleton-Century-Crofts, 1961, pp. 153–171.

Weiss, J. M. A. The suicidal patient. In S. Arieti, eds., *American Handbook of Psychiatry,* Vol. III. New York: Basic Books, 1966, pp. 115–130.

Wittenborn, J. R. Depression. In B. B. Wolman, ed., *Handbook of Clinical Psychology.* New York: McGraw-Hill, 1965, pp. 1030–1057.

Zilboorg, G. Differential diagnostic types of suicide. *Archives of Neurology and Psychiatry,* **35**:270–291, 1936.

Zilboorg, G. Considerations on suicide, with particular reference to that of the young. *American Journal of Orthopsychiatry,* **7**:15–31, 1937.

CHAPTER 6

School Phobia

The term "school phobia" does not appear in the traditional nomenclature of psychological disorders, and it is usually regarded as a problem more of childhood than adolescence. Yet adolescent school phobia merits major attention in any consideration of adolescent psychopathology. In a great many adolescent youngsters brought for professional help in connection with anxiety, phobic, and conversion or psychophysiologic reactions (especially headache, abdominal pain, diarrhea, nausea, and vomiting) refusal to attend school has been the event that crystallized parental concern. Clinical data furthermore indicate that school phobia is a significant precursor of work phobia in adults (see Pittman, Langsley, and DeYoung, 1968) and constitutes a clearly definable psychological disorder:

"The clinical findings, both my own and most of those in the literature, seem to show that school refusal is a definite and specific pattern of human behaviour, well definable in its symptomatology, and so circumscribed that it is possible to state differential-diagnostic criteria that enable one to separate it from other disorders of similar appearance" (Clyne, 1966, p. 34).

Because school phobia embraces a broad range of neurotic symptom formation as manifest in young people, the clinician who works with disturbed adolescents needs to recognize, understand, and treat it. This chapter first outlines the clinical manifestations of school phobia and delineates the patterns of family interaction that usually participate in its genesis and course. Several illustrative cases are then presented, leading to a discussion of major issues in the treatment of this disorder. The psychopathology of school phobia is for the most part identical in children and adolescents, and much of the following material has emerged from studies involving school-phobic youngsters of all ages; wherever relevant, however, significant areas of divergence between childhood and adolescent patterns of school phobia are explicated.

CLINICAL MANIFESTATIONS

As reviewed by Eisenberg (1958a,b); Millar (1961); Waldfogel, Coolidge, and Hahn (1957); and others, clinical studies of school-phobic youngsters have yielded a fairly distinct picture of this disturbance. School phobia consists essentially of some degree of psychological inability to attend school. This inability may range from partial reluctance to total refusal to remain in school, primarily in response to intense feelings of anxiety, dread, and panic associated with the school setting:

"Those of us who have watched children flee from school or stand paralyzed in approaching the building are impressed by their acute state of panic. They all show some of the following manifestations of fears: extreme pallor, trembling, nausea, inability to move, or feeling impelled to flight. Above all, they are subject to a feeling that a powerful force has control over them" (Talbot, 1957, p. 290).

Published case reports summarized by Leventhal and Sills (1964) suggest that boys and girls develop school phobia with approximately equal frequency. Most commonly the youngster achieves his school refusal through somatic complaints that persuade his parents to keep him at home or the school nurse to excuse him from the classroom. Headaches, abdominal pain, nausea, vomiting, and diarrhea are the major somatic concomitants of school phobia, although in some instances the school-phobic youngster merely anticipates the onset of such symptoms; he may, for example, admonish his parents that he is certain to become nauseated and vomit in class if they send him to school.

Whatever the youngster's somatic complaints, they generally subside within a few hours if he is excused from attending school. Should his parents drag him to school, his symptoms are likely to increase to such an extent that he must be sent home. If he is allowed to remain at home in the morning with the understanding that he will leave for school as soon as he is feeling better, his complaints are likely to persist until he is assured that there will be no further attendance pressure put on him that day.

Some school-phobic youngsters present in addition to, or instead of, somatic distress a variety of specific fears or concerns by which they seek to justify their school refusal—the teacher is unfair, the students are unfriendly, the work is too difficult, and so forth. In the school-phobic youngster virtually all such complaints are flimsy rationalizations that have little direct relation to his school aversion. Attempts to correct the protested situation—as by changing his teacher, finding him friends, or easing his assignments—typically have no lasting salutary effect on his reluctance to go to school.

School phobia differs sharply from situations that foster realistic fears of going to school. The youngster who has been threatened with a thrashing by the school bully or who faces an examination he expects to fail may become visibly apprehensive about attending school; were the bully expelled or the examination canceled, his qualms would quickly fade. Whereas this youngster may need help to cope with the bully or the examination, his fears do not necessarily reflect a neurotic conflict, in which the major sources of anxiety remain unconscious: "There is a world of psychologic difference between the occasional 'normal' use of somatic complaints to avoid an unwelcome task and the phobic child's uncontrollable psychophysiological symptoms" (Eisenberg, 1958b, p. 645).

In addition to differentiating school phobia from reality-based apprehensions about school that readily yield to superficial environmental manipulations, it is also important to distinguish between school phobia and truancy. One of the first clinical descriptions of school phobia appears in a paper addressed by Broadwin (1932) to "the study of truancy." Broadwin reviews his experience with youngsters who were consistently absent from school for extended periods of time, during which they remained at home with their parents' knowledge. These youngsters could offer no comprehensible reason for their school refusal, other than the fact that they were manifestly fearful and unable to function in school; at home, on the other hand, they remained happy, content, and symptom free.

Subsequent clinical and research reports indicate that such a pattern of school refusal has little in common with typical truancy (see Eisenberg, 1958a; Hersov, 1960). The truant youngster usually dislikes or does poorly in school, absents himself from classes on an irregular basis as the fancy takes him, and spends his truant time in pleasurable activities away from home without his parents' knowledge or consent. The majority of school-phobic youngsters, in contrast, linger at home with their parents' consent if not their approval, earn average or better grades, and profess to like school and to value academic pursuits.

School Phobia as a Diagnostic Label

In elaborating the distinctions among school phobia, truancy, and reality-based concerns about school attendance a number of writers have debated the implications of "school phobia" as a diagnostic label. School-phobic anxiety has traditionally been considered a neurotic disturbance from both intrapsychic and intrafamilial points of view, and many clinicians liken school phobia to classical phobic symptom formation (see Malmquist, 1965). As first elaborated in Freud's (1909) discussion of Little Hans, phobias derive from the externalization of frightening impulses and their displacement onto a previously neutral object that then becomes aversive. Waldfogel et al. (1957) and Sperling (1961), among others, regard school phobia as similar to other phobias in this respect, with anxiety being shifted from some basic source to the school. These writers accordingly consider school phobia to be a definite and appropriately labeled clinical entity, and they stress that the various patterns of dread, psychophysiological reaction, and rationalization displayed by the school-phobic youngster are identical to classical phobic and phobic-equivalent symptoms.

Sperling (1967) adds that school phobia qualifies as a true psychoneurosis on three significant grounds: (a) it is based on unconscious conflicts, (b) the school-phobic youngster remains unaware of the real origins of his anxiety, and (c) the reasons he gives for remaining at home are rationalizations. She further stresses that recognition of school phobia as a traditional symptom neurosis is important to adequate treatment planning. To regard it as something less than a full-blown neurosis, she continues, is to run the risk of overlooking the depth of its dynamics and instituting superficial treatment procedures that have little enduring effect (see p. 237).

Among clinicians who would agree that this disturbance is a symptom neurosis, some doubt that it is truly a phobia and prefer to designate it otherwise; for example, Johnson et al. (1941) and Estes, Haylett, and Johnson (1956) argue that a youngster's terror at being in school has at least as much to do with fears of being separated from his home and parents, especially his mother, as it does with any fears of school, and they minimize the significance of displacement in the development of school aversion. Johnson and her co-workers regard this disturbance as a particular form of anxiety neurosis, rather than a phobia, and they recommend the label "separation anxiety" instead of "school phobia" to describe it.

Millar (1961) also challenges the "school phobia" designation for this disturbance. He too discounts displacement as an integral feature of school aversion, inasmuch as some school-aversive youngsters do not express any fears of school. Furthermore, he continues, since the school-aversive youngster remains anxious about being separated from his home and mother, the disturbance fails to achieve the psychic economy classically associated with phobic symptom formation; that is, of reducing the anxiety in relation to the original objects or situations from which anxiety has presumably been displaced.

Turning to treatment implications, Millar expresses concern that the "phobia" label focuses inordinate attention on the youngster's anxiety and intrapsychic dynamics to the neglect of maladaptive parent-child relationships that almost always participate in such school nonattendance.

Not only is the "school-phobia" designation likely to distract the therapist from crucial interpersonal aspects of the disorder, Millar continues, but it may also evoke undue hesitation about returning the youngster to school; that is, to interpret the nonattendance primarily as phobic anxiety may foster unnecessary concerns about precipitating panic by encouraging early return. Millar accordingly advocates "school refusal" rather than "school phobia" as the preferable term for this disorder.

Kahn and Nursten (1962) likewise prefer to term problems in school attendance as "school refusal" rather than "school phobia." They emphasize that psychologically determined breakdowns in school attendance are "not confined to phobic conditions but can occur in any type of neurotic or psychotic disorder in children and adolescents" (p. 707). In their opinion "school phobia" is too specific a label to denote such attendance difficulties.

On closer examination none of these criticisms of "school phobia" as a diagnostic label appears to provide compelling reasons for discarding it. Although "separation anxiety" appropriately focuses attention on intrafamilial pathology that often contributes to school-phobic tendencies, it fails to encompass the many school-phobic youngsters for whom school-related problems are demonstrably more troublesome than anxiety about separation. Thus Glaser (1959) notes that distress at being in school and anxiety about being away from home usually overlap in school phobia, and either may be the more central. The teenage boy with unconscious concerns about homosexuality who displaces anxiety from a threatening locker-room situation to his previously neutral classrooms, for example, may develop a school-phobic reaction that has little primary relationship to separation anxiety. Furthermore, the inability to separate from the home is far from ubiquitous in school phobia. The case reports reviewed by Leventhal and Sills (1964) include many youngsters who maintained numerous social activities outside the home despite an otherwise unequivocal school-phobic reaction (see also p. 209).

As for Millar's arguments, the fact that a youngster expresses no fears of school does not necessarily imply that he experiences none and is therefore not employing displacement mechanisms. A sense of panic or onset of somatic distress associated with school attendance adequately demonstrates such fears, arrived at by displacement, whether or not the youngster can specify them. Furthermore, the school-phobic youngsters who are persistently anxious about being away from home often remain comfortable and relaxed so long as they are allowed to stay at home or in their parents' presence. Such comfort amply attests the psychic economy expected to accompany a phobic neurosis; if phobic mechanisms were not operative, with displacement to the school of anxiety originally experienced in relation to the parents, these youngsters might well exhibit continuing fears of imminent disaster despite being permitted to remain at home.

Finally, Kahn and Nursten's endorsement of a broad view of school refusal seems inadvisably to blur differential diagnostic and treatment considerations. The youngster who cannot bring himself to attend school because of, for example, depressive lethargy or schizophrenic apprehensions of the outside world may manifest few of the defining characteristics of school phobia outlined in the preceding pages. Rather, his inability to attend school could constitute a relatively nonspecific symptom of his depressive or schizophrenic disorder that will respond to adequate treatment of the primary disorder.

On the other hand, it is possible for a schizophrenic or depressed youngster additionally to develop phobic or conversion symptoms that carry specific dynamic and therapeutic implications in their own right. Thus a depressed adolescent may refuse school not only because he is enervatingly lethargic but also because he becomes acutely anxious or somatically upset in the school setting. In such instances the inability to attend school is likely to comprise the particular phenomenological and dynamic constellations that are associated with school phobia, and psychotherapeutic intervention must be addressed specifically to school phobia as well as to depression.

Whereas school phobia is best conceived as neurotic symptom formation, in other words, it may occur in the absence of any other psychological disturbances or in combination with various neurotic, characterological, or psychotic disorders. For adequate treatment planning it is therefore essential not to lump together all instances of school refusal but rather (a) to differentiate carefully between phobic nonattendance and nonattendance that is a nonspecific derivative of some other personality disorder, and (b) to determine what, if any, other pathological conditions coexist with the school phobia.

Acute and Chronic School Phobia

The extent to which school phobia occurs in combination with other psychological disturbances provides the basis for categorizing it into its *acute* and *chronic* forms. These subcategories of school phobia were first delineated by Coolidge, Hahn, and Peck (1957) as the "neurotic crisis" and "way of life" patterns of school phobia. The acutely disturbed school phobics whom Coolidge et al. saw at the Judge Baker Guidance Center were primarily youngsters whose psychological difficulties had arisen suddenly and were limited to their phobic anxiety about attending school. Their school phobia had appeared in conjunction with an upsurge of uncharacteristic clinging, whining, and uncooperative behavior, but their overall personality integration had remained intact and their general cognitive and social development had proceeded apace despite their neurotic aversion to school: "In spite of this change [school phobia], the children generally continued to function well in other areas; intellectually and socially they did not lose ground, generally remaining active in their many friendships and peer groups" (Coolidge et al., 1957, p. 297).

In the youngsters with chronic school phobia studied by Coolidge et al., in contrast, the school refusal tended to be imposed on underlying characterological disturbances. These youngsters demonstrated a long history of behavior problems of one kind or another, and their avoidance of school had neither commenced abruptly nor been accompanied by marked personality change. In further contrast to the youngsters with the "neurotic crisis" type of school phobia, this characterological group typically displayed improverished, constricted personality functioning and a deteriorating social adjustment. Frequently their fears of school had mounted gradually and been diffusely generalized to the environment, so that over the years they had become increasingly reluctant to attend school, uncomfortable in interpersonal or unfamiliar situations, and inclined to cling to their mothers at the expense of maintaining peer-group activities and friendships.

As elaborated by Coolidge et al. (1960) and Levenson (1961), it is generally the case that, the older the school-phobic youngster, the more likely he is to demonstrate the chronic rather than the acute form of the disorder. Thus the school-phobic adolescent tends primarily to present with gradual development of his school aversion and accompanying withdrawal from social and peer-group activities. In the experience of Coolidge et al., furthermore, the school-phobic adolescent has invariably experienced some earlier episode of school-phobic anxiety. Unlike the acute, readily remediable school phobia that is typical of the elementary school child, they conclude, "In the older group . . . one encounters chronic, deeply imbedded problems that yield slowly to treatment, and in which the prognosis is anything but bright" (p. 599).

Levenson reports a similar history of onset in 10 sixteen- to twenty-year-old boys who became anxious about attending school and withdrew into their family group. In each case he was able to unearth some previous instance of phobic symptom formation and regressive behavior related to school attendance. These earlier episodes had typically occurred at age seven or eight and then been followed by several years consistent school attendance prior to the adolescent recurrence.

Eisenberg (1958b) and Sperling (1967) have similarly found that the school-phobic anxiety that arises in the older child is especially likely to coexist with other psychological difficulties, and Sperling has elaborated further the differing implications of traumatic and gradual onset in school phobia. She notes that some episodes of school refusal develop in the context of clearly precipitating circumstances and others do not, and she suggests that, the more gradual the onset, in the absence of apparent traumatic events, the more significantly family pathology can be assumed to have contributed to the disorder.

The traumatic events that trigger a rapidly arising school phobia typically reflect the underlying psychodynamics of the youngster's school-aversive propensities. Where concern about separation is the primary dynamic element, precipitous school phobia usually follows on the heels of events that exacerbate separation anxiety: an illness or surgical procedure involving the youngster or his parents; absence of the parents on vacation or of the mother to give birth; moves to a new home, neighborhood, school, grade, or classroom; and the like. In youngsters who do not appear to be particularly prone to separation anxiety sudden onset of school phobia can usually be traced to some specific humiliating or anxiety-provoking experience in the school setting: the youngster's classmates mock his appearance, the gym teacher publicly denigrates his athletic ability, and so forth.

The less apparent such identifiable precipitating events are in the onset of a school phobia, the more likely the phobia is to have developed gradually out of interlocking family pathology. Whereas parent-child relationships always influence the origin and duration of a school-phobic reaction, it is only when the interacting neurotic needs of the significant family members are particularly potent that a youngster's school refusal is likely to be tolerated in the absence of any precipitating event that provides the family some basis for rationalizing the absence.

Many of these differential considerations are summarized by Kennedy (1965) in a list of diagnostic guidelines he proposes for distinguishing between acute and chronic school phobia: acute school phobia is the more likely diagnosis when the present episode is the first episode; when the onset has been acute and occurred on a Monday after an illness the previous Thursday or Friday; when the child is relatively young, concerned about death, and worried about his mother's health; and when the parents are relatively well adjusted, in good communication with each other, and readily able to understand the dynamics of their youngster's difficulties. Conversely, in an older youngster who has had previous episodes of school phobia and presents a gradual onset in which Monday, illness, and concerns about death play no observable part, and whose parents manifest psychological disturbances of their own and are relatively difficult to work with, the indicated diagnosis is in all probability chronic school phobia.

PATTERNS OF FAMILY INTERACTION IN SCHOOL PHOBIA

Clinical studies of school-phobic youngsters have identified characteristic patterns of family interaction that typically participate in the genesis and course of this disturbance. Susceptibility to a school-phobic reaction following psychological stress appears rooted in the concurrence of certain kinds of neurotic needs in the parents and certain types of concerns and coping styles in the child. The following description of these family patterns is drawn from the author's clinical work and the extensive experience reported by Coolidge et al. (1957, 1962), Eisenberg (1958a,b), Johnson et al. (1941), Talbot (1957), and Waldfogel et al. (1957).

The Role of the Mother

The mothers of school-phobic youngsters tend to be dependent women who are only partially emancipated from their own mothers. They often compare themselves unfavorably to their mothers, who in turn usually reinforce their daughters' self-derogating beliefs. The grandmother of the school-phobic youngster typically dominates his mother and depreciates her sense of competence as a person, wife, and parent with patronizing advice and constant criticisms of her child-rearing and home-managing practices. The mothers of school-phobic children often resent having had to sacrifice their own dependent needs to the nurturant requirements of their children, while at the same time they have little confidence in their capacity to provide them adequate mothering. These mothers additionally tend to be uncomfortable with aggressive impulses, and they seek to avoid experiencing hostile feelings or provoking them in others.

Such personality dynamics lead the typical mother of a school-phobic child to overprotect him from early in life. She strives incessantly to gratify her youngster's needs, guard him against deprivation and frustration, and curry his love and affection. By such solicitousness for her child the mother attempts both to deny her negative feelings toward him and to forestall any anger or resentment he might otherwise feel toward her. At the same time, by identifying herself with the child for whom she is so devotedly caring, the mother may vicariously assuage some of her own unfulfilled dependent longings.

Yet even the most solicitous mother inevitably encounters unrealistic demands from her child and infantile rage when these demands cannot be met. The mothers of school-phobic children characteristically sow the seeds for school refusal by their inability to deal incisively with such situations. These women are quick to back away from angry confrontations, and their accession to excessive or unreasonable requests has unfortunate consequences for both mother and child. The mother, already burdened by her limited sense of competence, feels overwhelmed and exploited by her child and experiences increased resentment toward him: "Why should he treat me this way after all I've done for him?" Then, aghast at her upsurge of hostile impulses, she tends to pursue with renewed vigor the same maladaptive, overcompensatory solicitousness that brought the difficulty to pass. The child—observing that his foot stamping, breath holding, crying, and the like can triumph over adult authority, power, and reason—is encouraged to further manipulations of his parents by such means and develops inflated confidence that with intemperate outbursts he can bend all situations to his will.

Typically, then, these are mothers who excessively foster their children's dependence; cushion them from discomfort; discipline them by bribes, appeals to reason, and pleas for consideration; and prefer to keep them physically and psychologically close. When a school-phobic tendency first threatens, the mother usually responds in a manner that compounds rather than eases the situation. If her youngster grumbles about a situation in school, she is inordinately quick to commiserate with him and agree that a few days at home might be the best thing for him. If he complains of headache or stomach pain, she seldom doubts the necessity of his remaining at home.

These mothers are transparently ambivalent toward the school-phobic pattern once it has been established and toward the efforts of any therapist whose counsel they seek. While paying lip service to the necessity of prompt return, the mother covertly communicates to her nonattending child that she enjoys having him at home and will not resort to drastic action should his refusal continue: "You're supposed to go back to school today, but it looks like rain, and I don't want you catching cold; so let's wait until the weather clears." To the therapist she appeals urgently for help in altering her child's nonattendance and dependence on her, but her words and actions suggest that she unconsciously wishes that little be changed.

Often the mother's mixed feelings concerning treatment for her school-phobic youngster impede therapeutic efforts from the very beginning. The therapist may find the mother huddled close to her child in the waiting room, as if preparing him for the worst. She may promptly advise the therapist that he will have difficulty in getting the youngster to leave her side, even as she clutches him firmly or by the tone of her voice reveals that she does not want to surrender him to another's care. In the older adolescent, where such blatant infantilizing is rare, at least in public, it is still common for the mother to intrude on the interviewer's initial efforts to introduce himself to the youngster, as if to ensure that any diagnostic or therapeutic transactions will proceed through her. These mothers customarily expect and prefer to be interviewed first and to have their youngster interviewed only in their presence.

Should the youngster respond eagerly to the therapist's overtures, these mothers often exhibit obvious disappointment and hurt. If the therapist, at his insistence or in response to the youngster's demonstrated readiness, takes him alone into the office, the mother may remain vigilantly on the threshold, ever-ready to rush in and soothe the anguish she anticipates or hopes her child will experience when thus separated from her. In a joint interview these mothers usually dominate the conversation to such an extent that the therapist has little opportunity to engage the youngster directly or begin to kindle a positive treatment relationship.

The Contribution of the Father

The fathers of school-phobic children also contribute conspicuously to their youngster's susceptibility to this disturbance. In most instances the father intensifies the problematic mother-child relationship by failing to provide any counteractive balance to his wife's overprotective, infantilizing approach and by undermining her already limited sense of competence. Generally two kinds of men exert such paternal influences, and the fathers of school-phobic children usually demonstrate one or the other of the following two personality styles.

Many of these fathers are passive, dependent men with a weak sense of masculine identification whose needs are very similar to those of their wives. They overprotect and cater to their children, attempt to promote their dependency and unflagging adoration, and avoid as much as possible any negatively toned family interactions. Like their wives, they retreat from angry confrontations and yield to their child's demands at the slightest hint of pending unpleasantness. Often they will absorb outrageous abuse from their child, physical as well as verbal, with no firmer response than an appeal for mutual love and respect. At some point these men may explode into unreasonable, childish fits of anger, perhaps crying in frustration or breaking one of their own valued possessions, but such outbursts serve only to evoke subsequent guilt and increased manipulability on their part. Since fathers of this kind usually compete with their wives for the maternal role in the home, their youngsters confront not one but two parents whose neurotic needs foster the dependency, inflated self-confidence, and manipulative proclivities that are associated with susceptibility to school phobia.

These fathers also share their wives' ambivalent attitudes toward the school-phobic pattern and its treatment. They exhort their youngster to return to school, and they express to the therapist their unqualified support for whatever measures are necessary to resolve the attendance difficulty. Yet these men show a striking inclination to seize on reasons for delay ("Maybe we should wait until the beginning of next week rather than tomorrow to take him back, sort of give him the weekend to prepare himself"); to capitulate to blatant manipulation ("But, Doctor, she says she'll tear the house apart if we make her go back as we agreed on, and we wouldn't want to let things get that far out of hand, would we?"); and directly to dilute or sabotage the treatment ("I know he's supposed to see you today, but I've got this important meeting that came up, and my wife doesn't like to drive when it's raining out, and there's no other way to get him there, so maybe we could let it go for this week").

In contrast to this passive, maternally competitive type of father, many others are vigorously or even hyper-masculine, minimally invested in family affairs, and far removed from any rivalry with their wives. These are men whose wives and children command only secondary attention relative to their work, hobbies, or engagements with other people. Such a man is rarely sufficiently informed or interested to intrude constructively on a potentially maladaptive relationship between his wife and child. Not unusually this type of school-phobic father remains unaware that his youngster is missing school until the nonattendance is brought directly to his attention—he calls home during the day and his child answers, or the school principal contacts him to discuss a prolonged absence.

Such obliviousness often reflects not only this type of father's detachment from his family but also a pact between his wife and child to keep the attendance problem as their "secret." These pacts usually develop from the mother's attempts to cultivate her child's tractability at home by bribing him with the promise not to tell the father he is out of school; the youngster in turn capitalizes on this opportunity to trade his good behavior at home for the pledge that his father, whom he expects to be unsympathetic and less manipulable than his mother, will not be informed. When this type of father finally learns of the school-phobic situation, he usually becomes furious and blames the problem on his wife. Should the school-phobic reaction persist, he tends to vacillate between berating his wife for her inept motherhood and "washing his hands" of the whole business; in either case his behavior serves only to intensify the previously existing difficulties.

Concerns and Coping Behaviors in the School-Phobic Youngster

The school-phobic youngster generally displays certain characteristic concerns and coping styles that complement his parents' neurotic needs.

Most commonly he shares with his mother and sometimes his father major concerns about expressing aggression and asserting independence. The school-phobic youngster has usually come to resent his mother's overprotectiveness. He correctly construes her smothering solicitousness as an attempt to damp or deny his developing capacities, and he often senses the hostility that in part underlies and motivates her excessive ministrations. Yet, because she is manifestly devoted to him and continually sacrifices her overt needs to his, any anger he feels toward her tends to generate considerable guilt. Often the school-phobic youngster has handled such guilt by externalizing his hostile impulses, with the result that he frequently anticipates harm to himself or his parents and is apprehensive about being separated from his family.

Regarding independence, many school-phobic youngsters have recognized that their mothers were obstructing their individuation by discouraging them from the expanding privileges and responsibilities being enjoyed by their peers. Whereas the typical school-phobic youngster tends therefore to become particularly intent on pressing for independence, the extent to which he has been overprotected has usually left him poorly prepared for independence. He is subject to considerable anxiety in situations that challenge him to affirm his independence, and he preferentially responds to such threats with a regressive withdrawal to the dependent comforts and solace he has known at home under his parents' wing. In these respects the school-phobic youngster exemplifies many of the general characteristics of phobic disturbance, including exaggerated dependency, which is perceived as incompatible with self-reliance, and exaggerated avoidance of difficult, fear-evoking situations. Both these patterns are usually learned as an individual adapts to the expectations of overprotective parents (see Andrews, 1966).

Coexisting pressures for independence and regression are particularly prominent in the adolescent school-phobic youngster. Cultural expectations generally identify puberty as the threshold of major developments in the capacity for independence, and specific school events emphasize such expectations. With entrance to junior and particularly senior high school, boys and girls surrender their single classroom and a primary relationship with one teacher for multiple classrooms and teachers. They change classes several times daily, under minimal supervision, and they are given increasing responsibility for budgeting their time, organizing their studying, and even choosing their subjects. Whatever his strivings for independence, the youngster who is ill-prepared for autonomous action may experience a marked upsurge of anxiety when his relatively structured elementary school program gives way to the more ambiguous junior and senior high school settings.

Concurrently with the diminishing support and dependent gratification provided by the formal aspects of his school setting, the pubescent young-ster must also withstand pressures that are related to sexual maturation. In respect to physical characteristics, for example, the girl who is embar-rassed by menstruation or the size of her breasts, or the boy who is dismayed by a delayed growth of pubic hair or the unpredictable pitch of his voice quickly identifies the school as the main locus in which these aspects of physical development are exposed to his or her peers. The menstruating girl must make frequent trips to the lavatory, and the squeaky voiced boy is required with the rest of his classmates to recite in class. Mandatory gym classes, with specified gym- and swim-suits for the girls and unsequestered locker and shower facilities for the boys, further restrict the youngster's opportunity to keep his physical attributes private.

For the adolescent with actual or fantasied deviations in pubescent physical development such constant exposure may imbue the school with considerable anxiety-provoking potential. Many youngsters can weather such concerns without becoming phobic about attending school; for the teenage youngster with preexisting conflicts around individuation and a proclivity to regress in the face of stress, however, the anxiety that is en-gendered by this lack of privacy may trigger a school-phobic reaction. Clinical experience attests the frequency with which distress about gym, swimming, and locker-room situations precipitates reluctance to attend school in early adolescent youngsters.

Psychosexual aspects of adolescent development also contribute to the vulnerability of many teenage youngsters to school-phobic reactions, par-ticularly in middle and late adolescence when young people are expected to establish more definite sexual identities and roles than they have previ-ously achieved. The youngster whose poor preparation for individuation includes uncertainty about his sexual identity or fears of heterosexual relationships may experience especially acute anxiety in school when his peers begin to structure their school life in boy-girl terms. The youngster who cannot move comfortably with his classmates into the world of dating, parties, and proms may become unable to sustain his self-image as an adequately maturing person, and he may withdraw from this confrontation with failure by developing an aversion to school. Case material presented by Adams, McDonald, and Huey (1966) indicates that fears of attending school may be particularly acute in youngsters whose earlier confusion in their sexual identity makes it difficult or impossible for them to adopt the clearly defined sex roles being assumed by their peers.

To compound these problems of individuation and independence many school-phobic youngsters have responded to their parents' reluctance to discipline or frustrate them by developing an inordinate sense of mastery. Often the youngster has been able to exert extensive control over household affairs, legislating not only how his time will be spent but even such matters as when meals will be served and when and with whom his parents will socialize. Should his parents demur, he tyrannizes them with tantrums, threats, and physical complaints until they bow to his demands, as he has come to expect they will.

Despite becoming expert at exploiting his parents' guilts and uncertainties, the school-phobic youngster has usually had limited opportunity for a realistic appraisal of his environmental mastery. As noted above, his parents have typically handled difficult problems for him and shielded him from frustration as much as possible. Beyond his hollow victories over his parents, he has seldom experienced the satisfaction of turning failure into success through self-initiated determination and perseverance. He therefore approaches the school situation with an unjustified belief in his own powers and little adaptive self-assurance to fall back on should his privileged position be seriously challenged:

"We believe that, regardless of other features, what is relevant to the school refusal behavior is that these children commonly overvalue themselves and their achievements and then try to hold onto their unrealistic self-image. When this is threatened in the school situation, they suffer anxiety and retreat to another situation where they can maintain their narcissistic self-image. This retreat may very well be a running to a close contact with mother" (Leventhal and Sills, 1964, p. 686).

Additional clinical reports by Jackson (1964), Suttenfield (1954), and Levenson (1961) confirm that adolescent school-phobic youngsters tend to be excessively dependent on overprotective parents and prominently concerned about separation, individuation, and capacity to meet challenge. Levenson notes that the youngsters he studied (see p. 209), during the several-year period between their early school-phobic problems and their late adolescent decompensation, had performed industriously and with considerable attainment in their studies. The onset of their symptoms had come as a surprise to these late adolescent youngsters, who tended to view themselves as highly effective and successful persons. Levenson's further investigation revealed that their early difficulties had been denied or overlooked by these students and their families and that a family fiction, comparable to the narcissistic self-image described by Leventhal and Sills, had evolved that ignored any possibility of failure or difficulty.

These same patterns of school-phobic reaction have been observed among late adolescent college students. Hodgman and Braiman (1965) describe four college freshmen who, despite good academic performance and avowed satisfaction with the college setting, became panicky about remaining in school and patently rationalized their anxiety in unconvincing terms of problems with teachers, classmates, courses, or assignments.

Interviews with these college students and their parents disclosed the same patterns of interdependence and resistance to separation that accompany childhood school phobia. In the new college situation these young people quickly developed regressive yearnings for the protective bosom of their family, and the families promptly exploited these regressive tendencies, apparently to fill their own needs. The parents of Hodgman and Braiman's students typically responded to their youngster's distress wth an immediate decision to take him out of school and back home. Sometimes they were temporarily dissuaded from this clinically unnecessary course of action, but three of the students eventually withdrew from school with their parents' approval, and the fourth mother was prevented from precipitously withdrawing her daughter only by the active intervention of a psychiatrist with whom she was independently in treatment.

These college students further demonstrated typical school-phobic coping styles by desperately seeking out multiple dependent relationships while at the university. These youngsters were well known to the college psychiatrist, the dean, the dormitory advisor, their professors, and their classmates, to all of whom they had repetitively turned for advice, reassurance, and support almost from the day of their arrival on the campus. Hodgman and Braiman suggest that such urgent quests for succor differentiate the school-phobic college student from other drop-outs, who more commonly tend to keep their own counsel or share their concerns with only a few close friends or advisors.

In concluding this section it should be emphasized that such reconstructions of family and intrapsychic dynamics are rarely unique to any single pattern of disturbance. Not every set of parents of an apparently school-phobic youngster will display the full range of neurotic difficulties outlined in the preceding discussion, nor will every school-phobic youngster demonstrate all of the personality characteristics that have been described here. Moreover, it is possible for a family constellation of a dependent and overprotective mother, a passive or detached father, and a clinging, manipulative, and overconfident youngster to be associated with a variety of pathological states or with no psychopathology at all.

Furthermore, the onset of an overt school-phobic reaction requires the interaction of predisposing family patterns with more or less apparent external events that intensify concerns about leaving home or attending school; for example, a predisposed youngster who is moved frequently from one school to another or who experiences repetitive illnesses or accidents in himself or his family will be more likely to develop school phobia than a youngster with similar predispositions who seldom encounters such threats to his sense of security. On the other hand, an adolescent who is not disposed to retreat to his family's bosom in the face of stress may endure repetitive external threats without becoming school phobic, even though he may develop other psychological symptoms in response to the threats. These qualifications notwithstanding, the family patterns outlined in this section will be found to characterize most instances of school phobia.

CASE ILLUSTRATIONS

The following four cases are presented in some detail to illustrate the typical clinical manifestations, patterns of family interaction, and clinical course in school phobia. The case material covers a broad age range and includes instances both of acute school phobia with rapid remission and chronic disturbance in which lengthy treatment was necessary to effect return to school. These youngsters and their families exemplify many of the interpersonal orientations described in the preceding section, and these excerpts additionally depict a variety of treatment approaches that are elaborated in the final section of the chapter.

Case 1

Beverly, a 12-year-old sixth-grade student, flatly announced to her parents on a Monday morning that she would no longer attend school. When pressed for her reason, she referred only to having been humiliated in class the previous Friday when several boys had laughed at her inability to answer a question. When she persisted in her refusal, the parents consulted their pediatrician, who elicited from Beverly her promise that she would return to school the following day. The next day, however, she reaffirmed her refusal to the tune of a tantrum that again sent the parents to their pediatrician for help. After three repetitions of this sequence of events a psychological consultation was arranged for Monday of the next week.

At that time the parents reported that, although Beverly's school refusal had arisen suddenly, she had been a behavior problem for them since her menarche several months earlier. After the onset of her menses she had grown increasingly irritable, short-tempered, and insistent on having her own way. In contrast to her domestic cantankerousness, however, she had become markedly ingratiating with her peers, catering to their wishes whatever the inconvenience to herself or to her parents. Yet, although deploring Beverly's lack of consideration and respect, her parents also described her as a conscientious girl who expressed considerable guilt whenever they became noticeably upset at her misbehavior.

Beverly, a large, well-developed girl who looked older than her 12 years, exuded conciliation and remorse during her first interview. She was obsequiously pleasant and agreeable, and she apologized profusely for having troubled her parents in the week past. She denied any problems or concerns, stated she missed being with her friends, and professed a readiness to return to school. Since nothing in Beverly's history or interview behavior suggested major psychological difficulties other than the school nonattendance, it was decided initially to accept her statements at their face value. The therapist accordingly supported her expressed readiness, and her return to school was planned for the following day.

The following evening the therapist received a telephone call from Beverly's father, during which her screaming was clearly audible in the background. She had convinced her mother to allow her to remain at home that day, and, when her father had arrived home and protested her continuing refusal, she had responded with infantile rage, yelling and breaking dishes until he had backed down. Further discussions with the family a few days later clarified the extent to which Beverly kept her parents constantly on the defensive with insistent demands, rapid changes of mind, and well-timed tantrums. She was an acutely sensitive girl who had become enormously adroit at exploiting her parents' desires to placate her and their fears of doing the wrong thing, and they in turn readily rose to the bait of her manipulative provocations.

During this second interview the parents were encouraged to take a strong stand with Beverly and to insist that she follow their dictates, including an edict that she return to school. Beverly herself was again contrite, compliant, and manifestly eager to return to school, and it was agreed that she would attend school the next day. That same night her father again placed an urgent call to the therapist. Beverly had disavowed her promise to return to school, a violent argument had unsued, and she had begun to beat on her father with her fists. This situation had rendered him totally impotent; to the therapist's suggestion that he restrain Beverly from striking him, he replied, "I don't know, she's a strong girl, I don't know if I could do it"—this despite his being a large man with no physical infirmities. At this point the therapist insisted as gently and supportively as he could that the father act as a man, that he use his paternal status and his adequate physical strength to prevent Beverly from any further destructive behavior, and that he proceed with unshakeable resolve to implement fully the recommendations of the previous interview.

Beverly returned to school the next day without incident and attended without complaint throughout the week. After the second telephone conversation the parents had been able to modify their behavior. During the week they had either ignored Beverly's provocations, refusing to get involved in disagreements or verbal battles with her, or had taken issue with sufficient vigor to impose their requirements on her. They later reported having felt guilty while they were treating her so "cruelly," but they had utilized the therapist's recommendations as sanction for persevering in their "hard line." They added with obvious pride and satisfaction that, once their resoluteness had been unequivocally established, Beverly's irascibility had given way to even-tempered acquiescence.

Discussion. The sudden onset of Beverly's school aversion following an identifiable precipitating event (the humiliation in class), the absence of other diagnosable psychopathology or withdrawal from peer-group activities, and her rapid remission after conservative therapeutic intervention identify her disturbance as acute school phobia. Although the basic sources of her school-phobic anxiety were not pursued, it is possible to speculate on the unconscious concerns that made school attendance temporarily threatening to her.

Considering that she was a somewhat early maturing girl whose behavior became problematic shortly after her menarche, it may be that she was uneasy about psychosexual matters and self-conscious about her advanced physical development. Because of her minimal self-confidence, as reflected in her fawning relationships with her peers, having to stand and recite in class, with all eyes fastened on her, might have sufficed to embarrass her; to have in addition her preadolescent male classmates titter as she was thus exposed could have evoked an intense wave of psychological distress that far exceeded what might have been associated solely with her failure to answer the question. Interestingly her report of the situation referred only to boys, although it is reasonable to suppose that some girls may have laughed as well. Thus her phobic reaction might have represented displacement of her aroused psychosexual anxiety onto the school, so that she had no conscious awareness of the real origin of her concern and could offer only the weak explanation that she had been humiliated at not responding correctly in class.

As for her family patterns, the limited reference to Beverly's mother in the above case excerpt reflects her subordinate role in this family; neither Beverly nor her father had much regard for her capacities to manage the home, and she in turn meekly submitted to the dictates of her husband and daughter. Beverly's father preempted many of his wife's roles, including leaving his job to bring Beverly for her appointments when his wife could have done so, but he too was basically a passive person who could exert authority only with accompanying anxiety and guilt. Both parents therefore presented dependent models to Beverly, and by their reluctance to stand up to her they encouraged her to manipulate them.

In view of these family patterns it is significant that at the time of acute crisis, when specific suggestions were forcefully made to Beverly's parents, they were able to modify their behavior in a constructive fashion. Their modifiability was consistent with the other indices that Beverly's was an acute school-phobic disturbance and it contributed heavily to her rapid remission.

Case 2

Dick was a 13-year-old seventh-grade student who, on the day he was to return to school after an incapacitating bout of asthma, began to vomit. The vomiting persisted with such frequency that Dick's pediatrician hospitalized him for intravenous feeding and an extensive diagnostic evaluation. Diagnostic studies did not reveal any organic basis for the vomiting, which gradually diminished during the 10 days Dick remained in the hospital. On the tenth day, after two full days without vomiting, Dick was informed by his pediatrician that he was ready to return home and to school. Within minutes of receiving this announcement he began again to vomit. He was nevertheless discharged from the hospital, but a psychological consultation rather than return to school was arranged for the following day.

Dick was a small, somewhat effeminate boy who was pale, weak, and visibly undernourished at the time of this first interview. Despite his poor physical condition, he related to the therapist in a warm, lively fashion and talked freely about his reluctance to attend school. Mostly he deplored the transition from sixth grade to junior high school, and he complained particularly that the frequent changing of classes created unsupervised interludes during which other boys could bully him. Further investigation strongly suggested that this complaint was only a remote derivative of his longing to hold on to the old ways. The "bullying" he described consisted of no more than the usual shoving, name calling, and miscellaneous indignities that early adolescent boys inflict on one another. In addition, it was learned that from the first day of the school year, before he had even experienced the new school situation, he had felt nervous, "with a tightening in my stomach," as he waited for the school bus. Despite his trepidation, however, his academic performance had been consistently excellent throughout the year.

As in the preceding case, it was the father who assumed the major parental role in the treatment. In contrast to Beverly's father, however, Dick's father was in the words of the referring pediatrician a "rigid executive type." A tall, good-looking, assertive man who spoke in clipped, unemotional tones, he conveyed little sympathy either with his son's disturbance or with the necessity for psychological assistance. He had taken charge of making arrangements only because his wife was inept at handling such matters, he stated in her presence, and he had appeared for the first interview only because of the therapist's insistence, which he professed not to comprehend. He resented having to take time away from his work because of what he regarded as his son's patent stubbornness, and he declared himself unaware of anything in Dick's or the family's history that could have contributed to emotional difficulties.

Since Dick's physical debility precluded any immediate return to school, it was decided to continue the psychological evaluation while his pediatrician managed the medical aspects of his condition. Only Dick's mother appeared with him for the second appointment one week later, and a private conversation with her yielded important additional information. She had a much closer relationship with him than her husband and was able and willing to discuss many more matters than he. She reported that Dick's total life experience away from his parents consisted of two abortive visits to summer camp. On the first occasion he had developed an asthmatic attack and returned home; the second time he had come down with pneumonia and spent the entire camp session in an infirmary bed. She added that physical symptoms frequently earned him reprieves from being alone or doing things for himself; for example, she admitted that he regularly induced her to read to him by complaining of a headache.

At the first interview the therapist had pointed out that, whereas early return to school would be a major focus of Dick's treatment, his physical status contraindicated pressure for immediate return. Since he had already missed two weeks of school, home tutoring was arranged to keep him abreast of his studies. During the week between the first and second appointments he had responded eagerly to the tutoring and also had been frequently visited by friends who encouraged him to come back to school. At the second interview Dick began to talk about missing these friends and being bored at home.

By the third session he had gone two weeks without vomiting, had pretty much recovered his physical strength, and was able to talk about some mixed feelings he had toward his parents. He was seeing his friends regularly and increasingly missing their companionship at school, and it began to appear that his successful return to school was imminent. Unfortunately, however, his father could wait no longer. Early Monday morning after the third session he called the therapist to announce that Dick was obviously healthy again, the "foolishness" had gone far enough, Dick was being taken to school that morning, and no further interviews were desired. The therapist in response acknowledged Dick's progress and impending school readiness, but he cautioned that additional work might be necessary to ensure a lasting resolution of his school-attendance problem. He encouraged the father to inform him of subsequent developments.

The very next morning Dick's father, noticeably cowed, called to report that the previous day's events had proved disastrous. Dick had vomited several times at school and returned home at noon, after which his symptoms abated. In the evening, after arriving home to learn that his plans had failed, the father had become furious. He had castigated Dick for "letting me down," whereupon Dick had complained that his stomach was beginning to hurt again and that he was about to vomit. At this point the father had completely lost his temper. He had accused Dick of throwing a tantrum, forced him under a cold shower, and then ordered him to run in place to "work it out of his system." Dick had then been put to bed, where he promptly vomited on his bedclothes and explained that he had been unable to get up in time.

Part of this episode was related during the telephone conversation and the rest when Dick and his mother were seen later that same day. Dick was fairly calm by then; he had, after all, succeeded in driving both his parents to distraction and he was still out of school. His mother, however, was tearfully distraught. She had been helpless to moderate the previous evening's uproar, and she lamented her growing conviction, shared by her husband, that Dick was essentially a diabolical, unmanageable boy whose personality was deteriorating.

Given Dick's actual personality assets and the progress he had been making prior to this paternally induced crisis, the therapist felt it was now necessary to direct active attention to the parents' role. He accordingly declared to the mother that the family had become disastrously engaged in psychological warfare and that, as long as she and her husband continued to devastate Dick with their heavy parental artillery, he would retaliate with the most effective weapon available to him, namely, his vomiting. It was emphasized that Dick was moving toward school attendance, but that they could not expect peremptorily to legislate his symptoms out of existence. Whereas further treatment would emphasize return to school, she was told, immediate return was not the only satisfactory indication of progress.

Dick's mother was able to appreciate and accept this view of the situation, and his father had been sufficiently chastened by recent events to concur temporarily with a "hands off" policy and allow the therapy to proceed. As for Dick, he reported during this fourth interview that he had not been particularly apprehensive about attending school the previous day. As the morning had progressed, however, he had become uncomfortable at the curiosity of many of his classmates, who wondered about his long absence, and at being behind in his work. He had missed just enough material to interfere with his understanding of class discussions ("It was like they were speaking a foreign language") and he had become worried about his ability to catch up.

Two subsequent therapy sessions dealt with Dick's discomfort about these aspects of getting back into the swing of things, and at the same time additional home tutoring was directed toward exposing him to exactly the same subject matter his classmates were studying. Within the next two weeks, in the absence of any further pressure from his parents, he decided that he very much wanted to return to school. With the therapist's encouragement he set his return for the day after the sixth session, and at a final session one week later he indicated that he was back in school and enjoying it.

Discussion. Dick's symptom formation clearly represents an instance of acute school phobia. Like Beverly, he demonstrated a sudden onset of school refusal after a readily identifiable precipitating event (his asthmatic illness), and his school aversion was not accompanied by other diagnosable psychopathology or any diminution of his social interests. He too had a fairly rapid remission, although his actual physical debility and the unsympathetic attitude of his father contributed to a somewhat longer absence than Beverly experienced. It is nevertheless noteworthy that Dick's parents, in common with Beverly's, were able to modify their attitude at the therapist's suggestion.

In several other respects, however, Dick presented a combination of characteristic school-phobic patterns that was different from the case of Beverly. Whereas Beverly complained only of vague apprehensions about school, Dick developed pronounced and debilitating gastrointestinal distress when he was in school or threatened with school attendance. Furthermore, whereas her attendance problems appeared primarily related to anxiety-provoking aspects of being in school, his concerns about school, as crystallized by the change from elementary to junior high school, seemed mainly to reflect underlying fears of being away from home. Relevant in this regard is his history of physical decompensation each time he had been away from home (the two abortive camp sessions). It is not unlikely that he had utilized his teacher as a parental surrogate to still his separation anxiety during the elementary grades and found such reassurance no longer available to him in the multiple-teacher set of junior high school.

Dick's father, like Beverly's, was the dominant parent about whom most was learned during the brief treatment contact. Yet he presented much more the detached rather than the dependent type of school-phobic father. When critical events forced him to become more involved in family affairs than was his custom, he responded with angry bluster, resistance to any approach but hard-line common sense, and attempts to abrogate the disturbance by fiat rather than understanding.

Case 3

Mary, age 16, became nervous and upset on the first day of her junior year at the parochial school she had previously attended without difficulty. She attributed her nervousness to "just being around" her classmates and to a lack of confidence that she could perform adequately in her subjects. The latter was particularly striking in view of the 90 average she had regularly maintained. She came home at midday, and her parents did not insist that she return. After she had sat out the entire first week of school, however, they consulted their family physician. He suggested a trial return to school on a half-day basis, which Mary attempted but found too anxiety provoking to continue. At this point the physician—who had meanwhile become concerned about Mary's apparent lethargy, retarded thought processes, and lack of emotional response in his interviews with her—recommended psychological assistance.

In the initial psychological consultation Mary was so anxious about attending school that even thinking about being in a classroom caused her overt distress. Yet there was no discernible event that had precipitated her phobic aversion other than her returning to school to begin the fall term. During the two weeks she had been out of school prior to the first interview she had not ventured from her home or made any attempt to contact her friends, some of whom had called to find out where she was. When asked why she was not socializing with her girlfriends, especially those who lived right in her neighborhood, she responded, "It wouldn't be right, not when I'm not going to school with them."

In addition to her school aversion, Mary was unquestionably a depressed and withdrawn girl, and the therapist had considerable initial difficulty in establishing a relationship with her. She sat slumped in her chair, her chin planted firmly on her chest and her coat clutched tightly around her. She responded relevantly to questions, but she offered no spontaneous comments and maintained a somber affective tone throughout the sessions. Subsequent psychological examination helped to rule out the possibility that her withdrawal and limited affective response represented an incipient schizophrenic reaction, and the course of her treatment clarified that her initial difficulties represented concurrent depression and school-phobic anxiety.

A subsequent interview with Mary's mother revealed two significant aspects of her history. First, during the fourth grade her convalescence from a mild midwinter illness had extended to the end of the school year. The parents had not encouraged her to return to school ("You can't rush these things") and had arranged for a medical exemption and home tutoring. Second, during the summer that preceded the onset of school phobia she had been dating a 21-year-old fellow. Although the parents had disapproved of this young man, primarily because of his age, they had not interfered with Mary's seeing him as frequently as two or three times a week. Near the end of the summer they had overheard Mary call this boy and tell him she wanted nothing more to do with him.

This sketchy report from the parents suggested that some embarrassing or guilt-provoking sexual encounter with this young man might have contributed to the onset of Mary's depressive and phobic symptoms, and her subsequent treatment course tended to support such a hypothesis.

From the initial diagnostic evaluation it appeared that Mary had little prospect of being able to function in school in the immediate future and would require ongoing psychotherapy both for her school aversion and her depressive reaction. Weekly therapy sessions and home tutoring were therefore arranged. The first six months' treatment saw painfully slow progress that seriously taxed the therapist's perseverance. Through much of this period Mary was essentially uncommunicative in the sessions, answering questions summarily and rarely commenting spontaneously on her thoughts and feelings. The therapist carried the ball during this time by arduously inquiring about the details of her daily life, encouraging gradual increases in the level and scope of her activity, and trying to foster a genuine emotional relationship with her.

In the first 25 sessions virtually nothing was learned about the origins of Mary's depressive and school-phobic disturbances, and she remained incapable of thinking or talking about school without becoming markedly anxious. Some positive changes in her life pattern and interview behavior did occur during this phase of the treatment, however. Initially she had given only perfunctory attention to her tutoring and complained that she became too fatigued by her assignments to complete them; she had evinced no interest in having anything to do with her friends and had resisted social overtures to the point where they no longer came her way; and she had disregarded all suggestions that she leave her house for any purpose. As the first six months of treatment progressed, however, she began to pursue her studies with some vigor, to call her friends to catch up on local gossip, and to accompany her mother on shopping trips and to the movies. In her therapy sessions she began to sit more erectly in her chair, occasionally to look and even smile at the therapist, to remove her coat, and to talk about such things as girlfriends and dating.

During the 25th session Mary spontaneously reported that she had been thinking about going to summer school to ensure being adequately prepared for her senior year in the fall, and she admitted to conscious concerns about what questions her peers might ask when she rejoined them in academic and social activities. These comments stirred some optimism that the previous treatment efforts were coming to fruition and that Mary was now on her way to recovery. The very next session confirmed this impression and also provided a dramatic breakthrough of material that cast considerable light on the development of her disturbance.

Mary began this 26th session by talking freely and with obvious pleasure about some recent shopping trips with her mother and about having accepted an invitation from a girlfriend to attend a play at her school. The therapist decided to take advantage of her sense of well-being and apparent readiness to talk by probing some areas he knew to be sensitive. Specifically, he broached the fact that she remained persistently prone to anxiety attacks when she accompanied her family to church, even though her concern about leaving home for most other activities had greatly diminished. The following exchange ensued in regard to her previous Sunday's experience:

THERAPIST: What was it that you were feeling in church?
PATIENT: (Pause) I don't think you'll believe me.
THERAPIST: Try me.
PATIENT: Well, this sounds crazy, but I just felt dirty, terribly dirty, and I couldn't wait to get home and take a bath, and I scrubbed myself until I was purple.

This report suggested to the therapist that Mary was struggling with strong underlying guilt feelings, very possibly in relation to her previous summer's dating experience as was initially suspected. He accordingly next asked her to tell him more of the events of the past summer. Although she did not then relate exactly what these events had been, she was able to elaborate the nature of her relationship with the older boy she had been dating. She began by describing him as "dangerous," and her clarification of this epithet left little doubt that he was a sexually aggressive young man whom she was constantly having to fight off. As this session closed she spontaneously commented, "You know, I've really got to do something about this school problem; it's been a terrible burden on my parents."

Mary's behavior changed dramatically after this interview. She retained consistently good spirits, actively sought out her girlfriends, and passed the word that she would be receptive to dates. She became increasingly bored at home and decided that, instead of waiting for summer school, she would return to her classes and try to finish out the year with her classmates. She returned at the beginning of May and was able with minimal distress to resume her full peer-group membership and to earn adequate grades in her subjects. Regular treatment was terminated by mutual agreement at the close of the school year, and a follow-up appointment during the summer revealed that she was continuing to lead an active and enjoyable life. She had a part-time job for the summer, was dating several different boys, and was eagerly looking forward to her senior year in the fall.

Discussion. Although Mary's school-phobic reaction arose suddenly and in combination with marked personality change, her disturbance differed in several respects from that exhibited by Beverly or Dick. First, there was no identifiable precipitating event other than the beginning of the fall term, which did not present Mary with any objective changes in the school environment to which she had previously adjusted comfortably. Second, her personality change did not comprise the upsurge in manipulative or clinging behavior that often accompanies acute school-phobic reactions, but rather reflected a depressive syndrome coexisting with her phobic aversion to school. Finally contrasting with the previous two cases were the parents' lack of insistence that Mary return to school and the history of an earlier episode in which both Mary and her parents had tolerated an unnecessarily prolonged absence from school.

These features of Mary's disturbance exemplify the chronic, characterological patterns of school-phobic reaction that are frequently observed in older adolescents who become aversive to school. Her previous long absence from school that had apparently never been identified as a problem, her concurrent depressive disturbance, and her pronounced social withdrawal precluded any remission of the school phobia until ongoing treatment had proceeded to the point described above.

Although the treatment was directed almost exclusively toward Mary, with minimal engagement of her parents, the parents' role in her disturbance was clarified during the therapy. It emerged that her mother, a former nurse, had always been gratified by having Mary at home and under her care. In this vein the encouragement that Mary received during the treatment to reinvest herself in social contacts and activities outside the home came almost entirely from the therapist and seldom from her mother. Mary's father was a self-employed man who spent long hours at his business. He failed to join his wife and daughter for the initial consultation, as he had agreed to do, he was never known to express interest in the therapist's views or in the course of his daughter's treatment, and he was rarely mentioned by Mary during her sessions. This family, then, appeared to include a disinterested, uninvolved father and a nurturant mother who consistently communicated to Mary that her continued presence at home was welcome.

These family patterns had probably predisposed Mary to withdraw to her home whenever she felt threatened, and she seemingly had never had to develop any manipulative techniques in order to guarantee her mother's permission to remain there. The most likely basis for her depressive reaction was feelings of guilt and worthlessness she developed in the course of her relationship with the sexually aggressive boy she had been dating. It is therefore possible that her school aversion was precipitated by her return to school because she was then faced with day-long interactions with her peers, of whom she apparently felt unworthy ("It wouldn't be right," she had said when asked about keeping in touch with her friends). It is also possible that her sudden discomfort in the presence of her peers was intensified by feelings of being exposed, as if the others were aware of or could sense her real or imagined transgressions. This formulation is strengthened by the facts that she was from a strictly religious family, was attending a parochial school, and had been subject to particularly acute distress while attending church.

Case 4

Seventeen-year-old Nora was halfway through her senior year in high school when she received a notice from the principal that her graduation was contingent on an improved attendance record. For Nora this was only another chapter in a history of school-phobic reactions that dated back to the seventh grade. She recurrently suffered headaches, abdominal cramps, and bouts of fatigue that typically had their onset as she awoke in the morning and disappeared shortly after it was established that she would spend the day at home. During her junior and senior high school years she had averaged little better than 50% attendance. During her numerous extended absences she had made good use of tutorial opportunities, however, and had always managed to return for a superlative performance on the final exams. She had never attributed her nonattendance to problems in school but in each instance had merely insisted that her physical malaise was too great for her to leave the home.

Nora's parents, primarily at her father's insistence, had sought professional help for her at the time of her first school refusal. After several months of unsuccessful efforts to find a therapist she would consent to see they were able to arrange treatment with a psychologist whose efforts helped Nora through the eighth and ninth grades with diminishing phobic tendencies. The family then moved to a distant community, and Nora's school phobia reassumed major proportions during her tenth and eleventh grades. Some tentative efforts were made to find a therapist in the new community, but Nora's repetitive rejections of potential therapists had transcended her parents' persistence until the principal's ultimatum brought her into the present treatment.

The most striking feature of the first interview with Nora was her apparent immaturity and withdrawal. Although her physical development had proceeded normally, she was a short, very slight girl who looked 13 or 14 rather than 17. Much as a young child, she had to be prompted by her mother to answer the therapist's greeting and accompany him to his office. After glancing nervously around the room she curled up in her chair, stared fixedly at her knees, and greeted with complete silence the therapist's initial attempts to engage her in conversation. The therapist considered at this point that Nora might be a very disturbed, potentially schizophrenic youngster. However, acting on the alternative possibility that she was just a socially immature, frightened girl who had been forced into a threatening situation against her will, he managed the following exchange:

THERAPIST: It seems difficult for you to talk.
PATIENT: M-m-m-m (with head nodding agreement).
THERAPIST: How can I make it easier?
PATIENT: Ask questions.

So he asked questions, and extensive therapist activity became the hallmark of Nora's subsequent treatment. Nora in turn was eventually able to express herself with sufficient freedom to clarify that her initial appearance of possible schizophrenic withdrawal reflected tremendous shyness, abysmal lack of self-confidence, and extremely limited social experience. The course of the therapy revealed that she had never had a semblance of an adequate social life. She had very few friends and was terrified at the thought of making social overtures to her classmates. She had never been on a date or even considered that a boy might be attracted to her. Despite her exemplary grades and the fact that she was basically a very attractive girl, she thoroughly disparaged both her intellect and her looks.

Most of her time out of school she spent at home, where she would read, paint, and keep up with her studies. She would occasionally accompany her mother on a shopping trip or to a concert, but she had never so much as gone to the corner drugstore by herself. On the other hand, she had maintained active friendships with two girl cousins her age, whom she had known all her life, and it was only in sustaining these relationships that she had utilized her underlying capacity for good object relatedness.

Nora's mother deplored not only Nora's imminent expulsion from school but also her persistent clinging and her failure to develop typical teenage social patterns. The mother was also distressed that her husband, after initially being the moving force behind seeking treatment for Nora, no longer wanted even to hear about her problems. He reportedly ignored Nora's school nonattendance and social inertness as much as possible and held his wife responsible for any of her problems that were called to his attention.

The long and almost unbroken history of Nora's school phobia, the combination of her mother's tolerance and her father's disregard for her nonattendance, and her minimal peer-group engagement suggested that ongoing psychotherapy would be necessary both to resolve her school refusal and to catch up on her delayed social maturation. At the present writing Nora has been engaged for 18 months in an ongoing psychotherapy that has ranged widely in scope and content. Initially there was a heavy emphasis on reviewing her daily activities on a superficial level and encouraging independent behavior outside the home. As she became increasingly comfortable in her relationship with the therapist, the sessions dealt more extensively with her attitudes toward her parents, her perceptions of herself as a person and a girl, and the enormous gulf between her social and academic aspirations and her progress toward them.

Over time Nora displayed gradual behavior change and began increasingly to utilize resources that had apparently long been dormant. She applied herself to her studies and, without the therapist's direct urging, attended school frequently enough to satisfy the school authorities. The principal in the meantime was prevailed upon to approve home tutoring for those periods when her physical complaints recurred. She managed to earn excellent grades on her final examinations and to graduate with her class. During the summer she took an additional course to satisfy college-entrance requirements, and in this summer course she established for the first time in six years a consistent attendance record. Her steady attendance and excellent academic performance have continued throughout her freshman year in college.

Concurrently with these developments she began to reach out for social activities. By the end of her freshman year an objective observer would still have regarded her as a shy, quiet girl without too much self-confidence, but she nevertheless was going out on dates, engaging in the informal social life of the campus, and even traveling by herself to visit out-of-town relatives, all of which she enjoyed immensely.

Discussion. Nora's disturbance, like Mary's in the previous case, demonstrates the pattern of chronic school phobia that tends to replace the acute forms of this disorder as the adolescent grows older. Unlike Beverly and Dick in the first two cases, Nora did not present a recent onset of school phobia in response to a readily identifiable precipitating event, nor was she free from other adjustment difficulties. Rather, she had a long previous history of school refusal and major accompanying problems of social immaturity and withdrawal. Furthermore, the combination of her mother's overprotection and her father's detachment had created an atmosphere in which retreat to the home had been a constantly available recourse. Unlike Mary, however, Nora's major source of anxiety appeared to lie not in being in school in the company of her peers but in being away from home and separated from her mother.

TREATMENT

This final section reviews briefly some major issues in the treatment of school phobia and presents some therapeutic guidelines for the individual case. Above all, the treatment plan will depend on whether the therapist prefers to defer the youngster's return to school until he has achieved some insight into his difficulties or opts for early return to prevent crystallization of the disorder. These contrasting treatment strategies and the differential indices for each are discussed below.

Deferred Return

Traditional approaches to school phobia have emphasized insight into the problem as necessary to its amelioration. Johnson et al. (1941) in their classic paper defined the successful treatment of the school-phobic youngster as a resolution of the conflicts that contribute to his anxiety symptoms and of his basic neurotic dependency as well. As elaborated by Talbot (1957), this treatment approach views return to school as a long-range goal that can be meaningfully achieved only after insight-oriented psychotherapy has progressed sufficiently to provide the youngster with a full understanding of his difficulties.

More specifically, Talbot maintains that the essential first step in the treatment of school-phobic youngsters at any age is to relieve all pressures on them to attend: "When the 'tug of war' is over, treatment can begin" (p. 292). The therapist should intercede as necessary with the parents and the school to guarantee such relief, she continues, and the youngster's return must be delayed so as to follow, rather than precede, his full readiness. This stage of readiness is seldom reached before a good treatment relationship has been established, Talbot concludes, and in the meantime the youngster should be exempted from school, with home tutoring, for as long as necessary.

Talbot describes 24 five- to fifteen-year-old school-phobic youngsters who were treated with this approach in weekly therapy sessions, 20 of whom had resumed regular school attendance by the time of her report. In addition to stressing these positive results Talbot cautions that attempts to return a youngster to school prior to definitive psychotherapy may minimize the importance of treatment in the parents' eyes and also lead to symptom substitution: "If it is possible to maneuver the environmental situation so that a child is able to go to school without treatment, he may be making an adjustment within his neurotic involvement by projecting his anxieties onto other objects than the school" (p. 293).

Waldfogel et al. (1957) have developed a similar treatment approach in their work with school-phobic youngsters at the Judge Baker Guidance

Center. They advise against any interpretive focus on the youngster's concerns about school and separation until a therapeutic relationship has been solidified, and they encourage the therapist to resist pressures that he work toward early return of the child to school at the expense of appropriate attention to more basic problems:

"The child's return to school, although an important achievement in itself, is in reality only the relief of the symptom, and . . . the real therapeutic aim is to correct the disturbances in the family relationship . . ." (pp. 764–765).

Coolidge, Brodie, and Feeney (1964) report a 10-year follow-up of 49 school-phobic youngsters, age 4 to 11, who were treated at the Judge Baker Guidance Center within this frame of reference. Of these 49 patients, 47 had returned to school and had either graduated or were still attending high school. Hersov (1960b) also describes the successful outcome of school phobia in youngsters treated with an emphasis on intensive psychotherapy. Of 50 seven- to sixteen-year-old patients in his sample, 34 returned successfully to school within 12 months, 24 of them during the first 6 months of treatment. Hersov endorses the traditional expectation that "return to school without a concomitant improvement in social relationships, fears, and anxiety symptoms makes a relapse likely" (pp. 141–142).

Early Return

The early return approach to the treatment of school phobia was prompted by Klein's (1945) report of a 9-year-old girl who, despite working through a number of neurotic problems in intensive psychotherapy, remained so fearful of school that she could not tolerate even its mention. In Klein's view the decision to remove this youngster from the phobic object during the treatment and to arrange home tutoring actually impeded her progress, partly because she adjusted extremely well to the tutoring and partly because there was no ongoing school-related feedback with which to work in the therapy sessions:

"If the child remains out of school for a while, there is a quick development of primitive regressive fear, in young children of an oral character, in older ones of a paranoid nature simulating schizophrenia. . . . This regression can be prevented by getting the child back to school promptly. . . . The treatment is greatly speeded up if the child maintains even a fragmentary daily contact with the school from the start. . . . The school anxieties may remain quite inaccessible as long as he is not in any contact with the object of his dread" (pp. 266 and 267).

Several writers have elaborated Klein's impressions into treatment programs that stress immediate resumption of at least partial school attendance; for example, Millar (1961) argues that normal psychological maturation is impossible as long as a youngster remains out of school, and he recommends any reasonable strategy that avoids such absences. He impresses on the parents that their school-phobic child's interests will not be served by nonattendance; he informs the youngster that his problems will not be solved by remaining at home, that return to school is obligatory, and that he will meet with him to discuss any difficulties he encounters on returning; and he discourages the school authorities from any special curricular provisions other than the regular classroom requirements.

Eisenberg (1958a,b) agrees that early return to school is essential to the continuing psychological growth of the school-phobic youngster. He endorses impressing on the youngster that his attendance is mandatory, even to the extent of scheduling a hearing in juvenile court, and he encourages getting him back into the school building as soon as possible even if his mother has to sit in the classroom with him. Eisenberg cautions against any arrangements that legalize the absence from school. In his view a home teacher renders the situation too comfortable for all concerned, whereas firm emphasis on compulsory school attendance mobilizes the necessary anxiety for concurrent psychotherapeutic work. Eisenberg does add, however, that so long as a youngster is making perceptible progress it is appropriate for the therapist to intervene to lessen any penalties that might otherwise be imposed on him by his school. As for achieving a symptomatic cure without resolving the underlying disturbance, Eisenberg (1958a, p. 717) levels the following rejoinder:

"It is essential that the paralyzing force of the school phobia on the child's whole life be recognized. The symptom itself serves to isolate him from normal experience and makes further psychological growth almost impossible. If we do no more than check this central symptom, we have nonetheless done a great deal. Furthermore, we have been impressed with the liberating role of this accomplishment in opening avenues for rapid progress in both child and parents in subsequent treatment."

Leventhal et al. (1967) concur that early return to school, implemented over the school-phobic youngster's objections if necessary, considerably enhances the possibilities for effective psychotherapy. They regard the therapeutic task in school-phobic situations as one of reducing the youngster's resolve and strengthening his parents' control of him. Since school phobia usually represents the youngster's intimidation and manipulation of his school and parents, they continue, an enforced return to school usually highlights the existing power struggle and makes it available for discussion in the therapy. Leventhal et al. prefer to avoid a pitched battle of wills, however, and they encourage the youngster as much as possible to make his own decision to return to school.

Behavior therapy techniques have also been employed to achieve rapid, forced return to school. Garvey and Hegrenes (1966) describe a youngster who had realized a generally improved adjustment, increased self-confidence, and a good relationship with his therapist during six months' "conventional" psychotherapy but had made no progress in conquering his phobic anxiety about school. At this point a desensitization program of gradually increasing exposure to the school setting was instituted. The desensitization schedule included such steps as sitting in the car in front of the school, getting out of the car and approaching the curb, stepping to the sidewalk, going to the bottom of the steps to the school, and so forth. This progressive procedure was carried out in 20- to 40-minute sessions for 20 consecutive days, by which time the youngster had returned to regular class attendance and had no subsequent manifestations of phobia over a two-year follow-up.

Regarding the effectiveness of a treatment approach emphasizing early return to school, Rodriguez, Rodriguez, and Eisenberg (1959) report that 29 (71%) of 41 school-phobic youngsters seen in brief psychotherapy at the Johns Hopkins Children's Psychiatric Service resumed regular school attendance. Three-quarters of these youngsters were in treatment less than four months, and insistence on early return was an integral aspect of the therapeutic strategy. Significantly, however, return to school was achieved by 23 of their 27 children who were less than 11 years old at the onset of the school phobia (89%) but by only 5 of their 14 youngsters age 11 or older (36%). They conclude from this finding that the older youngsters in their sample were probably more disturbed than their younger patients.

The Rodriguez et al. data may additionally indicate that the prognosis is generally poorer for the older school-phobic youngsters and/or that a focus on early return is less effective in the treatment of the older child with phobic aversion to school. To the extent that older youngsters are more likely to present with chronic rather than acute forms of school phobia (see p. 209), furthermore, it may be that the data of Rodriguez et al. imply a more guarded prognosis for chronic than for acute school phobia, particularly if the treatment is restricted to a focus on school return.

Clinical experience appears to support such a hypothesis. Kennedy (1965) describes the treatment of 50 acutely school-phobic youngsters, mostly in the elementary grades, with forced school attendance and brief supportive psychotherapy aimed primarily at keeping them in school as comfortably as possible. This brief treatment approach successfully returned all 50 of these young, acutely school-phobic children to school, and follow-up contacts extending up to eight years indicated no evidence of substitute symptom formation. In contrast, of six chronic school-phobic youngsters treated at the same clinic during the study period, one was hospitalized, one was sent to a training school, and only two of the remaining four were able to return to school.

Coolidge et al. (1960), despite their emphasis on deferred return (see p. 233), nevertheless attempt to get the school-phobic youngster back in school as soon as possible to prevent his becoming chronically incapacitated. Yet in their experience at the Judge Baker Guidance Center the school-phobic adolescent, even more so than the younger child, has required extended psychotherapy to achieve even relatively modest goals. Because disturbed adolescents cannot as rapidly as younger children mobilize sufficient resources to cope with the reality tasks that confront their age group, they point out, the therapist of a school-phobic adolescent must be prepared to accept a longer absence from school than he would with a younger child. Accordingly, the older the school-phobic youngster, the less his treatment will focus directly on getting him back to school and the more it will emphasize ongoing psychotherapy and such ancillary measures as tutoring, special school placement, and vocational training.

Interestingly, other clinicians who consider return to school to be secondary to therapeutic progress in the treatment of school phobia also endorse the importance of early return. For example, Sperling (1961) argues that results achieved by manipulating, persuading, punishing, or reasoning with school-phobic youngsters are short lived and foster undesirable pathological reactions. Yet she regards school phobia as an emergency situation and recommends intensive psychotherapeutic efforts to unearth the basic conflict that underlies the youngster's phobia, in order that he might be able to return to school with minimum delay.

Chapel (1967) advocates treatment progress before return to school, but in the context of behavior therapy techniques aimed at rapid symptom removal. He relates the case of an 11-year-old acutely school-phobic boy who was initially treated with forced return to school and thrice-weekly psychotherapy. Despite some initial improvement, his psychological distress in the classroom later mounted to such disturbing proportions that the school authorities felt compelled to suspend him. At this point the boy was hospitalized and treated with daily sessions of hypnotic relaxation and reciprocal inhibition based on hierarchies involving solely his fears of separation. After six weeks of this treatment, during which his anxiety rapidly subsided, the boy pronounced himself ready to return to school and shortly thereafter resumed regular school attendance.

Greenbaum (1964) similarly urges that the school-phobic youngster judge his own readiness to return to school. He describes his treatment of eight 7- to 14-year-old school-phobic youngsters who were seen in ongoing psychotherapy with the understanding that they were not to return to school until they had made the decision, together with their therapist, that they were ready to do so. Tutoring was arranged for these patients to enable them to return to school at grade level when such a decision had been made. Greenbaum reports that seven of these youngsters returned to school, six of them shortly after they had been able to express and explore with the therapist their anger toward their mothers.

Greenbaum concludes from his experience that, whereas rapid return to school is admirable where it can be successfully accomplished, there is no inevitable pitfall in preceding return with some definitive psychotherapy where indicated. He observes that the oft-stated anticipation that a youngster's prolonged absence from school will promote regression and chronic incapacitation has not been documented in the literature since Klein's single case report (see p. 234), and he emphasizes that none of his eight patients demonstrated further regression during the treatment, nor in any did the phobia become a fixed pattern that resisted routine therapeutic progress. In his one unsuccessful case regression took place only after the youngster had returned to school.

Planning for the Individual Patient

In considering the effectiveness of various treatment approaches to school phobia it is important to examine not only return to school but also a youngster's subsequent social and academic course. The available information in this area is unfortunately sparse, and the data leave little to choose from in arguing for the greater efficacy of one or another treatment approach. In the Coolidge et al. (1964) follow-up of the school-phobic youngsters treated in the Judge Baker frame of reference half of their 47 "successful" subjects were still manifesting academic and social concerns related to the original phobia. Despite having returned to school, they had remained persistently apprehensive about matters of attendance or achievement, were frequently absent from school for minor physical ailments, and expressed more than ordinary concern about leaving home or approaching new situations. Furthermore, 43% of the group were performing below the academic level that would have been predicted from their intelligence test scores. With respect to their overall emotional health and psychological development, only 13 were maturing satisfactorily and were considered normal, whereas 20 displayed definite limitations in their psychological growth, and 14 exhibited serious failure to progress toward psychological adulthood.

Thus a treatment approach that placed primary emphasis on definitive psychotherapy rather than return to school actually achieved an extremely impressive rate of return to school (47 of 49) but only a modest assurance of satisfactory psychological adjustment and development after return (13 of the 47 "successes"). Equally perplexing are the long-term results of the Johns Hopkins sample of school-phobic youngsters who were treated with a primary emphasis on early return to school. As already noted, only 20 of the 41 school-phobic youngsters followed by Rodriguez et al. (1959) had achieved regular school attendance at follow-up three years after their initial clinic contact. Yet 23 of these 29 successful cases were also making satisfactory academic and social progress on follow-up. Hence, the approach that stressed immediate return to school appears to have done less well in actually returning youngsters to school than the approach used at the Judge Baker Guidance Center, but it seems to have achieved more meaningful and complete success with those youngsters whom it did return.

It is further of interest to note that comparable outcomes have been reported for school-phobic youngsters who received neither outpatient psychotherapy nor encouragement to immediate return but were instead hospitalized for residential treatment. A 5- to 10-year follow-up of 14 school-phobic youngsters admitted to the Hawthorn Center revealed that 11 (79%) had returned to school and 10 (71%) had subsequently maintained an "excellent" or "good" overall adaptation (Weiss and Cain, 1964; Weiss and Burke, 1967).

These data are far too sketchy to allow any definitive comparisons of alternative treatment approaches to school phobia. The published reports leave the comparability of the subject groups uncertain and the uniformity of the outcome criteria indefinite. Moreover, although the deferred return and early return treatment approaches have been contrasted here for purposes of discussion, it is not in fact known to what extent the actual treatment experience of the individual youngsters differed from one setting to the next (i.e., the Judge Baker Guidance Center, Johns Hopkins, and elsewhere). It has long been recognized that the actual behavior of competent, experienced therapists may be more similar than their expressed allegiance to polar theoretical conceptualizations would suggest (e.g., Fiedler, 1950).

On the other hand, the literature reviewed in this chapter seems to indicate clearly that the outcome of school phobia, in respect both to resumed attendance and subsequent psychological maturation, depends on the appropriateness of a particular treatment approach to the youngster with whom it is used. The emphasis, in other words, needs to be less on treating school phobia than on treating the school-phobic youngster.

Sperling (1967) is one of the few writers in this area who specifies differential treatment programs for school-phobic youngsters according to their age and the particular form of their disturbance.

With regard to age Sperling suggests that, the older the school-phobic youngster, the more his treatment should focus directly on him. Whereas in younger children primary attention to the parents with only limited contact with the youngster can yield excellent results, she continues, by later adolescence only minimal contact with the parents is preferable, and the treatment can be directed almost entirely toward the primary patient.

As for the form of a youngster's school phobia, Sperling regards the distinction between acute and chronic school phobia as vital to the appropriate timing of return to school. Although she regards psychological insight rather than purely symptomatic treatment as necessary to effective treatment of school phobia, she nevertheless views acute school-phobic reactions as emergencies and stresses early return as helpful in averting what may be an insidiously developing neurosis. She reports from her experience that one or a few interviews in which the therapist is able to recognize and interpret to the youngster the unconscious significance of the events precipitating his school-phobic reaction may suffice to return him to school (Sperling, 1967, p. 378).

Where chronic school phobia is diagnosed, however, Sperling points out that the therapist must direct his efforts less toward quick return to school and more toward ameliorating the personality and character disturbances associated with chronic school phobia:

"This differentiation is of dynamic importance because in cases of common chronic school phobia it is obviously unwise to attempt the removal of the school phobia before working on the latent personality disturbance. In these cases the removal of the presenting symptom without sufficient therapeutic work endangers the precarious balance that is maintained with the help of the school phobia" (1967, p. 393).

The case reports in this chapter reflect the present author's similar commitment to a variable treatment approach, planned according to initial diagnostic impressions. Virtually all of the apparently contradictory views of treatment reviewed in the preceding pages can be found in the treatment of the four youngsters described on pages 219–232. Beverly, a 12-year-old with a delimited, acute school-phobic reaction, was treated primarily through the counseling of her parents and insistence that she return to school immediately. Dick, a 13-year-old with an acute school phobia who was additionally physically debilitated and struggling with anger against his detached, authoritarian father, was treated through a few conversations with his parents, a brief period of home tutoring, and several treatment sessions in which he was helped to recognize and express his anger, after which he was encouraged to return to school. Mary, a 15-year-old seriously depressed girl was exempted from school for several months and seen in ongoing psychotherapy that did not include her parents. And Nora, a 17-year-old with characterological problems but no incapacitating symptoms other than her phobic-equivalent physical complaints, was seen in intensive psychotherapy over an extended period in which both home tutoring and periodic returns to school, as frequently as she felt able, were employed.

In summary, then, the younger the adolescent school-phobic youngster and the more his difficulties are limited to the school-attendance problem, the more appropriate it is to include the parents in the treatment, to emphasize early return, and to work with the youngster only as intensively as necessary to effect his comfortable return to school. The older he is and the more his psychological difficulties extend beyond phobic anxiety about attending school, the more necessary it is to focus directly on him, to engage him in ongoing psychotherapy, and to view return to school as one of the outcomes, rather than an essential prerequisite, of successful treatment.

REFERENCES

Adams, P. F., McDonald, N. F., and Huey, W. P. School phobia and bisexual conflict: A report of 21 cases. *American Journal of Psychiatry*, **12**:541–547, 1966.

Andrews, J. D. W. Psychotherapy of phobias. *Psychological Bulletin*, **66**:455–480, 1966.

Broadwin, I. T. A contribution to the study of truancy. *American Journal of Orthopsychiatry*, **2**:253–259, 1932.

Chapel, J. L. Treatment of a case of school phobia by reciprocal inhibition. *Canadian Psychiatric Association Journal*, **12**:25–28, 1967.

Clyne, M. B. *Absent: School Refusal as an Expression of Disturbed Family Relationships*. London: Tavistock, 1966.

Coolidge, J. C., Brodie, R. D., and Feeney, B. A ten-year follow-up study of sixty-six school-phobic children. *American Journal of Orthopsychiatry*, **34**:675–684, 1964.

Coolidge, J. C., Hahn, P. B., and Peck, A. L. School phobia: Neurotic crisis or way of life? *American Journal of Orthopsychiatry*, **27**:296–306, 1957.

Coolidge, J. C., Tessman, E., Waldfogel, S., and Willer, M. L. Patterns of aggression in school phobia. *Psychoanalytic Study of the Child*, **17**:319–333, 1962.

Coolidge, J. C., Willer, E. L., Tessman, E., and Waldfogel, S. School phobia in adolescence: A manifestation of severe character disturbance. *American Journal of Orthopsychiatry*, **30**:599–607, 1960.

Eisenberg, L. School phobia: A study in the communication of anxiety. *American Journal of Psychiatry,* **114**:712–718, 1958a.

Eisenberg, L. School phobia. *Pediatric Clinics of North America,* **5**:645–666, 1958b.

Estes, H. R., Haylett, C. H., and Johnson, A. M. Separation anxiety. *American Journal of Psychotherapy,* **10**:682–695, 1956.

Fiedler, F. E. A comparison of therapeutic relationships in psychoanalytic, non-directive, and Adlerian therapy. *Journal of Consulting Psychology,* **14**:436–445, 1950.

Freud, S. (1909). Analysis of a phobia in a five-year-old boy. *Standard Edition,* Vol. X. London: Hogarth, 1955, pp. 5–147.

Garvey, W. P., and Hegrenes, J. R. Desensitization techniques in the treatment of school phobia. *American Journal of Orthopsychiatry,* **36**:147–152, 1966.

Glaser, K. Problems in school attendance: School phobia and related conditions. *Pediatrics,* **23**:371–383, 1959.

Greenbaum, R. S. Treatment of school phobias—theory and practice. *American Journal of Psychotherapy,* **18**:616–634, 1964.

Hersov, L. A. Persistent non-attendance at school. *Journal of Child Psychology and Psychiatry,* **1**:130–136, 1960a.

Hersov, L. A. Refusal to go to school. *Journal of Child Psychology and Psychiatry,* **1**:137–145, 1960b.

Hodgman, C. H., and Braiman, A. "College phobia": School refusal in university students. *American Journal of Psychiatry,* **121**:801–805, 1965.

Jackson, L. Anxiety in adolescents in relation to school refusal. *Journal of Child Psychology and Psychiatry,* **5**:59–73, 1964.

Johnson, A. M., Falstein, E. I., Szurek, S. A., and Svendsen, M. School phobia. *American Journal of Orthopsychiatry,* **11**:702–711, 1941.

Kahn, J. H., and Nursten, J. P. School refusal: A comprehensive view of school phobia and other failures of school attendance. *American Journal of Orthopsychiatry,* **22**:707–718, 1962.

Kennedy, W. A. School phobia: Rapid treatment of fifty cases. *Journal of Abnormal Psychology,* **70**:285–289, 1965.

Klein, E. The reluctance to go to school. *Psychoanalytic Study of the Child,* **1**:263–279, 1945.

Levenson, E. A. The treatment of school phobia in the young adult. *American Journal of Psychotherapy,* **15**:539–552, 1961.

Leventhal, T., and Sills, M. Self-image in school phobia. *American Journal of Orthopsychiatry,* **34**:685–695, 1964.

Leventhal, T., Weinberger, G., Stander, R. J., and Stearns, R. P. Therapeutic strategies with school phobia. *American Journal of Orthopsychiatry,* **37**:64–70, 1967.

Malmquist, C. P. School phobia: A problem in family neurosis. *Journal of the American Academy of Child Psychiatry,* **4**:293–319, 1965.

Millar, T. P. The child who refuses to attend school. *American Journal of Psychiatry,* **118**:398–404, 1961.

Pittman, F. S., Langsley, D. G., and DeYoung, C. D. Work and school phobias: A family approach to treatment. *American Journal of Psychiatry,* **124**:1535–1541, 1968.

Rodriguez, A., Rodriguez, M., and Eisenberg, L. The outcome of school phobia: A follow-up study based on 41 cases. *American Journal of Psychiatry,* **116**:540–544, 1959.

Sperling, M. Analytic first aid in school phobias. *Psychoanalytic Quarterly,* **30**:504–518, 1961.

Sperling, M. School phobias: Classification, dynamics, and treatment. *Psychoanalytic Study of the Child,* **22**:375–401, 1967.

Suttenfield, V. School phobia: A study of five cases. *American Journal of Orthopsychiatry,* **24**:368–380, 1954.

Talbot, M. Panic in school phobia. *American Journal of Orthopsychiatry,* **27**:286–295, 1957.

Waldfogel, S., Coolidge, J. C., and Hahn, P. B. The development, meaning, and management of school phobia. *American Journal of Orthopsychiatry,* **27**:754–780, 1957.

Weiss, M., and Burke, A. A five- to ten-year follow-up of hospitalized school phobic children and adolescents. *American Journal of Orthopsychiatry,* **37**:294–295, 1967.

Weiss, M., and Cain, B. The residential treatment of children and adolescents with school phobia. *American Journal of Orthopsychiatry,* **34**:103–114, 1964.

CHAPTER 7

Academic Underachievement

According to Lichter et al. (1962, p. 2) 40% of all children in the United States fail to complete high school, and of these school drop-outs more than half possess at least average intellectual ability. This tragic waste of youthful potential highlights the social importance of academic under-achievement, and learning difficulties have been observed to participate prominently in the psychological disturbances of the young.

Gardner and Sperry (1964), for example, report that the parents of as many as 40% of all youngsters referred to the Judge Baker Guidance Center have as a major concern "failure to learn in school." Ross (1966) found poor school achievement to be the primary reason for referral in 39 (30%) of 129 consecutively seen youngsters at the Philadelphia Child Guidance Clinic, and academic difficulties were an important secondary reason for referral in an additional 40 (31%) of these youthful patients. As for the older adolescent, Blaine and McArthur (1961) indicate that difficulty with studying is the most frequent complaint for which college students seek psychological assistance, and they estimate that worries about studying and grades account for over 50% of student requests for counseling or psychotherapy.

Academic underachievement is traditionally defined as "a significant and sustained disparity between capacity and performance, which . . . obtains when measured intelligence contradicts class tests, achievement tests, and teachers' impressions" (Brower, 1967, p. 299). This definition appropriately distinguishes the underachiever from the youngster whose mediocre or failing academic performance reflects a limited intellectual endowment, and the clinician should routinely review available data concerning a failing youngster's intellectual capacity.[1] Nevertheless, since the aptitude-testing programs of most schools adequately identify instances

---

[1] Jordan (1966, Chapters 6, 9, and 10) and Robinson and Robinson (1965, Parts 5 and 6) review the psychodiagnostic assessment of mental retardation and its application to therapeutic and educational planning for the defective youngster.

of academic difficulty due to low intelligence, the vast majority of academically unsuccessful young people referred for clinical attention will be underachievers.

The able youngster who cannot or will not utilize his intellectual potential may irretrievably surrender educational and occupational attainments that would otherwise be within his grasp. Data from the Fels Research Institute confirm a high positive correlation between involvement in intellectual activities at age 10 to 14 and achievement behavior in the adult years 20 to 29 (Moss and Kagan, 1961). Hess (1963), who assessed boys and girls as high school seniors and again eight years later, similarly found a significant positive association between academic achievement in high school and subsequent occupational level and upward mobility.

In addition to considering such long-range implications of academic underachievement it is important to recognize that underachieving patterns may emerge early in a youngster's school career and be firmly entrenched by the time he reaches adolescence. In a study of equally bright achieving and underachieving high school students who had been classmates from the first grade on Shaw and McCuen (1960) found that the underachieving boys had tended to receive lower grades than the achieving boys beginning in the very first grade. The underachieving boys had dropped to a significantly lower performance level by grade 3 and had demonstrated increasingly poorer achievement in each consecutive year up to grade 10. A similar but later developing pattern was found for the underachieving girls, who began to receive lower grades than those of the achieving girls in grade 6 and declined to a significantly lower performance by grade 9.

The apparently progressive nature of underachievement has also been noted by Marcus (1966), who observed numerous cumulative effects of learning difficulty in bright 12- to 14-year-old youngsters he studied. The poor background of these students in subject matter they had previously failed, their depreciated image of themselves as students, and their loss of motivation and pleasure in learning had contributed to progressively larger gaps between capacity and performance as their underachievement persisted from one year to the next.

Failure to achieve commensurately with intellectual capacity derives from one or a combination of several determinants. Comprehensive categorizations of the various origins of learning difficulty outlined by Eisenberg (1966), Pearson (1952), and Rabinovitch (1959) suggest that the sources of academic underachievement can be meaningfully classified under the broad headings of organic, sociocultural, and psychological determinants. Whereas the presence and extent of academic underachievement can be readily assessed by comparing a youngster's measured intellectual capacity with his demonstrated scholastic attainment, the complex and multiple etiology of learning difficulty necessitates careful differential diagnosis and treatment planning, particularly in respect to the relative participation of organic, sociocultural, and psychological influences. This chapter first discusses these three major determinants of academic underachievement, then elaborates on the especially significant psychological pattern of passive-aggressive underachievement, and finally outlines general guidelines for the treatment of underachieving adolescents.

ORGANIC DETERMINANTS

Most overt among the organic determinants of academic underachievement are the broad range of grossly incapacitating physical limitations; for example, the student who is debilitated by disease or chronic invalidism often cannot muster the energy necessary to achieve the academic goals of which he is intellectually capable. The existence of uncorrected sensory deficits may similarly impair a youngster's performance in his studies. Eisenberg (1966) notes, for example, that low visual acuity, poor discrimination of speech sounds, and defective intersensory integration have each been found associated with aspects of underachievement. Although modern medical practice and school health programs make it unlikely that an underachieving youngster referred for psychological assistance will be suffering from an undiagnosed physical illness or a previously undetected visual defect or hearing loss, such possibilities must be kept in mind. As a general rule the therapist's diagnostic study of an underachieving adolescent should include a full report from his physician concerning his physical status.

In the absence of overt physical handicaps the organic factor that is most commonly implicated in underachievement is some pattern of minimal brain dysfunction that prevents a youngster from fully utilizing his intellectual capacity. The adverse effect of brain dysfunction on academic performance proceeds through one or more of the following three manifestations:

1. Gross behavioral disturbances (especially distractibility and hyperactivity) that interfere with effective concentration.

2. Specific cognitive deficits—particularly in capacity for memory, abstract thinking, visual organization, and perceptual-motor coordination—that selectively handicap a student in subject areas heavily dependent on these skills.

3. Specific learning disabilities, of which the most common are inability to read at grade level, special problems with language usage, and relative inability to master science and mathematics.

Before considering further the phenomenology and differential diagnosis of such organically determined underachievement it is useful to review briefly the development and clinical significance of the concept of minimal brain dysfunction, especially in relation to its appearance in adolescence.

The Concept of Minimal Brain Dysfunction

The concept of minimal brain dysfunction—as distinct from such severe brain syndromes as cerebral palsy, epilepsy, mental retardation, and gross sensory deficits—developed primarily from the work of Werner and Strauss (1941) (see also Strauss and Werner, 1942). These writers described a group of children in whom organic impairment could not be objectively demonstrated but whose history suggested a high probability of brain injury (see p. 250) and whose behavior was marked by hyperactivity, emotional lability, perceptual disorder, impulsiveness, distractibility, rigidity, and perseveration. This behavior pattern, arising in the absence of demonstrable brain pathology, came to be considered the clinical picture of the brain-damaged child.

Many clinicians who use "brain-damaged child" as a diagnostic label nevertheless have misgivings about it (see Birch, 1964; Clements, 1966). Among its other shortcomings, the "brain-damaged" designation is easily confused with gross brain damage and implies specific brain lesions even though none can be demonstrated. Yet Birch argues cogently that the children to whom this diagnosis is applied constitute such an important clinical grouping that the label's semantic unclarity should not be allowed to obfuscate the condition it denotes. Clements attempts to resolve the problem by reserving the term "brain dysfunction" for the severe and demonstrable brain syndromes and using the term "minimal brain dysfunction" to designate only the particular behavior patterns described by Strauss, Werner, and others. Actually the term "minimal brain dysfunction" was anticipated by Gesell and Amatruda (1947, pp. 240–248) and Strauss and Lehtinen (1947, p. 128), who used the terms "minor brain damage" and "minimal brain injury," respectively, to describe children in whom minimal neurological impairments appeared to be subtly affecting learning and behavior without diminishing general intellectual capacity. Clements (1966, pp. 9–10), noting that almost 40 other terms have been used to denote this condition, provides a summary definition of minimal brain dysfunction that captures the intended meaning of the term in this chapter:

"The term 'minimal brain dysfunction syndrome' refers . . . to children of near average, average, or above average intelligence with certain learning or behavior disabilities ranging from mild to severe, which are associated with deviations of function of the central nervous system. These deviations may manifest themselves by various combinations of impairment in perception, conceptualization, language, memory, and control of attention, impulse, or motor function. Similar symptoms may or may not complicate the problems of children with cerebral palsy, epilepsy, mental retardation, blindness, or deafness. These aberrations may arise from genetic variations, biochemical irregularities, perinatal brain insults, or other illnesses or injuries sustained during the years which are critical for the development and maturation of the central nervous system, or from unknown causes. During the school years, a variety of learning disabilities is the most prominent manifestation of the condition which can be designated by this term."

Available data indicate clear sex differences in the incidence of such organically determined learning difficulties. Bentzen (1963) observes that learning disorders are generally found to occur from 3 to 10 times more frequently in males than in females of the same age, and Eisenberg (1966) reports a male-to-female ratio greater than 4:1 for the incidence of specific reading disability. The studies to which these writers refer do not consistently distinguish between organically and nonorganically determined learning problems; however, it is generally well established that organic brain dysfunction is many times more frequent in boys than in girls (Gruenberg, 1964), whereas there appears to be comparatively little relation to sex in the incidence of personality patterns associated primarily with underachievement (see p. 275). It thus seems logical to infer that the higher relative frequency of learning disability in boys is due largely to the higher incidence of organically determined underachievement in boys.

Turning specifically to the adolescent youngster, it is important to stress that, whereas minimal brain dysfunction represents neurologic deficits that generally have existed since infancy or early childhood, by adolescence many of its characteristic features are no longer present or apparent. Although some minimally brain-damaged adolescents display the same impulsiveness, hyperactivity, irritability, distractibility, social incompetence, and cognitive deficits that have usually marked their childhood behavior, for most the cumulative effect of developmental processes operates to disguise or suppress clear-cut manifestations of organic impairment. The increased emotional control, enhanced social facility, and improved cognitive skills that attend development from childhood to adolescence benefit the brain-damaged as well as the normal youngster. Thus the child who is emotionally, socially, or cognitively handicapped by minimal brain dysfunction will frequently manifest fewer and less severe direct effects of his disorder in adolescence than in childhood.

In addition, the advent of adolescence in the youngster with minimal brain damage often evokes behavior problems that further cloak the essentially organic origin of his difficulties. The increasing requirements for independent judgment, abstract thinking, and interpersonal communication during adolescence sorely tax his capacities. Because adolescence also brings with it enhanced awareness of limitations relative to one's peers and heightened sensitivity to being "different," the boy or girl with minimal brain damage is highly susceptible to psychological decompensation after puberty. Most commonly decompensation takes the form of antisocial or withdrawn behavior, both of which can readily obscure a previously undetected neurologic deficit.

The frequency with which minimal brain dysfunction in the adolescent youngster masquerades as a personality disorder characterized by defiant and unmanageable behavior, immaturity, poor judgment and planning, and social unrelatedness has been noted by Anderson and Plymate (1962), Laufer (1962), and other writers. Laufer presents interesting data to confirm that, with the usual disappearance of the childhood behavior picture in the youngster with minimal brain damage during the second decade of life, problems in learning tend to be the sole manifestation of the disorder that persists consistently into the adolescent years. In 20 minimally brain-damaged adolescents he studied the only symptom that was common to all was poor school performance despite adequate intellect. Among the various other complaints that brought these organically impaired youngsters for help were "nervousness," social withdrawal, recalcitrance. stealing, assaultive behavior, and suicide attempts.

Diagnosing Minimal Brain Dysfunction

Inasmuch as academic underachievement is the most consistently persistent consequence of minimal brain damage, the possibility of organic impairment should be considered whenever an adolescent presents with learning difficulty. The identification of subtle organic bases for academic underachievement in the adolescent youngster requires detailed attention to his developmental history, current behavior patterns, and performance on psychological and neurological examination.

Developmental History. Several types of developmental events increase the likelihood that a youngster has suffered damage to his brain. These include the following:

1. Prenatal and natal complications—especially viral illnesses, bleeding, and premature contractions in the mother during her pregnancy and prematurity, anoxia, and obvious trauma at birth.

2. Failure to achieve important developmental landmarks—for example, sitting up, standing, walking, and talking—within normal age limits.

3. Childhood problems of poor motor coordination, difficulty in learning to read, and reversals in speaking and writing ("was" for "saw," "d" for "b," etc.) that persist beyond the ages at which such problems normally occur.

4. Instances of prolonged high fever, encephalitis, or major head injury.

Any of these elements in the history of an adolescent with learning problems should alert the clinician to possible minimal brain dysfunction and focus his attention on psychological and neurological test findings that might corroborate this possibility.

Current Behavior Patterns. Although adolescent development may mitigate the characteristic behavioral manifestations of minimal brain dysfunction, certain adolescent behavior patterns are nevertheless frequently associated with the persistent inroads of organic impairment on personality functioning. Significant in this regard are the following:

1. Rigid, stereotyped, habit-dominated behavior patterns.

2. Limited ambiguity tolerance, with prominent susceptibility to anxiety in unstructured situations.

3. Social behavior marked by inability to discriminate between important and trivial considerations, difficulty in grasping abstract and complex aspects of interpersonal relationships, and frank unmanageability or acting out.

Although these indices of rigidity, anxiety, poor judgment, and impulsiveness are by no means unique to organic brain syndromes, their occurrence in the underachieving youngster whose history indicates a high probability of damage to the brain strongly suggests minimal brain dysfunction as the likely source of the behavior disturbance.

The underachieving youngster's academic profile may also provide important current clues to possible organic origins of his difficulty. No single pattern of cognitive deficit or intellectual impairment uniformly accompanies organic brain dysfunction (see Yates, 1966, pp. 111–123), and virtually any pattern of specific learning difficulty can reflect psychological as well as organic influences. Yet certain types of learning disability are both frequently associated with minimal brain dysfunction and more likely to indicate organic than functional disturbance.

Three subject areas in which relatively poor performance has particular implications for possible brain dysfunction are science and mathematics, language, and reading. The brain-damaged youngster's impaired capacity for conceptual thinking frequently prevents him from earning science and mathematics grades that are equivalent to those he is able to achieve in subjects more tied to everyday interpersonal events, such as social studies. As for language, the conceptual and memory skills that are necessary to master spelling and writing and to learn a foreign language may be unavailable to the minimally brain-damaged youngster. In respect to reading, it has been widely noted that a significant discrepancy between a youngster's measured intelligence and the level of his reading achievement often reflects the subtle disturbances in neurological organization that characterize minimal brain dysfunction (Eisenberg, 1966; Rabinovitch, 1962).

It should be emphasized that the origin of reading disability in brain dysfunction is easily overlooked, partly because of the appeal of certain psychodynamic interpretations of reading difficulty (see p. 263) and partly because of the frequency with which retarded readers also display overt emotional disturbance. Yet Eisenberg (1962, p. 5) relevantly points out that "emotional disorder is almost inevitably a consequence of the repeated frustration entailed in trying, but being unable, to read," and no subsequent data challenge Gates' (1941) earlier estimate that in 75% of youngsters who manifest both reading disability and personality disturbances the emotional problems result from, rather than cause, the reading problem. Recent symposia edited by Flower, Gofman, and Lawson (1965) and by Money (1962) elaborate the significance of reading retardation for brain dysfunction, and for a full discussion of this and other specific learning disabilities the reader is also referred to Johnson and Myklebust (1967) and three volumes compiled by Hellmuth (1965, 1966, 1968).

Psychological and Neurological Examination. Neurological consultation should always be considered for the underachieving adolescent, especially when his developmental history or current behavior patterns contains any hint of possible brain dysfunction. Although electroencephalographic and gross neurological examinations often fail to detect minimal brain dysfunction, subtle neurological indices that are apparent to the specialist may combine with suggestive data from other sources to support a diagnosis of organic impairment (see Clements and Peters, 1962).

On psychological examination, test performances that reflect relative impairments of attention, concentration, memory, abstract thinking, visual organization, and perceptual-motor coordination generally suggest organic brain dysfunction. The standard psychodiagnostic test indices of these impairments, as outlined by Burgemeister (1962), Pope and Scott (1967, Chapter 7), and Ross (1959, Chapters 13 and 14), will not be elaborated here. It should be noted, however, that the already noted maturational factors (see p. 249) may complicate the psychodiagnosis of organic impairment in adolescents; that is, cognitive impairments that are due to minimal brain dysfunction may be harder to detect with such standard psychodiagnostic tests as the Wechsler and Bender-Gestalt in adolescents than they are in children. Greenberg (1967) and others have accordingly been working to develop improved methods for identifying adolescent brain dysfunction with a variety of specialized conceptual, perceptual, and motor tests.

In summary, then, the clinican must take care to avoid premature commitment to psychogenic interpretations of academic underachievement in the absence of full diagnostic attention to historical data, current behavior patterns, and neurological and psychological test findings that might reflect minimal brain dysfunction. Such caution is especially advised for those situations in which apparently obvious and compelling psychodynamic hypotheses tend to suppress adequate consideration of organic alternatives. Daryn (1961), who worked with children in an outpatient clinic, Pollack (1967), who studied adolescents at the Hillside Hospital, and Hartocollis (1968), who examined 15- to 25-year-old patients at the Menninger Foundation, have presented impressive documentation that careful assessment of psychological, neurological, and historical data frequently yields suggestive evidence of minimal brain dysfunction in patients whose difficulties had previously been considered to be entirely psychogenic.

Case Illustration

The following case illustrates the probable contribution of minimal brain dysfunction to academic underachievement in a teenage boy in whose case organic impairment had not previously been considered.

> Evan was 15 years old and nearing the end of his freshman year when his school recommended clinical assessment of his academic decline. Whereas he previously had received average or somewhat below average marks, he was failing his ninth grade English, social studies, and arithmetic courses, and his teachers were convinced that reading retardation was contributing to his difficulties in at least the first two subjects.
>
> Evan had been delivered without incident after a normal pregnancy and had achieved normal developmental landmarks during his preschool years. As a second grader, however, he had been seriously ill with scarlet fever for several weeks and, according to his pediatrician, had run a 104 to 105°F fever for at least two days. After this illness he had been noticed to have a reading problem, and a private tutor was retained to help him with his reading for the remainder of the second and the third grades. Although Evan consistently earned marks in the 75 to 85 range, he was observed again

in the fifth grade to be reading below grade level, and he had additional remedial reading in the fifth and sixth grades.

On neurological consultation Evan's EEG and performance on gross neurological examination were considered to be within normal limits. However, the neurologist stated that indices of cross-dominance, hesitant right-left discriminations, and slow eye-hand coordination, together with the history noted above, were in his opinion consistent with minimal brain dysfunction and specific reading disability. Psychological examination indicated a WISC (Wechsler Intelligence Scale for Children) full-scale IQ of 97, in the low average range, and a profile of cognitive strengths and weaknesses that was generally consistent with brain dysfunction. Relative to his overall capacity Evan demonstrated slight impairment in ability to concentrate and remember, and he performed noticeably less well in these areas than when he was asked to specify items of information or to make judgments about social situations.

In addition to his distractibility, Evan demonstrated on such tests as the Bender-Gestalt and Graham-Kendall Memory for Designs subtle difficulties in visual recall and perceptual-motor coordination. His performance on tests of reading skill yielded a reading age of 11.4 years and a reading grade of 5.5, compared to his actual age of 15 and grade of 9. His reading retardation, in combination with the psychodiagnostic evidence of mild difficulties with attention, concentration, memory, and perceptual-motor coordination, seemed sufficient to suggest minimal brain dysfunction as a major determinant of his school difficulties.

Noteworthy in Evan's history is the fact that, despite the earlier problems with reading, his apparent brain dysfunction did not noticeably impair his academic achievement until the ninth grade. Eisenberg (1959) has observed that the intelligent youngster with a reading handicap is often able to compensate adequately for his deficiencies in the early school years, only to have his grades plummet in junior and senior high school as his coursework becomes increasingly dependent on reading proficiency. The onset of Evan's underachievement seemed indeed to reflect the combined influence of his cumulative handicap and the difficulty of his coursework; it simply became impossible for him any longer to maintain adequate grades in the face of his retarded reading skills.

Evan was thus a 15-year-old boy with a recent onset of failing academic performance who had no previous record of underachievement, had not previously been considered to have any organic impairment, and also had no history of hyperactivity, unmanageability, or social incompetence.

His situation was precisely the type in which there is a high probability that some readily available psychogenic explanation for the sudden academic failure will discourage comprehensive diagnostic studies and thus prevent consideration of an underlying brain dysfunction that has only recently begun to impair academic achievement. In Evan's case a careful study of his history and the psychological and neurological examinations it prompted turned up evidence of organic deficit that might otherwise have been missed.

SOCIOCULTURAL DETERMINANTS

For many underachieving adolescents the discrepancy between their academic performance and their intellectual capacity reflects social and cultural influences that have little to do with individual organic or psychological disturbances. Following Rabinovitch (1959) the sociocultural determinants of academic underachievement can be roughly classified under the headings of *motivation* and *opportunity*.

Motivation

Sociocultural motives influence academic performance primarily through the attitudes and orientations the young person brings to his academic pursuits. The youngster whose behavior is guided primarily by nonintellectual values and nonacademic goals is minimally motivated to exercise his scholastic talents. The association of such motivational variables with underachievement has been demonstrated in a number of empirical studies; for example, Pierce and Bowman (1960), in comparing equally bright high-achieving and low-achieving 10th and 12th grade boys and girls, found that (a) on an interview measure the achievers were rated significantly higher on strength of educational motivation than the underachievers, and (b) on a semantic differential the concepts *school, work,* and *imagination* were valued significantly more highly by the achievers than by the underachievers.

Hathaway and Monachesi (1963, p. 115) similarly report that, of 824 male and 671 female high school drop-outs they studied, 33% of the boys and 21% of the girls gave "lack of interest" as their main reason for quitting school. The only reason given more frequently by either sex was marriage or illegitimate pregnancy, which was given by 53% of the girls. In contrast, failing grades were mentioned as the main reason for dropping out by only 12% of the boys and 5% of the girls.

Noneducational values and goals typically originate in certain demonstrable patterns of parental and peer-group influence. The youngster whose parents depreciate the relevance of education to occupational attainment or success in life, view the school as an essentially foreign or hostile institution, and neither praise his scholastic successes nor deplore his failures is unlikely to develop much intrinsic achievement motivation relative to school. Such parental influences have been confirmed in studies (Morrow and Wilson, 1961; Wilson and Morrow, 1962) of achieving and underachieving high school boys of equal intelligence and socioeconomic status, which demonstrated (a) that the parents of the achievers were generally more encouraging with respect to achievement, (b) that the families of the achievers more actively fostered intellectual interests in their sons and a positive attitude toward teachers and toward the school, and (c) that the achievers were less inclined than the underachievers to express negative attitudes about school or to view their teachers as unreasonable or unsupportive.

Whereas lower class and certain minority group families may explicitly depreciate education and distrust the school as a middle class institution (see Katz, 1967), it is not unusual for lower class and especially middle class parents of underachieving adolescents overtly to espouse educational values while covertly communicating to their youngster that his underachievement makes little difference. Typical in this regard is the self-made man who, having succeeded in the business world despite minimal schooling or a poor academic record, berates his son for his low grades and distaste for school but nevertheless considers him a "chip off the old block." Such tacit approval of academic underachievement by a youngster's parents seldom fails to find expression in subtle but clear messages that reinforce the adolescent's disdain for the benefits of scholastic diligence.

The experienced clinician is familiar with the frequency with which parents of teenage youngsters complain, "He just doesn't take any interest in his studies; how do we get him motivated?" In some instances of this type the youngster's failure to become invested in his school work may reflect individual psychological difficulties, as discussed in the next section. Relative to value systems, however, this particular parental complaint often reveals that the parents, despite lip service to intellectual values, nourish an underlying antipathy or even scorn that they have conveyed to their youngster. In this regard Bledsoe (1959) has demonstrated an inverse relationship between the likelihood of a youngster's dropping out of high school and the amount of schooling his parents had received, and he also found that children of unskilled, unemployed, or retired parents drop out in disproportionately high numbers in relation to children of professional, managerial, sales, and clerical workers.

Although academically unmotivated youngsters may take pains to avoid the inconvenience and embarrassment of frank failure, they see little reason to exert themselves beyond what is necessary just to get by. Their life experience has yielded no associative links between academic achievement and inner satisfaction, expectation of reward, or a feeling of progressing toward meaningful long-term goals. Indeed Hummel and Sprinthall (1965) have observed that bright underachieving high school students are relatively unlikely to perceive their school work in terms of future consequences, whereas good achievers tend to regard academic tasks as a necessary route to their life goals and to approach them purposefully. Studies with college students by Todd, Terrell, and Frank (1962) have similarly confirmed that, particularly among male students, significantly fewer underachievers than normal achievers regard doing well in coursework as important to the attainment of their long-range objectives.

Participation in a peer group that endorses nonintellectual values further reinforces the effects of family attitudes that ignore or depreciate the importance of academic achievement. In a survey of several high schools Coleman (1960) found a clear relationship between the extent to which scholastic success was valued by the student body and the number of bright students among the top achievers; for example, in schools where athletic excellence was especially valued many good students appeared to avoid high achievement for fear that it might detract from their popularity.

Negative peer-group influence associated with lower class anti-intellectual values has been graphically depicted by Evan Hunter in *The Blackboard Jungle*. The youngsters in the school he describes utterly disdain discipline and learning in the classroom both because they cannot see education as benefiting them in any way and because they take shared pleasure in frustrating the efforts of their middle-class teachers to instruct them. The teacher hero of Hunter's novel is dumbfounded when he learns that some of his most apparently dull and exasperatingly inattentive students have demonstrated superior intelligence on aptitude measures.

Such peer-group influences may induce a youngster to neglect his studies despite strong family commitment to intellectual pursuits. Such a pattern of underachievement frequently results when an able youngster's conflicts with his family or unrewarding social relationships with his intellectual equals lead him to seek out companions whose values run counter to those of his parents or who are considerably less bright than he. As suggested by Braham (1965), furthermore, negative sanctioning of intellectual achievement by a youngster's peers may even operate to retard his actual cognitive development during adolescence. The pattern of underachievement that is brought about by these influences resembles that seen in youngsters with problems of individual development and psychopathology, which is discussed in the next section.

Another important sociocultural determinant of academic motivation is the prevailing definition of sex roles in the youngster's subculture. In some groups academic effort and attainment are viewed as essentially feminine, and the high school boy who is conscientious and successful in his studies risks being labeled not only as "brain" or "grind" but also as "sissy," "fairy," "teacher's pet," or some other pejorative that implies he is less than all boy. In this vein Wilson and Morrow (1962; see p. 206) found that underachieving boys explicitly regarded academic achievement as incompatible with being a "regular guy" or a "good Joe," and Hathaway and Monachesi (1963, p. 102) have demonstrated in fact that high school boys who do well in their studies are more feminine in their interests, as measured by the MMPI (Minnesota Multiphasic Personality Inventory), than their less academically successful peers.

In other groups, particularly during the late high school and college years, scholastic excellence and career-mindedness are considered masculine characteristics, and the girl who values her studies above her social life—especially if she is preparing to enter such predominantly masculine fields as engineering, law, and medicine—may find her femininity called in question by her family and friends. Parents who doubt the compatibility of femininity and academic striving often reserve their special pride for the intellectual achievements of their sons and take little interest or pleasure in their daughters' educational plans and accomplishments. The considerable negative reinforcement that is experienced by able girls in such circumstances frequently dulls their academic enthusiasm and results in underachievement.

Modern movements away from these traditional sex-role definitions appear to be abrogating their influences, however. The premium that is placed in contemporary society on maximum educational advancement for all talented people has done much to eliminate such earlier concepts as the "gentleman's C" and the essential restriction of career-minded girls to teaching, nursing, and social work. Nevertheless in the individual instance it is clinically relevant to explore the extent to which a youngster's reluctance to employ his or her full intellectual potential derives from some feeling that by so doing he will compromise his sexual identity.

Recent events have graphically demonstrated that institutional as well as family and peer-group influences may diminish student motivation to study and thus contribute to academic underachievement. In colleges and universities particularly there has been a precipitous increase in what Harris (1966) calls negative institutational transference. Harris' thesis is that a climate of impersonality or anonymity between faculty and administration and the student body may foster the students' transferring onto the school feelings of anger and rebellion they previously had directed toward their parents.

In this era of increasingly large and impersonal educational institutions it may be that the anger and rebellion Harris labels negative institutional transference is a potent factor in college demonstrations aimed specifically at achieving greater student participation in campus affairs. Such a view is consistent with the analyses of riotous behavior and student dissent presented by Braiman (1966) and Keniston (1967). Although Flacks (1967) reports that campus activists tend to be academically superior young people and rarely low achievers, it should be recognized that any activities that channel major portions of a youngster's time and energy away from his studies—whether to demonstrations, sports, hobbies, or just "goofing off"—may contribute to his achieving significantly below his potential.

Opportunity

Able youngsters who are otherwise motivated to achieve in school may be prevented from realizing their goals by sociocultural factors that impede their learning or hinder their studying. Among the most widely publicized of these factors is the failure of elementary education to prepare youngsters adequately for high school and college work. In an underequipped, understaffed school with crowded classrooms, taught by poorly trained, disinterested, or otherwise inadequate teachers, the child may lose irretrievable ground in developing the basic academic skills and study habits he needs to realize his academic potential. The youngster who gets to high school without having learned, for example, to multiply, read fluently, or take examinations and the late adolescent who enters college without ever having had to write a composition or conduct a laboratory experiment are ill-prepared to meet the educational demands that await them.

Even the youngster who has had the benefit of attending good schools may become inadequately prepared for educational advancement if illness or changes of school disrupt the continuity of his learning; for example, changing in midyear from one school where his class is about to embark on an intensive study of fractions to another school where the class has just finished fractions and is starting on decimals can leave a youngster chronically deficient in his understanding of fractions. In the bright youngster such a deficiency might well pass unnoticed until he suddenly fails algebra some years later.

Academic underachievement can also result from extracurricular circumstances that detract from a youngster's attention to his school work. The student who must work long hours at a job or assume burdensome responsibilities in the home may simply lack the requisite time and energy to do justice to his studies, even though he has the ability and the will to do well. Even the lack of a private or reasonably quiet place to study may determine a youngster's failure to maintain the grades of which he appears capable. Mundane as such matters seem, their potentially significant contribution to underachievement obligates the clinician to consider their possible role in academic underachievement before he presumes organic or psychological determinants.

PSYCHOLOGICAL DETERMINANTS

The major psychological determinants of academic underachievement, as elaborated below, comprise two somewhat different patterns of disturbance: (a) developmental and psychopathological states that have no specific relationship to learning but handicap a youngster's educational efforts by generally restricting his personality functioning and (b) specific learning aversions and psychological syndromes defined primarily by a reluctance or refusal to achieve.

Developmental and Psychopathological States

The developmental states that impair scholastic performance include several aspects of cognitive, physical, and emotional immaturity. An adolescent youngster's level of cognitive maturity influences his academic progress primarily in relation to his capacity for abstract thinking. This educationally significant aspect of cognitive maturation in adolescence was first elucidated by Piaget (Inhelder and Piaget, 1958, Chapter 18; see also Muuss, 1967), whose work demonstrated that important developments in cognitive functioning normally occur during adolescence.

Specifically, Piaget observed that not until the early teen years do most youngsters begin to advance from the primarily concrete operations that characterize the thinking of children to the formal operational thinking that typifies mature cognition. These cognitive developments greatly expand the youngster's capacity for abstract thinking: now he becomes able to manipulate relationships between ideas verbally, in the absence of concrete props; to deal with possibilities, hypotheses, and even contrary-to-fact ideas as well as with facts; to take his own thought as an object and reason about it; and to formulate and grasp notions of how things might be as well as how they are (see Ausubel and Ausubel, 1966; Elkind, 1967, 1968).

In concert with these developmental changes the academic demands that are placed on adolescents increasingly require them to assume such abstract attitudes. High school teachers generally formulate their methods of instruction, examination, and grading with the expectation that their students will possess such cognitive capacities. Consequently an otherwise normal adolescent whose cognitive maturation is lagging behind that of his peers may be handicapped in his studies by a temporary inability to abstract at grade-level.

The classroom problems of cognitively immature youngsters can be readily illustrated. The eighth-grader whose science teacher begins by saying, "Imagine that the earth is flat," cannot appreciate what follows if he is unable to progress beyond perplexedly recalling that in the sixth grade he was taught the earth is unquestionably round. Similarly, whereas a 10-year-old may define "time" specifically in terms of the clock—that is, in hours, minutes, and seconds—for the 15-year-old "time" becomes an abstract interval defined as "a measurement of space" (Gesell, Ilg, and Ames, 1956, pp. 63 and 247). Thus the 15-year-old whose recitation responses and examination answers reflect such relatively concrete orientations as "time is what the clock tells" is almost certain to receive lower grades than his equally intelligent peers whose more normal rate of cognitive development allows them to think abstractly of time as "an interval of space."

The association of delayed physical maturation with learning difficulty has been noted among others by deHirsch (1963), who reports that a significant proportion of the underachieving adolescents seen at the Pediatric Language Disorder Clinic of Columbia-Presbyterian Medical Center are passive and infantile youngsters who are physiologically immature and often appear young and small for their age. The negative impact of physical immaturity on academic performance is typically mediated through the anxiety that attends delayed or arrested growth. Delayed development of puberty usually generates sufficient dismay to disrupt a broad range of a youngster's personality functions, including his capacity to concentrate on his school work.

Considerable empirical data have confirmed the generally adverse personality effects of delayed puberty. Studies of several hundred adolescent boys by Schonfeld (1950), Mussen and Jones (1957, 1958) and Weatherly (1964) have demonstrated that late-maturing boys are more likely than their normally developing peers to suffer serious doubts as to their adequacy, to be personally and socially maladjusted during adolescence, and to have more difficulty in achieving the transition from childhood to adulthood. Jones and Mussen (1958) report that late-maturing girls similarly have a depreciated view of themselves. For girls, however, they also found considerable evidence that early as well as late maturation may be anxiety provoking. Particularly in early adolescence the rapidly developing girl may so outstrip her peers in height and secondary sexual characteristics that for a time she experiences a distressing sense of self-consciousness and isolation.

The role of emotional immaturity in poor school performance has been demonstrated primarily in relation to vocational attitudes, which constitute a meaningful index of maturity level (Crites, 1965). Available evidence suggests that an adolescent's failure to formulate appropriate long-range occupational goals, as a reflection of emotional immaturity, depletes his intrinsic motivation to achieve at capacity; for example, in the already mentioned Todd, Terrell, and Frank (1962) study of college students significantly more normal achievers of both sexes had decided on a specific vocational goal than had students whose grades were well below their placement on aptitude-test scores.

In related work with a large random sample of high school boys Douvan and Adelson (1958) found that psychological immaturity—as defined by infantile, dependent ties to parents, vulnerability to conflict, and under-developed capacities for judgment, impulse control, and delay of gratification—was associated with a likelihood of downward mobility. Specifically, immature boys more often than their peers aspired to levels of adult work ranking lower in the hierarchy of skills and status than their fathers' vocations.

Another area of relationship between emotional development and school performance is reported by Maurer (1964), who pursued the hypothesis that a youngster's emotional maturity is reflected in the nature of his anxiety about death and his defenses against such anxiety. Exploring attitudes toward death in high school seniors, he found that the youngsters who expressed more fear of death and a greater incidence of primitive beliefs about it tended to be the relatively poor achievers within their class; high achievement, on the other hand, was associated with greater sophistication and a less fearful acknowledgment of the inevitability of death.

With regard to psychopathological states, finally, it is important to recognize that any form of anxiety state, by disorganizing, distracting, and preoccupying a youngster, may vitiate his academic efforts:

"The natural learning impetus, of which curiosity and attention are a part, is frustrated by tensions in thinking and doing. It is a herculean task to direct one's energies in two directions. When one is self-absorbed and deeply concerned with internal anxiety which calls for constant vigilance, how can the natural impetus to learn be as free and resilient as it should be, and as it is in the secure individual?" (Liss, 1949, pp. 503–504).

Specific patterns of psychological disturbance—especially schizophrenic disturbance, depressive disorder, and school phobia (see Chapters 4–6)— are similarly likely to impede the adolescent's exercise of his intellectual capacity. Commonly the disturbed youngster's inability to function effectively in school serves to increase his level of distress and to intensify his primary disturbance, which in turn leads to even poorer performance. Thus the depressed youngster becomes more depressed as he deplores his declining grades, and the school-phobic adolescent becomes increasingly apprehensive about returning to school as he falls farther and farther behind in his studies. The brighter youngster is especially susceptible to such vicious circular relationships between academic underachievement and other psychological disturbances, since his is the more frustrating experience of wasted talent and unrealized aspirations (see Liss, 1955).

Specific Aversions and Syndromes

Specific aversions to the learning process typically reflect certain negative implications that are unconsciously associated by the individual with learning. The origin of academic underachievement in unconscious implications of the learning process has been elaborated mainly by psychoanalytic writers; for example, Fenichel (1945, p. 181) suggests that there are two major reasons "why an ego may be induced to keep its intellect permanently in abeyance": (a) a repression of sexual curiosity that blocks normal interests in thinking and knowing, and (b) the equation of thinking with sexual functions so that the inhibition of thinking has the meaning of castration or its avoidance.

Lorand (1961) has more recently explicated the role of mishandled childhood curiosity and sexual preoccupation in learning problems that arise after puberty. She notes that adolescents who are struggling with repressed or unsatisfied childhood curiosity about bodily and sexual functions may have particular difficulty in concentrating on such subjects as biology, even though their learning in other courses proceeds apace. As for adolescents who tend to become preoccupied with sexual fantasies or masturbatory impulses during solitary intellectual activity, she continues, the very process of studying, whatever the subject matter, may become so anxiety laden and inefficient as to bring their academic progress to a standstill.

Aggressive fantasies can also inhibit a youngster's application to his studies; for example, Sperry, Staver, and Mann (1952) note that a student with pressing concerns about aggression may have difficulty in understanding *Treasure Island* because its violence frightens him. Similarly a youngster who is uncomfortable with his aggressive impulses may panic at the dissection of animals and thus do poorly in biology, or be so appalled by warfare that he cannot concentrate on his history assignments or on Caesar's *Gallic Wars* in Latin class.

Other dimensions of specific unconscious handicaps to learning are discussed by Blanchard (1946) and Liss (1941a). In reviewing various psychoanalytic conceptions of academic underachievement Blanchard suggests that errors in school work, especially in reading, may serve as disguised ways of gratifying repressed impulses; that is, some aspects of inaccurate school work may derive from the same kinds of unconscious influence to which Freud (1901) attributed certain types of forgetting, mistakes in speech, reading, and writing, and erroneously carried out actions. Liss stresses that the learning process may take on sexual connotations that suffuse it with taboo implications, and he also points out that learning may carry with its unconscious implications for the responsibility of utilizing it that discourage academic attainment.

Although the inhibiting effects of such specific unconscious implications of learning are generally quite plausible to the dynamically oriented clinician and personality theorist, there are unfortunately no adequate data concerning how frequently they contribute to adolescent underachievement. The author's experience would suggest that even within the group of underachieving youngsters whose difficulties are primarily psychological rather than organically or socioculturally determined the vast majority of achievement problems can be adequately understood in terms of the maladaptive patterns of family interaction discussed in the next section, without hypothesizing specific unconscious implications of the learning process itself.

Nevertheless, the more general impact of sexual fantasies and masturbatory impulses on studying should be carefully considered in the evaluation of underachieving adolescents, especially boys. Such fantasies and impulses, together with the guilt and anxiety they often engender, may in some instances be the most important single cause of a youngster's inability to study and achieve. The role of masturbatory problems in underachievement is poignantly expressed in the following words of a bright 18-year-old college freshman boy who was in danger of flunking out of school:

"Whenever I sit down to study in my room, whether day or night, I get this tremendous urge to masturbate. If I fight it, I just don't get anything done; I find myself drumming my fingers, or looking out the window, or just staring at the page without seeing it. Sometimes I get up and walk around the room or even take a cold shower, but nothing relieves the pressure. Then, when I do finally masturbate, instead of feeling relieved I feel guilty and weak for not having any self-control, and I'm so preoccupied with being disgusted with myself that I still find it hard to concentrate."

Psychological syndromes consisting primarily of a reluctance or refusal to achieve commonly reflect maladaptive patterns of family interaction involving hostility, rivalry, and passive-aggressive behavioral styles. Each of these elements has been identified in clinical work with underachieving adolescents. Dudek and Lester (1968) and Parens and Weech (1966) present evidence that the focal conflict among underachieving young people usually involves anxiety engendered by aggressive wishes; Liss (1941b) elaborates the academically inhibiting effect of concerns about competing with parents or siblings; and Kotkov (1965) and Rubinstein, Falick, Levitt, and Ekstein (1959) describe their observations of specific learning-failure syndromes characterized by a youngster's utilization of passive-aggressive maneuvers to resolve his conflicts with his parents and to maintain control of aggressive desires he fears to express.

Considerable additional clinical and research data tend to confirm the roles of hostility, rivalry, and passive-aggressive behavior in psychologically determined underachievement. Although none of these elements is specific for learning problems, their combined impact is so frequently conducive to academic underachievement, especially in families that value education, that underachievement can often be predicted for youngsters in whom such problems coexist. Learning difficulties that are determined by unresolved hostile impulses toward family members, fears of competing with parents and siblings, and passive-aggressive proclivities thus constitute a fairly specific pattern of psychological disturbance, which for purposes of discussion can be labeled *passive-aggressive underachievement.*

PASSIVE-AGGRESSIVE UNDERACHIEVEMENT

This section draws on clinical and research literature to review more fully the manner in which hostility, rivalry, and passive-aggressive behavior operate to prevent young people from realizing their academic potential.

Hostility

Kirk (1952) has inferred from her counseling experience with underachieving college students that the passive-aggressive underachiever tends to be (a) expending considerable energy to avert any awareness or explicit expression of angry feelings, (b) struggling in particular with pronounced anger at family members who are demanding or expecting his success, and (c) utilizing academic failure as a means of indirectly aggressing against his parents. This association between restrained hostility and academic underachievement has been confirmed in studies by Sutherland (1952, 1953), Shaw and Brown (1957), and Shaw and Grubb (1958). In studies of bright underachieving high school boys with a variety of projective test, interview, teacher rating, and parental report measures Sutherland found that aggressive feelings were more frequently a source of guilt and anxiety for them than for a control sample and that they were significantly less able to give direct, effective expression to their negative feelings than the control youngsters. In the Shaw studies personality measures administered to high- and low-achieving college freshmen and high school sophomores, all of whom were at the 75th percentile or above on aptitude tests, demonstrated (a) more pronounced hostility among the underachievers and (b) the underachievers' preference to express their hostility in hypercritical attitudes toward others rather than in overt behavior.

Other studies of underachieving youngsters have located the particular origin of their anger in the resentment of parental authority they perceive as restrictive and unjust. Morrow and Wilson (1961) and Davids and Hainsworth (1967) report that low-achieving high school boys, more so than their equally intelligent but academically successful peers, describe their parents as restrictive, severe, and controlling:

"From our clinical experience working with these teenagers, we know that issues concerning control and discipline are of vital importance to them. Not only in casual conversations, but also in discussions recorded in group psychotherapy sessions, we have heard many of these boys describe their unresolved conflicts over yielding to adult authority or rebelling against it" (Davids and Hainsworth, 1967, p. 36).

Interestingly, however, questionnaire data provided by the mothers of Davids and Hainsworth's subjects revealed a fuller endorsement of controlling attitudes among the achievers' mothers than among the mothers of the underachievers. Drews and Teahan (1957) similarly found that the mothers of high-achieving junior high school boys and girls were more authoritarian and restrictive toward their children than the mothers of low achievers. These findings suggest that the passive-aggressive underachiever's resentment of parental control represents not so much a high level of parental authoritarianism as a disparity between the youngster's perception of what his parents' attitudes are and what he would like them to be.

Teahan (1963) has in fact demonstrated (a) that the mothers of underachieving college freshman girls are more strongly committed to domination and the use of discipline than are their daughters, (b) that the fathers of underachieving college freshman boys have more possessive and domineering attitudes than do their sons, and (c) that neither of these disparities characterizes the attitudes of normally achieving students and their parents. Comparable data are reported by Mutimer, Loughlin, and Powell (1966), who provide evidence that achieving girls identify more closely with their mothers than underachieving girls and that achieving boys are more completely identified with their fathers than underachieving boys.

Although incomplete parental identification is by no means specific to underachievement, its frequency among underachievers is consistent with one of the common precipitants of resentment and subsequent retaliatory underachievement: the parental imposition on a youngster of academic goals that he does not share. For example, the son of a lawyer or physician may be encouraged and expected to follow in his father's footsteps, despite his being uncertain of what he would like to do or perhaps preferring to become a history teacher or an architect. Even if he has no problem in identifying with the same-sex parent, a youngster may find himself unwilling or unable to accept his family's standards of behavior and success. A girl who is the only, the oldest, or the brightest child in her family may be selected to become their standard-bearer as a successful professional person, even though she would rather pursue a nonprofessional career or perhaps not even attend college. When such youngsters are unable to challenge or contravene their parents' demands openly, they frequently utilize underachievement to frustrate the parents' aspirations.

> Karen was a 15-year-old sophomore whose grades had dropped from an 80 to 85 average in junior high school to only a few points above failing. She was an attractive, personable girl who got along well socially and had never previously demonstrated any psychological disturbance. Her clearly stated ambition was to attend a business school after graduation from high school and to be trained as a legal secretary, a career her mother had happily pursued for many years. Her father, however, had other plans for her. He was determined that she be a top student and attend a "first-rate" liberal arts college. Significantly, Karen's only sibling was an older brother, a high school senior, whose mediocre grades made it unlikely that he would get into college.

> Karen was enrolled in a college preparatory program at the insistence of her father, who had steadfastly rejected her pleas and the school's recommendations that she be transferred to a less demanding curriculum consistent with her interests. Psychological examination indicated that Karen was sufficiently intelligent to earn passing grades in the college preparatory program if she wished to. However, deep resentment of her father's imposition of his values on her was clearly implicated in her declining performance, which represented an indirect aggressive weapon against him.

The passive-aggressive underachiever's discomfort with direct expression of hostility and resentment typically originates in three kinds of developmental experience that foster strong aversion to assertive or angry behavior. First, children who have been consistently punished for angry outbursts tend to become relatively passive youngsters who refrain from overtly assertive behavior. Having learned to fear the consequences of expressing anger directly, such youngsters frequently adopt a pervasive passive-aggressive stance in which inactivity is the hallmark of underlying anger.

In some instances, however, a youngster who is regularly punished for assertive or angry behavior may identify with the aggressor, his punishing parent (see Anna Freud, 1936, Chapter IX), and in some families a child may be chastised for aggressive behavior toward his parents but explicitly or implicitly encouraged to be assertive outside the home. In either of these circumstances a child may become generally active and assertive, rather than pervasively passive-aggressive, but in the specific area of his relationship to his parents he may resort to such passive means of expressing anger as unexpected school failure.

> Paul, a bright 14-year-old boy from a successful and socially prominent family, was about to be dismissed from boarding school because of his dismal academic record. His father, who had attended this same school and had gone on to an elite preparatory school and a distinguished university, had long planned that his son would follow in his footsteps. Discussions with Paul and his father revealed that the father was an emotionally cold, authoritarian figure who demanded outstanding accomplishment and absolute obedience from his son. Paul rankled under his father's constant criticism and lack of overt affection, but—although he was active and assertive with his mother, sister, and peers—the prospect of ever raising his voice against, or disagreeing with, his father was out of the question for him ("I'd just get clobbered"). When in the course of exploring Paul's scholastic debacle with him the therapist suggested that this seemed to be one area in which he could exert some control over his father, Paul smiled broadly, fully the Cheshire cat: "You said it; there's not a darn thing he can do about it; when he got the call from the headmaster he hit the ceiling, but he can't do a thing about it!"

The second type of experience that fosters aversion to assertive or angry behavior is the unintentional infliction of serious injury on a sibling or playmate at whom the child was angry. Often the child who has experienced this comes to fear his own destructive power, and the very experience of becoming angry threatens him with loss of control and dread consequences; as a result he develops a characterological, maladaptive aversion to any direct expression of anger. As in the case of Paul cited above, a youngster with this type of aversion to anger may express resentment toward his parents through poor school performance, especially if their investment in his education makes academic failure an apt mode of retaliation.

Third, aside from specific parental punishment or frightening experiences with the expression of hostility, an aversion to anger may be inculcated by a family atmosphere in which self-sacrifice precedes competitive striving as a guiding moral principle. A youngster whose parents impress on him the values of generosity, compassion, and humility to the exclusion of balancing concerns with his own self-realization may come to view competitive striving as an aggressive act that improperly deprives others of their chance for success. Sperry et al. (1958), in their studies of learning difficulty at the Judge Baker Guidance Center, comment in particular on how often the parents of underachieving youngsters are found to encourage their children to follow their own pattern of giving up success to the other person.

Rivalry

Problems with rivalry frequently contribute to inaction in achievement settings and avoidance of the competitive pursuit of excellence. Specifically, passive-aggressive underachievers typically suffer from fears of failing or fears of succeeding that generate a number of academically inhibiting defensive maneuvers. These characteristic defensive efforts can best be elaborated in relation to the fears of failure and success that prompt them.

Fear of Failure. Many passive-aggressive underachievers so doubt their own abilities that they erect elaborate defenses to buffer any possible confrontation with the experience of having failed. Most notably the youngster with a prominent fear of failure sets unrealistically high goals for himself and then works only half-heartedly to achieve them. In this way he provides himself two sets of rationalizations by which he can deny his limitations and dismiss any suggestion that he has actually been a failure. First, although his unrealistically high goals virtually guarantee his failure to reach them, to himself and others he can assert, "Of course I didn't do as well as I had hoped, but look at what I was aiming for—I can really be proud of myself for aspiring to such high goals, and I have no reason to feel embarrassed at not achieving them." Second, his abridged effort allows him to claim, "I didn't really put much time in on my studies, you know, and if I had really cared or worked hard, I could have done a lot better." Were such a youngster to set goals realistically within his grasp and work diligently toward them, he would then risk failure without having such excuses available to cushion the anxiety that would ensue.

The student who fears failure generally takes few such risks. He seldom risks being wrong, he seldom admits having worked hard even if he has, and he utilizes his purportedly limited effort to pride himself on what he has been able to accomplish without truly extending himself. As the insightful father of one underachieving boy put it, "I think he's afraid to work hard, because if he tried hard and still wasn't doing well, he would really have to feel terrible."

Berger (1961) has documented the association of such reaction patterns with underachievement among superior high school students who began to underachieve when they reached college, apparently in response to anticipating that they might no longer be able to maintain superior grades. Berger also selected a comparison group of college freshmen with similarly good high school records who, in contrast to the underachievers, seemed relatively able to accept their limitations: they denied extremely high standards, were willing to exert and acknowledge maximum effort even in the face of possible failure, and took pleasure in hard work. These latter students were found to earn significantly higher college grades than the comparably bright youngsters whose inability to accept their limitations indicated fear of failure.

Academically crippling concerns about competition frequently arise at transition points that confront a student with more difficult subject matter or more demanding academic standards than he has previously experienced. Thus for the able youngster who doubts his scholastic talents the transitions from grammar school to junior high school to senior high school to college may so enhance his fear of failure as to precipitate retreat from competitive effort and consequent underachievement. Similarly the youngster who transfers from one school to another and perceives his new classmates as brighter, more industrious, or better prepared than his former peers may be precipitated into underachievement at this point in his schooling.

The discouraging impact of the transition from high school to college has been elaborated by McArthur (1961), who describes the dilemma of the college student whose family and friends expect him to maintain the same relative excellence he displayed in high school, despite the fact that he is now competing only with students who had equally good high school records. Such youngsters often suffer what McArthur calls "big league shock" when they realize the nature of their competition, and their despair of ever being able to compete successfully in the college environment leads many of them to retreat from the competitive effort. In contrast the group of "competent" adolescents studied by Silber et al. (1961; see p. 53) generally acknowledged and were prepared for the fact that they probably could not expect to maintain the same grade-point average in college that they had earned in high school.

Intrafamilial concerns about competition are also characteristic in underachieving youngsters whose self-defeating approach to their studies reflects fear of failure. Whatever his potential, the youngster who fears failure has usually suffered from unfavorable comparisons with a successful parent or sibling whose abilities he cannot match. Directly stated or implied disappointment that a youngster does not live up to family standards often is involved in his eschewing the endeavor that would earn him grades commensurate with his ability ("What's the use of trying? I could never do as well as my brother did anyway"). In this context Coleman and Hewett (1962) found eight of their underachieving adolescent patients to have strong feelings of failure and inadequacy, and to have a problematic relationship with their father, who in each case was a highly successful man disappointed by his son's lackluster performance in school.

Case Illustration. The following case illustrates the manner in which resentment against parents, strong aversion to direct expressions of anger, fears of failure, and discouragement in the face of competition combine to produce academic underachievement.

> After two years in the sixth grade 13-year-old John was about to fail the seventh grade when his parents first sought psychological help for him. His low achievement had begun in the third grade and had been attributed by his teachers primarily to his being inattentive in class and neglecting his daily assignments. He had never presented any behavior problems in school, and current psychological testing indicated high average intelligence, with an approximate IQ of 110 and no suggestion of cognitive deficits associated with brain dysfunction.
>
> John's father, a teacher in the same school system where John was a pupil, displayed a constructive readiness to explore his own role in his son's difficulties. He spontaneously volunteered that he was known as an authoritarian, bossy person who "had a short fuse," yelled a lot, and was unpleasant to work with, and he added that perhaps he was too intolerant and punitive when his son did not behave exactly as he wanted him to. Although John did not overtly protest his father's treatment of him, he did appear to resent many of his parents' actions; for example, he reported with visible dismay that the previous Christmas his parents had received more presents than he had, and he quickly agreed with the interviewer's observation that it had probably seemed wrong to him for parents to receive more gifts than their children did.
>
> Yet it became clear in discussions with John and his parents that John was totally averse to any direct expression of anger or resentment. He consistently retreated from situations that involved verbal or physical aggression; for example, he had dropped out of the Boy

Scouts because they engaged in too much "roughhousing," and he reported that the boys in his class occasionally picked on him and tried to provoke him into fighting because, despite his good size and adequate strength, he had a reputation for being unwilling to defend himself. His teachers' reports and his interview behavior rounded out the picture of a shy, quiet, unassertive boy with little confidence in himself.

John's parents reported that he characteristically set perfectionistic standards for himself, became extremely upset over minor reverses, and avoided any situation in which he had once been a loser. Recently during a game of catch with his father and some other boys and their fathers he had become so humiliated at dropping the ball, even though it had been badly thrown to him, that he left the game and would not return. John himself could describe the inhibiting impact of his limited self-confidence and fear of failure on his academic efforts: his teachers incorrectly considered him inattentive in class, he said, when in truth he was just reluctant to volunteer or answer questions for fear he would say something wrong and give his classmates an excuse for laughing at him.

John also faced major problems in competing with his one-year-younger brother who, because of John's previous failure, was in the same grade. The brother was an outgoing, academically successful boy who at times participated in the teasing John received at school. John would say about his brother only that he was a "hood" with whom he had nothing in common. The scholastic attainments of his brother and teacher-father had intensified John's fears that he could never meet his family's standards and had discouraged him from fully utilizing what academic ability he possessed.

Fear of Success. Fear of success consists of the expectation that achievement will bring with it negative consequences far more distressing than the failure to achieve. Such paradoxical effects of success were first elaborated clinically by Freud (1916, pp. 311–331), who described patients apparently "wrecked by success." These people had become psychologically disturbed precisely upon the attainment of successes for which they had long and arduously labored. As more recently elaborated by Schuster (1955), the mental association of success with punishment and retaliation may not only prevent a person from enjoying what he has achieved but also induce him to abandon his aspirations or undo his successes.

It is through the abandonment of otherwise appropriate aspirations and the recourse to self-defeating maneuvers that the individual who fears success is likely to become an underachiever and never realize his innate potential. Although such aversion to success may develop in the setting of a family atmosphere that discourages aggressive striving (see page 269), fears of success that are powerful enough to result in academic under-achievement derive primarily from problems of intrafamilial rivalry. Specifically, a youngster who perceives his parents as dreading his competition and envying his attainments tends to expect disapproval, rejection, and retaliation in the wake of success. The degree of his distress and aversion to achievement depends on the degree to which he regards his parents as relatively unsuccessful or less able than himself. In this respect the underachiever who fears success differs markedly from the fear-of-failure youngster, whose difficulties have usually been intensified by unfavorable comparisons between himself and more successful members of his family.

Such fear-of-success patterns of family interaction have been frequently noted in clinical studies of academic underachievers. Sperry et al. (1958; see also p. 269) observed both prominent guilt and anxiety about competi-tive and acquisitive impulses in the boys they studied and a general family feeling that the father was something less than an unqualified success. Many of these fathers presented a superficial picture of having been suc-cessful in life but nevertheless considered themselves failures, primarily in relation to goals they had not realized, to the more significant accom-plishments of their friends, and to circumstances that threatened their self-image as breadwinners, such as their wives' working. Grunebaum et al. (1962) further note that the fathers of underachieving boys, in addition to depreciating themselves despite objective indications of their having been successful, tend (a) to view their sons as competitors, partic-ularly for their wives' support and admiration and (b) unconsciously and covertly to subvert their son's achievement strivings in an apparent effort to protect themselves from even greater feelings of having failed.

The characteristic approaches to achievement-related situations of youngsters who fear success contrast interestingly with the coping ma-neuvers employed by the student who is more prominently concerned with failure. The youngster who fears failure is likely to set very high goals and then, by exerting little effort to reach them, escape the anxiety of a near-miss, and he takes pains to impress on others that his ability is in reality much greater than his attainments would suggest. The under-achiever who fears success, on the other hand, publicly disparages his own abilities, even when they are considerable ("There's no sense in my trying to get into the advanced science section, I could never make it"); he sets very limited, unrealistically low goals for himself ("I'll be very happy to get a C average, and that's all I'm working for"); and he curtails his efforts as soon as he has reached his minimal goals ("I was lucky to get through high school; why should I try college and just flunk out?"). By such attitudes toward his work the youngster who fears success avoids the accomplishments that he feels might threaten his parents or endanger his own security and sources of affection.

The onset of fear-of-success underachievement in the late high school or early college years very commonly relates to mixed feelings about going to college and thereby surpassing high-school-educated parents. A boy whose father was prevented from reaching college by intellectual, financial, or other limitations, for example, may regard attending college as an aggressive triumph over his father that could undermine the father-son relationship. Familial preoccupation with what the father might have attained if he had had the chance for college exacerbates such anxieties, and a youngster may become particularly prone to disruptive fears of academic success if he regularly receives the paternal message, "Now you'll be able to do all the things I never could." Although such messages manifestly imply pride and encouragement, they can latently convey feelings of disappointment, envy, rejection, and even anger: "My way of life isn't good enough for you, so now you'll become a high-brow intellectual, and it will never be the same between us again."

Commonly in such situations a capable youngster, by sudden neglect of his studies, will either do poorly in college after a strong high school performance or tail off in his high school work sufficiently to compromise his chances of getting into college. On occasion the fear-of-success aversion to attending college involves nonacademic as well as academic areas in which a youngster is reluctant to surpass his parents. Thus for an athletic boy, college may mean opportunities for achievement in sports that his father never had, and for an attractive girl the campus life may represent social outlets never available to her mother. Youngsters with concerns in these areas may simply sabotage their chances for athletic or social success when they reach college, thus becoming athletic or social underachievers; or they may unconsciously utilize academic underachievement to keep themselves out of college, thereby resolving the conflict by leaving the field.

Passive-Aggressive Behavior

Passive-aggressive behavior consists of purposeful inactivity intended to vent underlying feelings of anger and resentment that cannot be expressed directly, save at the price of considerable anxiety. Most underachieving youngsters whose school problems are primarily psychological in origin demonstrate such behavior patterns, and, perhaps consistently with the notable incidence of academic underachievement (see p. 245) passive-aggressive personality is by far the most commonly diagnosed personality disorder among adolescents seen in outpatient clinics. Table 1 (see p. 82) indicates that 38% of the adolescent boys and 31% of the adolescent girls with personality disorders terminated from outpatient settings are diagnosed passive-aggressive.

As anticipated on p. 249, these data suggest that as a potential psychological source of academic underachievement the passive-aggressive personality is much less predominantly a male phenomenon than minimal brain dysfunction. Nevertheless, sociocultural factors probably influence more passive-aggressive boys than passive-aggressive girls to resolve their conflicts through academic underachievement rather than other means. Cashdan and Welsh (1966) have pointed out that societal and parental expectations concerning the roles of males in our culture may exert particular pressure on the talented boy to strive toward lofty career goals. Inasmuch as such pressure intensifies any preexisting fears of failure and also enhances the effectiveness of underachievement as a retaliatory weapon against the parents, these sociocultural factors are more likely to induce underachievement in boys than in the less pressured girls.

Furthermore, the literature on sex differences indicates that the achievement needs of boys tend to center around academic and vocational success, whereas girls are more oriented toward the attainment of social approval and personal recognition in their relationships with others (Garai and Scheinfeld 1968, p. 259). Hence underachievement among girls may frequently involve aspects of social and interpersonal success, whereas for boys underachieving tendencies are more likely to have implications specifically for academic decline. Yet it needs to be kept in mind that, as our societal values shift increasingly toward emphasizing maximum utilization of ability for girls as well as for boys, such attitudinal bases for differential rates of academic underachievement are likely to wane (see p. 258).

The passive-aggressive youngster, then, is one who is angry but fights back by inaction, rather than outwardly. He exerts control not by commission of disobedient acts, but by failure to do what is expected of him or what might please others. He frustrates and provokes the important people in his world by just sitting there. To his teachers and parents he seems lazy, distinterested, and unmotivated—a stubborn lump they would like to build a fire under.

This behavioral style determines the typical academic pattern of the passive-aggressive underachiever. Studies by Frankel (1960) and Wilson and Morrow (1962) substantiate that underachievers study less than their equally intelligent peers, delay completing their assignments, and reserve their enthusiasm for hobbies and activities that are unrelated to school. Underachievers "forget" to write down assignments, study the wrong material in preparation for examinations, turn in test papers in which they have "overlooked" a section or an entire page, sit silently through class discussions, and in dozens of similar ways compromise their chances of achieving commensurately with their abilities.

Such academic attitudes are typically reflected in the passive-aggressive underachiever's profile of intellectual functioning as measured by psychological tests. Specifically, the passive-aggressive underachiever characteristically performs less well on intellectual tasks that require previous school learning and concentrated effort than on tasks that can be handled with a relatively effortless application of general social knowledge or specific abilities unrelated to school learning.

Empirical findings that demonstrate this pattern of intellectual functioning are reviewed by Coleman and Rasof (1963), who also report supporting data from the WISC profiles of 126 underachieving youngsters they studied. Their learning-disorder population displayed a distinctive WISC pattern that did not appear in a group of overachievers they examined: the underachievers tended to score significantly below their overall intellectual level on subtests related to school-type learning, sustained concentration, and memory (Information, Arithmetic, Digit Span, and Coding) and to earn relatively high scores on subtests depending primarily on incidental learning and perceptual organization (Comprehension, Picture Completion, and Block Design).

Whereas such a profile of intellectual strengths and weaknesses may also be found among youngsters who are unmotivated or have had inadequate opportunities to learn in school, it distinguishes both the passive-aggressive and the sociocultural underachiever from the youngster with minimal brain dysfunction. The brain-damaged underachiever tends to do relatively well on measures of specific learned information and to fall down on such perceptual and abstract tasks as Picture Completion and Block Design (see p. 252). Accordingly in the absence of apparent sociocultural determinants an underachieving youngster's WISC profile may help to distinguish underachievement related to a passive-aggressive personality from that caused by organic impairment.

Case Illustration. The following case illustrates typical study patterns and intellectual functioning in an underachieving boy with passive-aggressive personality features who also demonstrated prominent concerns about hostility and competition.

Bob, an 18-year-old high school junior, had managed to get by in school with C grades through the ninth grade, at which point his parents, concerned that continuing mediocre performance would prevent him from getting into a prestigious college, had sent him against his wishes to a private boarding school in the hopes that he would improve his academic credentials. To the contrary, Bob had managed to fail every one of his courses. He had returned home, in disgrace, to repeat his sophomore year. After barely squeaking through this repeat of the 10th grade he was now on the threshold of failing in grade 11.

Bob stated flatly that he received low grades because he disliked studying and consistently avoided doing his school work. In contrast to his parents' educational aspirations for him, he was undecided about attending college, especially a demanding college that would require sustained diligence. Yet he was convinced that he could be an excellent student if he wanted to apply himself. As for his study habits, he reported that during the evening periods established by his parents as inviolable study hours he typically read widely—books, newspapers, magazines—but seldom studied his school assignments or absorbed course-related information that might help him elevate his grades.

Despite his lackadaisical neglect of his course work, Bob pursued numerous nonintellectual activities with industry and enthusiasm. He liked to hunt, fish, and camp and was an accomplished outdoorsman; he was a proficient carpenter and had completed a number of ambitious woodworking undertakings around his home; he enjoyed painting drawing, and ceramics, and during the previous summer had done very well in a special art course; and he had a reasonably active social life.

Bob's Wechsler data revealed superior intellectual abilities, with a functioning IQ in excess of 125. Yet, consistently with the already stated comments on cognitive functioning in the passive-aggressive underachiever, he fell down markedly on tasks related to specific school learning and persistent intellectual effort. His two lowest subtest scores occurred on Information and Digit Symbol, whereas he did best on Comprehension and Block Design, where his general social intelligence and capacity for perceptual organization (which probably also contributed to his artistic talent) facilitated very superior attainment.

TREATMENT

Treatment of the underachieving adolescent varies with the extent to which his academic efforts are handicapped by brain dysfunction, by commitment to sociocultural values that negate scholastic attainment, or by psychological disturbance. The following discussion outlines the major treatment emphases in clinical work with underachieving youngsters whose school difficulties derive from each of these sources.

Organically Determined Underachievement

Treatment of the underachieving adolescent with brain dysfunction typically must combine remedial education, family counseling, psychotherapy, and in some instances the use of drugs. Concerning remedial education, the brain-damaged youngster frequently needs special curricular attention to specific areas of deficiency that are hindering his academic progress. For younger children special class training in basic conceptual and perceptual-motor skills can often minimize the adverse effects of brain dysfunction on subsequent school learning. In most school settings, however, such special classes are not provided for the older youngster, partly because of limited facilities and partly because, to be maximally effective, such special training usually must begin in the early grades. The minimally brain-damaged adolescent whose difficulties have not been identified and treated early may therefore no longer be a candidate for special class placement.

However, most minimally brain-damaged adolescents can benefit from remedial classes or individual tutoring in reading, mathematics, or other subject areas in which they have become deficient as a consequence of their cognitive disabilities. Additionally, other aspects of a youngster's curriculum may be tailored to take maximum advantage of his strengths and to minimize the impact of his deficiencies; for example, in the case of a youngster with good verbal skills but limited ability to grasp abstract concepts the therapist may recommend that the school assign him to advanced English and social studies classes but encourage him to take a relatively undemanding general science course rather than attempt chemistry and physics. Such planning may significantly curtail the kinds of failure experience that would otherwise undermine the youngster's confidence and discourage him from studying.

Family counseling for the parents of the brain-damaged underachiever should be addressed to helping them recognize and accept their child's limitations. As documented by Marcus (1966), the families of underachievers generally hold unrealistic expectations of their youngster's potential, and, especially when a youngster is disabled in areas that have special significance in his family, parental disappointment may be compounding and entrenching his learning problem. Thus it may be difficult for an accountant or an engineer to face squarely the fact that his son cannot add and to feel for him the same fatherly warmth that he might feel for a son endowed more in his image. In a counseling relationship the parents can be assisted to understand and deal realistically with such reactions, and they can also be encouraged to endorse whatever curricular arrangements seem most appropriate to their youngster's abilities.

Individual psychotherapy is frequently indicated to help the brain-damaged underachiever deal with his inevitable emotional reactions to cognitive disability and academic reversals. A relationship with an adult who fully appreciates his limitations and can counsel him effectively concerning the social and academic impasses they engender can immeasurably bolster such a youngster's self-image and confidence and thereby spur him to fuller utilization of his abilities. The availability to the brain-damaged underachiever of other adults—parents, relatives, teachers—who can provide him this type of helping relationship determines the extent to which individual psychotherapy is necessary in his treatment.

The use of drugs in the treatment of the minimally brain-damaged adolescent becomes relevant primarily when childhood behavioral manifestations of organic impairment have persisted into the teen years. The adolescent who remains markedly hyperactive and distractible usually suffers in school not only from specific learning difficulties but also from his inability to pay attention in class and concentrate on his studies. Such drugs as the amphetamines, some phenothiazine derivatives, and some anticonvulsants have been reported to alleviate these behavioral consequences of brain dysfunction, and the medical reader is referred to Clements and Peters (1962), Fish (1968), and Levy (1959) for a specific description of drug treatment in such cases.

Socioculturally Determined Underachievement

Treatment of the underachieving adolescent whose minimal investment in school derives primarily from sociocultural factors that attenuate his motivation or limit his opportunities typically proves difficult. The underachieving youngster whose parents or peer group devalue academic achievement does not identify himself as having a problem. Unlike the brain-damaged or passive-aggressive underachiever, who usually endorses the value of good grades whatever his defensive protestations to the contrary, the sociocultural underachiever perceives little value in improving his scholarship. If he is seen at all in a professional setting he comes under duress, and, though he may be pleasant and superficially cooperative during an interview, he is patently disinterested in considering new ways of looking at things or of conducting his life.

Often the therapist can achieve psychological leverage with the socioculturally unmotivated underachiever only by convincing him of the potential advantages of scholastic attainment. The therapist who is adept at fostering mutual confidence, trust, and respect in his relationships with adolescents, even when they come to him unwillingly, may be able to help the unmotivated underachiever identify and aspire toward goals that are not shared by his parents or peers.

At first glance such a treatment prescription may appear to contravene the usual admonitions against a therapist's imposing his values on his patients. Yet helping a youngster to realize his potential through recognizing and adopting value systems that are more constructive than those to which he has previously adhered seems entirely consistent with good psychotherapeutic practice. Although the clinical literature in this regard is sparse, contemporary biography records numerous instances of bright young people who were influenced by certain experiences or a special relationship with some adult to discard the anti-intellectual value of their immediate sociocultural group and to achieve significant educational goals. In *Manchild in the Promised Land,* for example, Claude Brown vividly portrays the impact of his reform-school relationship with Ernst Papanek (see p. 327) in directing him away from his lower-class, delinquent, dropout subculture and toward college and law school.

When limited opportunity prevents an otherwise able and motivated youngster from utilizing his full academic potential, there may be little the individual psychological practitioner can do, except in his role as a public citizen. Problems of crowded schools, inferior instruction, and the necessity of long hours of afterschool work are essentially social problems that extend beyond the capacities of the psychotherapist to resolve.

Psychologically Determined Underachievement

In the youngster who is underachieving as a secondary consequence of schizophrenic disturbance, depressive disorder, school-phobic tendencies, or other psychopathology not directly related to learning, improved school work should accompany amelioration of the primary disturbance that impairs his functioning capacity. This discussion focuses on the passive-aggressive underachiever, in whom school difficulties constitute the primary manifestations of psychological disturbance. Although treatment of the passive-aggressive underachiever may take various forms, the therapy with few exceptions must be oriented toward the fact that his problem lies essentially in unexpressed anger and resentment toward his parents, against whom his inactive, self-defeating scholastic style is serving as an aggressive weapon.

When passive-aggressive underachievement is of recent onset and appears to be related primarily to a youngster's feelings that others' goals and values are being imposed on him, a relatively superficial, short-term counseling approach may prove sufficient to resolve it. If there is no other nascent psychopathology, the younger adolescent who begins to underachieve in such circumstances may be best helped by a brief evaluative contact with him and counseling for his parents. The parents should be apprised of their youngster's intellectual potential, which they may or may not have perceived correctly, they should be reassured that his declining grades do not presage inevitable failure, and they should be encouraged to relax whatever pressures they are placing on him for academic excellence. Relaxation of parental pressure frequently undercuts a youngster's motivations to passive-aggressive school failure; when they cease to decry his performance, he ceases to perceive poor grades as an effective retaliatory weapon against them.

Moreover in such instances it may be relevant to help the parents perceive their youngster's lack of intrinsic motivation to perform well in school as a developmental phenomenon that will give way to normal maturation; that is, they should appreciate the possibility that he may with age become increasingly able to plan constructively for his future and increasingly interested in working toward long-range goals. This entire approach of course presumes a careful diagnostic evaluation in which organic or sociocultural determinants of the youngster's underachievement have been ruled out along with any likelihood of serious psychological disturbance or a chronically entrenched pattern of school failure. Such a clinical contact may conclude with a recommendation that the family return for further discussion if the youngster's ensuing maturation does not bring with it increased academic motivation on his part and a return to his previous level of attainment.

In the older adolescent whose uncertainty about goals or about fulfilling the expectations of others contributes to sudden onset of underachievement, brief counseling can be effectively directed toward him rather than his parents. Such counseling should help the youngster recognize his abilities and interests, clarify his own value systems and preferred goals, and pursue his studies for his own sake rather than to meet the needs of others. This approach aims at speedy rehabilitation by focusing specifically on the youngster's conscious attitudes toward his academic goals and efforts and avoiding any penetrating or protracted exploration of his underlying feelings and personality style (see Goldburgh and Penney, 1962).

The therapist should in fact recognize that efforts to elicit unconscious material and implement personality reorganization may be contraindicated for the relatively well-integrated student who begins to underachieve primarily in reaction to being pushed toward goals that are not his own. The essentially stable young person who is struggling to establish his autonomy and affirm his own standards is very likely to view intensive psychotherapy as unnecessarily intrusive, particularly to the extent that it appears to challenge the rationality of his judgments. An attempt at uncovering therapy with such a youngster may accordingly lead him prematurely to withdraw from discussing his problems. On the other hand, without challenging such a youngster's current personality organization, the therapist can usefully clarify with him the nature of his values and the goals to which he would like to address his efforts. Group as well as individual counseling along such lines has proved successful with underachieving students at both ninth-grade (Broedel et al., 1960) and college levels (Gilbreath, 1968; Sheldon and Landsman, 1950).

For the youngster whose academic underachievement has persisted for some time and is related to significant problems with hostility and rivalry definitive psychotherapy rather than superficial counseling is frequently necessary to reverse his academic decline. Definitive psychotherapy in such instances is not inevitably long term, however. For many underachieving youngsters therapeutic help merely to recognize and express underlying resentments toward their parents proves sufficient to break up the underachievement pattern. Reversal of academic decline following the expression of resentment against parents has been noted among college students by Blaine and McArthur (1961), and Parens and Weech (1966) found in each of five underachieving youngsters they treated that an accelerated learning response followed directly upon some resolution or attenuation of the youngster's aggressive wishes toward his parents.

When the passive-aggressive youngster's parental resentments can be readily elicited and related to his academic efforts, he may within a few months' psychotherapy achieve a markedly improved school performance. Treatment beyond this point is then determined by the necessity for consolidating the scholastic improvement and the therapist's impressions regarding what other aspects of the youngster's personality functioning might benefit from psychotherapeutic exploration.

However, the more inaccessible an underachieving youngster's underlying feelings toward his parents and the more complicated his learning difficulties by major concerns about competition and success, the more likely it is that only extended psychotherapy will produce significant improvement. Such extended treatment usually involves detailed exploration of aspects of the youngster's personality dynamics that are only indirectly related to his scholastic difficulties and requires an explicit contract with the youngster to discuss broadly his underlying thoughts and feelings rather than to focus only on his grades and study habits (see McIntyre, 1964).

The therapist should be prepared for the fact that the passive-aggressive underachiever who requires such intensive treatment is seldom motivated to undertake it. He is rather likely to denote that he has any difficulties that call for professional attention and to doubt that talking about himself will serve any meaningful purpose. However, by repeated reference to imminent school failure and marked family discord, both of which can usually be demonstrated in the diagnostic evaluation of the passive-aggressive underachiever, the therapist can readily establish that things are not going as well as the youngster might like. If the therapist can convince the youngster at least to "give it a try," he can usually find abundant material in the initial sessions from which to point out the self-defeating nature of the youngster's defensive style and motivate him toward further recognition and expression of his maladaptive attitudes toward achievement.

REFERENCES

Anderson, C. M., and Plymate, H. B. Management of the brain-damaged adolescent. *American Journal of Orthopsychiatry,* **32**:492–500, 1962.

Ausubel, D. P., and Ausubel, P. Cognitive development in adolescence. *Review of Educational Research,* **36**:403–413, 1966.

Bentzen, F. Sex ratios in learning and behavior disorders. *American Journal of Orthopsychiatry,* **33**:92–98, 1963.

Berger, E. M. Willingness to accept limitations and college achievement. *Journal of Counseling Psychology,* **8**:140–144, 1961.

Birch, H. G. The problem of "brain damage" in children. In H. G. Birch, ed., *Brain Damage in Children.* Baltimore: Williams and Wilkins, 1964, pp. 3–12.

Blaine, G. R., and McArthur, C. C. Problems connected with studying. In G. R. Blaine and C. C. McArthur, eds., *Emotional Problems of the Student.* New York: Appleton-Century-Crofts, 1961, pp. 76–99.

Blanchard, P. Psychoanalytic contributions to the problems of reading disabilities. *Psychoanalytic Study of the Child,* **2**:163–187, 1946.

Bledsoe, J. C. An investigation of six correlates of student withdrawal from high school. *Journal of Educational Research,* **53**:3–6, 1959.

Braham, M. Peer group deterrents to intellectual development during adolescence. *Educational Theory,* **15**:248–258, 1965.

Braiman, A. Riotous behavior in the college: A psychosocial view. *Journal of the American College Health Association,* **14**:147–153, 1966.

Broedel, J. W., Ohlsen, M. M., Proff, F. C., and Southard, C. The effects of group counseling on gifted underachieving adolescents. *Journal of Counseling Psychology,* **7**:163–170, 1960.

Brower, D. Academic underachievement: A suggested theory. *Journal of Psychology,* **66**:299–302, 1967.

Brown, C. *Manchild in the Promised Land.* New York: Macmillan, 1965.

Burgemeister, B. B. *Psychological Techniques in Neurological Diagnosis.* New York: Harper and Row, 1962.

Cashdan, S., and Welsh, G. S. Personality correlates of creative potential in talented high school students. *Journal of Personality,* **34**:445–455, 1966.

Clements, S. D. *Minimal Brain Dysfunction in Children.* National Institute of

Neurological Disease and Blindness Monograph No. 3. Washington, D.C.: U.S. Department of Health, Education, and Welfare, 1966.

Clements, S. D., and Peters, J. E. Minimal brain dysfunctions in the school-age child. *Archives of General Psychiatry,* 6:185–197, 1962.

Coleman, J. C., and Hewett, F. M. Open-door therapy: A new approach to the treatment of underachieving adolescent boys who resist needed psychotherapy. *Journal of Clinical Psychology,* 18:28–33, 1962.

Coleman, J. C., and Rasof, B. Intellectual factors in learning disorders. *Perceptual and Motor Skills,* 16:139–152, 1963.

Coleman, J. S. The adolescent subculture and academic achievement. *American Journal of Sociology,* 65:337–347, 1960.

Crites, J. O. Measurement of vocational maturity in adolescence: I. Attitude Test of the Vocational Development Inventory. *Psychological Monographs,* 79 (whole No. 595), 1965.

Daryn, E. Problem of children with "diffuse brain damage." *Archives of General Psychiatry,* 4:299–306, 1961.

Davids. A., and Hainsworth, P. K. Maternal attitudes about family life and child rearing as avowed by mothers and perceived by their underachieving and high-achieving sons. *Journal of Consulting Psychology,* 31:29–37, 1967.

deHirsch, K. Two categories of learning difficulties in adolescents. *American Journal of Orthopsychiatry,* 33:87–91, 1963.

Douvan, E., and Adelson, J. The psychodynamics of social mobility in adolescent boys. *Journal of Abnormal and Social Psychology,* 56:31–44, 1958.

Drews, E. M., and Teahan, J. E. Parental attitudes and academic achievement. *Journal of Clinical Psychology,* 13:328–332, 1957.

Dudek, S. Z., and Lester, E. P. The good child facade in chronic under-achievers. *American Journal of Orthopsychiatry,* 38:153–160, 1968.

Eisenberg, L. Office evaluation of specific reading disability in children. *Pediatrics,* 23:997–1003, 1959.

Eisenberg, L. Introduction. In J. Money, ed., *Reading Disability: Progress and Research Needs in Dyslexia.* Baltimore: Johns Hopkins, 1962, pp. 3–8.

Eisenberg, L. Reading retardation: I. Psychiatric and sociologic aspects. *Pediatrics,* 37:352–365, 1966.

Elkind, D. Egocentrism in adolescence. *Child Development,* 38:1025–1034, 1967.

Elkind, D. Cognitive development in adolescence. In J. F. Adams, ed., *Understanding Adolescence: Current Developments in Adolescent Psychology.* Boston: Allyn and Bacon, 1968, pp. 128–158.

Fenichel, O. *The Psychoanalytic Theory of Neurosis.* New York: Norton, 1945.

Fish, B. Drug use in psychiatric disorders of children. *American Journal of Psychiatry,* 124:31–36, 1968.

Flacks, R. The liberated generation: An exploration of the roots of student protest. *Journal of Social Issues,* 23:52–75, 1967.

Flower, R. M., Gofman, H. F., and Lawson, L. I., eds. *Reading Disorders: A Multidisciplinary Symposium.* Philadelphia: Davis, 1965.

Frankel, E. A comparative study of achieving and underachieving high school boys of high intellectual ability. *Journal of Educational Research,* **53**:172–180, 1960.

Freud, A. (1936). *The Ego and the Mechanisms of Defense.* New York: International Universities Press, 1946.

Freud, S. (1901). The psychopathology of everyday life. *Standard Edition,* Vol. VI. London: Hogarth, 1960.

Freud, S. (1916). Some character-types met with in psychoanalytic work. *Standard Edition,* Vol. XIV. London: Hogarth, 1957, pp. 311–333.

Garai, J. E., and Scheinfeld, A. Sex differences in mental and behavioral traits. *Genetic Psychology Monographs,* **77**:169–299, 1968.

Gardner, G. E., and Sperry, B. Basic word ambivalence and learning disabilities in childhood and adolescence. *American Journal of Psychotherapy,* **18**:377–392, 1964.

Gates, A. I. The role of personality maladjustment in reading disability. *Journal of Genetic Psychology,* **59**:77–83, 1941.

Gesell, A., and Amatruda, C. *Developmental Diagnosis,* revised edition. New York: Hoeber, 1947.

Gesell, A. L., Ilg, F. L., and Ames, L. B. *Youth: The Years from Ten to Sixteen.* New York: Harper, 1956.

Gilbreath, S. H. Appropriate and inappropriate group counseling with academic underachievers. *Journal of Counseling Psychology,* **15**:506–511, 1968.

Goldburgh, S. J., and Penney, J. F. A note on counseling underachieving college students. *Journal of Counseling Psychology,* **9**:133–138, 1962.

Greenberg, E. S. The development of assessment techniques for the brain damaged adolescent. *American Journal of Orthopsychiatry,* **37**:214–215, 1967.

Gruenberg, E. M. Some epidemiological aspects of congenital brain damage. In H. G. Birch, ed., *Brain Damage in Children: The Biological and Social Aspects.* Baltimore: Williams and Wilkins, 1964, pp. 118–130.

Grunebaum, M. G., Hurwitz, I., Prentice, N. M., and Sperry, B. M. Fathers of sons with primary neurotic learning inhibitions. *American Journal of Orthopsychiatry,* **32**:462–472, 1962.

Harris, H. I. Drop-out and the negative institutional transference. *American Journal of Psychotherapy,* **20**:664–668, 1966.

Hartocollis, P. The syndrome of minimal brain dysfunction in young adult patients. *Bulletin of the Menninger Clinic,* **32**:102–114, 1968.

Hathaway, S. R., and Monachesi, E. D. *Adolescent Personality and Behavior.* Minneapolis, Minn.: University of Minnesota Press, 1963.

Hellmuth, J., ed. *Learning Disorders* (3 vols.). Seattle: Special Child Publications, 1965, 1966, 1968.

Hess, R. D. High school antecedents of young adult achievement. In R. E. Grinder, ed., *Studies in Adolescence.* New York: Macmillan, 1963, pp. 401–414.

Hummel, R., and Sprinthall, N. Underachievement related to interests, attitudes, and values. *Personnel and Guidance Journal,* **44**:388–395, 1965.

Hunter, E. *The Blackboard Jungle.* New York: Simon and Schuster, 1954.

Inhelder, B., and Piaget, J. *The Growth of Logical Thinking from Childhood to Adolescence.* New York: Basic Books, 1958.

Johnson, D. J., and Myklebust, H. R. *Learning Disabilities: Educational Principles and Practices.* New York: Grune and Stratton, 1967.

Jones, M. C., and Mussen, P. H. Self-conceptions, motivations, and interpersonal attitudes of early- and late-maturing girls. *Child Development,* **29**:491–501, 1958.

Jordan, T. E. *The Mentally Retarded.* Columbus, Ohio: Merrill, 1966.

Katz, I. The socialization of academic motivation in minority group children. *Nebraska Symposium on Motivation,* **15**:133–191, 1967.

Keniston, K. The sources of student dissent. *Journal of Social Issues,* **23**:108–137, 1967.

Kirk, B. A. Test versus academic performance in malfunctioning students. *Journal of Consulting Psychology,* **16**:213–216, 1952.

Kotkov, B. Emotional syndromes associated with learning failure. *Diseases of the Nervous System,* **26**:48–55, 1965.

Laufer, M. W. Cerebral dysfunction and behavior disorders in adolescents. *American Journal of Orthopsychiatry,* **32**:501–506, 1962.

Levy, S. Post-encephalitic behavior disorder—a forgotten entity: A report of 100 cases. *American Journal of Psychiatry,* **115**:1062–1067, 1959.

Lichter, S. O., Rapien, E. B., Siebert, F. M., and Sklansky, M. *The Drop-outs: A Treatment Study of Intellectually Capable Students Who Drop out of High School.* New York: Free Press of Glencoe, 1962.

Liss, E. Learning difficulties: Unresolved anxiety and resultant learning patterns. *American Journal of Orthopsychiatry,* **11**:520–524, 1941a.

Liss, E. The failing student. *American Journal of Orthopsychiatry.* **11**:712–717, 1941b.

Liss, E. The psychiatric implications of the failing student. *American Journal of Orthopsychiatry,* **19**:501–505, 1949.

Liss, E. Motivations in learning. *Psychoanalytic Study of the Child,* **10**:100–116, 1955.

Lorand, R. L. Therapy of learning problems. In S. Lorand and H. I. Schneer, eds., *Adolescents: Psychoanalytic Approach to Problems and Therapy.* New York: Hoeber, 1961, pp. 251–272.

McArthur, C. C. Distinguishing patterns of student neuroses. In G. R. Blaine and C. C. McArthur, eds., *Emotional Problems of the Student.* New York: Appleton-Century-Crofts, 1961, pp. 54–75.

McIntyre, P. M. Dynamics and treatment of the passive-aggressive underachiever. *American Journal of Psychotherapy,* **18**:95–108, 1964.

Marcus, I. M. Family interaction in adolescents with learning difficulties. *Adolescence,* **1**:261–271, 1966.

Maurer, A. Adolescent attitudes toward death. *Journal of Genetic Psychology,* **105**:75–90, 1964.

Money, J., ed. *Reading Disability: Progress and Research Needs in Dyslexia.*

Baltimore: Johns Hopkins, 1962.

Morrow, W. R., and Wilson, R. C. Family relations of bright high-achieving and under-achieving high school boys. *Child Development,* **32**:501–510, 1961.

Moss, H. A., and Kagan, J. Stability of achievement and recognition seeking behaviors from early childhood through adulthood. *Journal of Abnormal and Social Psychology,* **62**:504–513, 1961.

Mussen, P. H., and Jones, M. C. Self-conceptions, motivations, and interpersonal attitudes of late- and early-maturing boys. *Child Development,* **20**:243–256, 1957.

Mussen, P. H., and Jones, M. C. The behavior-inferred motivations of late- and early-maturing boys. *Child Development,* **29**:61–67, 1958.

Mutimer, D., Loughlin, L., and Powell, M. Some differences in the family relationships of achieving and underachieving readers. *Journal of Genetic Psychology,* **109**:67–74, 1966.

Muuss, R. E. Jean Piaget's cognitive theory of adolescent development. *Adolescence,* **2**:285–310, 1967.

Parens, H., and Weech, A. A. Accelerated learning responses in young patients with school problems. *Journal of the American Academy of Child Psychiatry,* **5**:75–92, 1966.

Pearson, G. H. J. A survey of learning difficulties in children. *Psychoanalytic Study of the Child,* **7**:322–386, 1952.

Pierce, J. V., and Bowman, P. H. Motivation patterns of superior high school students. *The Gifted Student.* Washington, D.C.: Cooperative Research Monograph No 2, U.S. Department of Health, Education, and Welfare, 1960.

Pollack, M. Early "minimal brain damage" and the development of severe psychopathology in adolescence. *American Journal of Orthopsychiatry,* **37**:213–214, 1967.

Pope, B., and Scott, W. H. *Psychological Diagnosis in Clinical Practice.* New York: Oxford University Press, 1967.

Rabinovitch, R. D. Reading and learning disabilities. In S. Arieti, ed., *American Handbook of Psychiatry,* Vol. I. New York: Basic Books, 1959, pp. 857–869.

Rabinovitch, R. D. Dyslexia: Psychiatric considerations. In J. Money, ed., *Reading Disability: Progress and Research Needs in Dyslexia.* Baltimore: Johns Hopkins, 1962, pp. 73–80.

Robinson, H. B., and Robinson, N. M. *The Mentally Retarded Child: A Psychological Approach.* New York: McGraw-Hill, 1965.

Ross, A. O. *The Practice of Child Clinical Psychology.* New York: Grune and Stratton, 1959.

Ross, D. C. Poor school achievement: A psychiatric study on classification. *Clinical Pediatrics,* **5**:109–117, 1966.

Rubinstein, B. O., Falick, M. L., Levitt, M., and Ekstein, R. Learning impotence: A suggested diagnostic category. *American Journal of Orthopsychiatry,* **29**:315–323, 1959.

Schonfeld, W. A. Inadequate masculine physique as a factor in personality development of adolescent boys. *Psychosomatic Medicine,* **12**:49–54, 1950.

Schuster, D. B. On the fear of success. *Psychiatric Quarterly,* **29**:412–420, 1955.

Shaw, M. C., and Brown, D. J. Scholastic underachievement of bright college students. *Personnel and Guidance Journal,* **36**:195–199, 1957.

Shaw, M. C., and Grubb, J. Hostility and able high school under-achievers. *Journal of Counseling Psychology,* **5**:263–266, 1958.

Shaw, M. C., and McCuen, J. T. The onset of academic underachievement in bright children. *Journal of Educational Psychology,* **51**:103–108, 1960.

Sheldon, W. D., and Landsman, T. An investigation of non-directive group therapy with students in academic difficulty. *Journal of Consulting Psychology,* **14**:210–215, 1950.

Silber, E., Hamburg, D. A., Coelho, G. V., Murphey, E. B., Rosenberg, M., and Pearlin, L. I. Adaptive behavior in competent adolescents: Coping with the anticipation of college. *Archives of General Psychiatry,* **5**:354–365, 1961.

Sperry, B. M., Staver, N., and Mann, H. E. Destructive fantasies in certain learning difficulties. *American Journal of Orthopsychiatry,* **22**:356–365, 1952.

Sperry, B. M., Staver, N., Reiner, B. S., and Ulrich, D. Renunciation and denial in learning difficulties. *American Journal of Orthopsychiatry,* **28**:98–111, 1958.

Strauss, A. A., and Lehtinen, L. *Psychopathology and Education of the Brain Injured Child.* New York: Grune and Stratton, 1947.

Strauss, A. A., and Werner, H. Disorders of conceptual thinking in the brain-injured child. *Journal of Nervous and Mental Disease,* **96**:153–172, 1942.

Sutherland, B. K. The sentence-completion technique in a study of scholastic underachievement. *Journal of Consulting Psychology,* **16**:353–358, 1952.

Sutherland, B. K. Case studies in educational failure during adolescence. *American Journal of Orthopsychiatry,* **23**:406–415, 1953.

Teahan, J. E. Parental attitudes and college success. *Journal of Educational Psychology,* **54**:104–109, 1963.

Todd, F. J., Terrell, G., and Frank, C. E. Differences between normal and underachievers of superior ability. *Journal of Applied Psychology,* **46**:183–190, 1962.

Weatherly, D. Self-perceived rate of physical maturation and personality in late adolescence. *Child Development,* **35**:1197–1210, 1964.

Werner, H., and Strauss, A. A. Pathology of figure ground relation in the child. *Journal of Abnormal and Social Psychology,* **36**:58–67, 1941.

Wilson, R. C., and Morrow, W. R. School and career adjustment of bright high-achieving and under-achieving high school boys. *Journal of Genetic Psychology,* **101**:91–103, 1962.

Yates, A. J. Psychological deficit. *Annual Review of Psychology,* **17**:111–144, 1966.

CHAPTER 8

Delinquent Behavior

Delinquent behavior, defined as the violation of legally established codes of conduct, may consist of a single delinquent act, a single episode of multiple illegal acts, occasional but repetitive delinquent exploits, or commitment to a consistently delinquent way of life. Delinquent acts themselves may range from major crimes against persons and property (assault, theft) to relatively minor misdemeanors (public intoxication, reckless driving), and they also include behavior that is illegal only by virtue of the subject's youth (purchasing liquor, leaving home). The outcomes of delinquency are as variable as the behaviors that define it. The perpetrator of a delinquent act may be brought before a court and either adjudged delinquent or not, he may come to the attention of some agency (police, clinic, school) that responds in a nonadjudicating manner, he may be detected by persons who do not refer him to any agency, or he may go completely undetected. These categories have been formally labeled by Carr (1950, p. 90) as "adjudged," "alleged," "agency," "detected," and "legal" delinquency, respectively.

Because delinquent behavior has such varied outcomes, its incidence among young people cannot be reliably estimated. The Children's Bureau reports that approximately 2.1% of the 10- to 17-year-old population appeared in United States juvenile courts for other than traffic offenses in 1966 and that the number of such appearances has increased more rapidly than the population of this age group in almost every successive year since 1949 (*Juvenile Court Statistics,* 1967, p. 2). Yet these and similar incidence data are seriously impugned by uncontrolled factors that determine whether a youngster who commits a delinquent act ever becomes an agency, alleged, or adjudged delinquent.

Available evidence indicates, for example, that a detected delinquent's prospects of being arrested, referred to a social agency or clinic, or let go often depend on his sex and socioeconomic status, and on the availability of social agencies and juvenile courts. Boys and lower class youngsters appear more likely to be arrested than girls and middle class or upper class youths who commit the same offense. Accessibility to social agencies tends to decrease the number of youngsters who are arrested but, on the contrary, the existence of a juvenile court in a youngster's locale often increases the likelihood of his being arrested for a given delinquent act (Wirt and Briggs, 1965), perhaps because police are less reluctant to arrest a teenager when they know there are special facilities available for dealing with him. Thus the increase in juvenile court cases noted by the Children's Bureau may be attributable at least in part to expanding juvenile court facilities rather than solely to more frequent delinquent behavior. These and other unquantifiable influences on whether a delinquent youngster is detected, referred, alleged, or adjudicated justify Vedder's (1963, p. 19) statement, "The expression 'the figures speak for themselves' does not apply to juvenile delinquency statistics or even suggest an hypothesis."

Most writers on delinquent behavior acknowledge these statistical vagaries but nevertheless concur that both the number of delinquent offenses and the incidence of delinquent behavior in the teenage population are growing: "A grave concern for what appears to be a continuous increase in juvenile delinquency is felt in nearly all countries" (Sellin and Wolfgang, 1964, p. 1). There is furthermore little question that the number of adolescent youngsters who commit delinquent acts far exceeds the number who come to public attention.

The prevalence of this "hidden" delinquency was first demonstrated in landmark studies by Porterfield (1943) and by Murphy, Shirley, and Witmer (1946). Porterfield compared the previous delinquencies admitted by 337 male and female college students with the delinquent acts of some 2000 juvenile court youngsters. He found almost universal prevalence of previous delinquent acts among the collegians, similar in kind and seriousness to those with which the court youngsters had been charged. The delinquency patterns of the two groups differed significantly only in that the college students appeared to have committed delinquent acts less frequently than the court youngsters and had rarely been alleged or adjudicated delinquent.

Murphy et al. followed 114 boys who were part of the counseling and service program of the Cambridge-Somerville Youth Study.[1] During a five-year period in which these boys had been in the treatment program all but 13 had been involved in some delinquent activity. Yet, of the

---

[1] In this study 650 mostly 9- to 11-year-old boys who were considered to have some kind of "difficulty" were divided equally into a nontreatment control group and a treatment group that participated in an ongoing counseling and service program (Powers and Witmer, 1951).

6416 infractions of the law they had committed, only 95 had led to legal complaints involving the police or the courts.

More recently the studies of modal adolescents by Offer, Sabshin, and Marcus (1965; see p. 51) have demonstrated the high prevalence of delinquent acts even among middle class, suburban youngsters who have not been identified as having "difficulties." Of their 84 representative 14- to 16-year-old boys, 75% had either participated in one or more delinquent acts or had associated with known delinquents. Commenting on these and similar data concerning the extent of hidden delinquency, Marwell (1966) concludes that delinquent acts are "endemic" within the adolescent population and that adolescence by itself seems to be a good predictor of whether or not a person will commit some delinquent act.

However accurate such a conclusion may be, it should not be invoked to resurrect the conception of adolescence as a particular age of normative emotional turbulence (see Chap. 2). Marwell notes in his paper that, although a disproportionate number of arrests seem to involve adolescents, there is no convincing evidence that the proportion of adolescents who commit illegal acts is greater than that of adults. Furthermore, the commission of an illegal act is hardly tantamount to chronic delinquency. None of the youngsters studied by Offer et al. was repeatedly delinquent, and the kinds of delinquent acts that appear to be endemic among teenagers include many that have few implications for criminality or psychological disturbance; for example, the offenses recorded by Offer et al. included such behavior as tipping over garbage cans after a football game.

On the other hand, repeated and serious delinquent acts often reflect behavior disturbances that require careful clinical attention. The long-term psychopathological implications of delinquent behavior patterns have emerged clearly in Robins' (1966) already cited work, *Deviant Children Grown Up* (see p. 114). In this 30-year follow-up of 524 child guidance clinic patients initially seen at a median age of 13 the primarily neurotic children were found as adults to resemble closely 100 control subjects, whereas the primarily antisocial children were notable as adults for their high frequency of arrests, alcoholism, divorce, poor job histories, child neglect, dependency on social agencies, and psychiatric hospitalization:

"Antisocial behavior in childhood not only predicts the full-blown picture of antisocial behavior that is diagnosed sociopathic personality, it also predicts the level of antisocial behavior in adults whose psychiatric picture is preempted by psychosis or who have less antisocial behavior than that required for a diagnosis of sociopathic personality. Antisocial behavior in childhood, then, seems to be an excellent predictor of one particular psychiatric syndrome, sociopathic personality, and also of the

advent of adult antisocial behavior that cuts across diagnostic lines"
(Robins, 1966, p. 158).

Robins' work confirms the importance of adequate treatment for the
repeatedly or seriously delinquent youngster and of careful attention to
the youngster whose occasional antisocial act may presage progression
to serious delinquency. In pursuing these treatment efforts the clinician
needs to keep the following two distinctions in mind:

1. Delinquent acts of whatever frequency and severity vary in the extent
to which they derive primarily from sociological or from psychological
determinants.

2. Youngsters whose delinquent acts derive primarily from psychological disturbance comprise some whose antisocial behavior is symptomatic
of intrapsychic or intrafamilial conflict, some whose delinquency represents
a characterologically asocial orientation, and some whose delinquent tendencies derive from psychotic or organic disturbance.

This chapter first reviews distinctions between sociological and psychological patterns of delinquency in relation to studies of adaptive and maladaptive delinquency, social and solitary delinquency, and lower and middle class delinquency. Later sections then discuss and illustrate the patterns
of neurotic, characterological, and psychotic and organic disturbance that
are found in primarily psychological delinquency. The final portion of
the chapter is devoted to the treatment of these various types of delinquent
behavior.

SOCIOLOGICAL AND PSYCHOLOGICAL DETERMINANTS

Variations in the nature and essential motives of delinquent acts have
stimulated numerous efforts to categorize delinquent behavior along social-psychological lines.[2] Three important dichotomies of delinquent behavior emerging from this work contrast adaptive with maladaptive delinquency, social with solitary delinquency, and lower class with middle class
delinquency. Although these dichotomies do not represent truly discrete
behavior patterns, the data concerning them clarify the major distinctions
between sociological and psychological determinants of delinquency.

Adaptive and Maladaptive Delinquency

Jenkins (1955, 1957) has defined adaptive delinquency as motivated,
goal-oriented behavior involving learning from experience; and maladap-

---

[2] Ferdinand (1966) reviews in detail most of the published typologies of
delinquency.

tive delinquency as frustration-induced behavior that is rigid, stereotyped, and refactory to punishment. Using the terms "socialized delinquent behavior" and "unsocialized aggressive behavior" to denote the adaptive and maladaptive patterns, respectively, Jenkins (1957, pp. 534–535) summarizes their essential differences as follows:

"With socialized delinquency, we have a predatory minority subculture in which acquisitive desires for what is most easily achieved by theft may be reinforced by the prestige which attaches to successful delinquency—or the contempt, loss of status and social rejection which may attend a refusal to participate. We are dealing with planful, normally motivated, easily understandable behavior. With the unsocialized aggressive, on the other hand, we have a gross failure of conscience or inhibitions of any sort in a highly frustrated individual with a low frustration tolerance, unrestrained impulsiveness and bitter resentments and hostilities."

Jenkins derived this distinction from data collected on 500 youngsters seen at the Michigan Child Guidance Institute, 300 delinquent boys committed to the Warwick, New York, training school, and 300 youngsters admitted to the Child Psychiatry Service at the University of Iowa. In the original Michigan study, done in 1941, three clinically meaningful clusters of youngsters were identified: 70 who manifested such characteristics as bad companions, gang activities, cooperative stealing, furtive stealing, habitual school truancy, running away, and staying out late at night and were called *socialized delinquents;* 52 who displayed such behavior as assaultive tendencies, starting fights, cruelty, defiance of authority, malicious mischief, and indequate guilt feelings and were labeled *unsocialized aggressive* children; and 73 marked by seclusiveness, shyness, apathy, worrying, sensitiveness, and submissiveness who were classified as *overinhibited* (Jenkins, 1964). Jenkins found relatively little overlap among the behaviors associated with these three categories, and most of the 300 delinquent boys in the initial Warwick study also proved readily classifiable as socialized delinquent, unsocialized aggressive, or emotionally disturbed (Jenkins and Glickman, 1947).

Jenkins' distinction between the socialized delinquent and unsocialized aggressive patterns, which has been incorporated into the recently revised psychiatric nomenclature (*Diagnostic and Statistical Manual of Mental Disorders,* 1968), also extends to background factors that appear to differentiate the two groups. Both the Michigan data (Jenkins, 1957, 1966) and observations in the Iowa sample (Jenkins, NurEddin, and Shapiro, 1966) suggested a relationship between unsocialized aggressive behavior and developmental problems related to maternal rejection from infancy or early childhood on. The unsocialized aggressive youngsters seemed never to have experienced a sense of being loved or wanted by their mothers. The socialized delinquent boys and girls, on the other hand, were not as likely to have experienced deficient mothering during their early years as inadequate parental care in their later childhood. Socialized delinquency was generally associated with unsupervised development in a disorganized home located in a deteriorated, high-delinquency neighborhood, with neither parent providing much in the way of direction or guidance during the preadolescent and adolescent years.

In a recent reanalysis of the Warwick data Jenkins and Boyer (1968) confirmed the distinctive significance of behavior clusters designated *socialized cooperative delinquency* and *unsocialized aggressive delinquency,* and they also identified a pattern of *runaway delinquency* consisting of staying out late, running away from home, furtive stealing, stealing in the home, and passive homosexuality. The cooperative delinquents appeared to have the most normal personality of these three groups and to come from the most normal home situation, whereas the runaway delinquents seemed to have the least well-organized personality and to have experienced even a greater degree of parental rejection than the unsocialized aggressive delinquents. Shinohara and Jenkins (1967) similarly conclude from MMPI data collected at the Iowa State Training School that socialized delinquents have less personality disturbance and better family relationships than either unsocialized aggressive or runaway delinquents.

Although the particular patterns of runaway delinquency are not elaborated here, it is pertinent to note that other clinical studies (Leventhal, 1963; Robey et al., 1964) have confirmed significant psychological disturbance and severe family problems in boys and girls who run away: "In contrast with lay and even many professional notions concerning the seemingly benign nature of running away, the findings here suggest severe pathology" (Leventhal, 1963, p. 127). It should also be noted, however, that such personal and family disorganization appears much less likely to characterize the one-time, short-term runaway who returns home voluntarily than the youngster who runs away repetitively, stays away a few days or longer, and has to be found and returned to his home (Shellow et al., 1967).

Social and Solitary Delinquency

The distinction between social and solitary delinquency was suggested by Lindesmith and Dunham's (1941) differentiation between *socialized* and *individualized* criminality: the socialized delinquent collaborates with others to commit criminal acts that are endorsed by his subculture and earn him status and recognition within it, whereas the individualized delinquent acts alone for personal and private reasons to perpetrate crimes that violate codes of acceptable behavior within his social milieu. According to Lindesmith and Dunham, the social delinquent is usually a psychologically normal person who shares antisocial values with his subcultural group, whereas the individual criminal is most often psychologically disturbed.

Subsequent work has tended to confirm such differences between social and solitary delinquent youngsters; for example, Randoph, Richardson, and Johnson (1961) found significantly higher scores on eight of the nine clinical scales of the MMPI among individually delinquent than among socially delinquent boys. Cowden (1965) reports that individual delinquent girls experience significantly higher levels of guilt and anxiety than girls whose delinquency has involved participation in delinquent peer-group activities. And Brigham, Ricketts, and Johnson (1967) obtained more deviant descriptions of maternal behavior, indicating disturbed relations with female authority figures, from solitary than from social delinquents.

These data indicate a close parallel between the social-solitary dimension of delinquency and Jenkin's adaptive-maladaptive continuum. Social and adaptive delinquency both constitute primarily sociological problems in which the antisocial norms of a deviant subculture generate delinquent behavior in its loyal, well-integrated, relatively stable members. Solitary and maladaptive delinquency, in contrast, emerge as essentially psychological problems in which delinquent behavior derives from individual disturbance in the absence of ostensible subcultural support.

Although most writers subscribe to such a distinction between primarily sociological and primarily psychological patterns of delinquency, this dichotomy has typically been couched in imprecise terms. From a broad sociological perspective most cooperative delinquency is neither adaptive nor independent of frustration. Concerning adaptation, some behavioral scientists do regard group delinquency largely as normative lower class behavior that represents a consistent, adaptive adherence to norms and values at variance with middle class standards and is thus coincidentally, rather than intentionally, antisocial (Kvaraceus and Miller, 1959; Miller 1958). Yet most emphasize that delinquent subcultures are deviant within any social class and serve no adaptive function beyond the immediate confines of the gang:

"Many of the delinquent behaviors of adolescents seem totally devoid of a social purpose which could be understood or accepted by adults. . . . The behavior of the delinquent is incongruent with the goals of the middle classes and can be considered a mockery or perversion of such goals. It is also at times alien to the goals of the lower class adult population, who are sometimes as disturbed as middle class adults by the unreasonable nature of juvenile crime" (Halleck, 1967, p. 116).

Data from the already mentioned Robins (1966) study further challenge the adaptive value of antisocial behavior among lower class youngsters. The significant relationship she observed between youthful antisocial conduct and adult behavior disturbances obtained as much for the lower class as for the middle class youngsters in her sample. Robins cogently points out that this equal predictability of adult disturbance from childhood antisocial tendencies in lower and upper classes seriously questions the notion that such tendencies serve adaptive functions in the lower class (p. 199).

As for frustration, the major sociological analyses of gang and subcultural delinquency stress the role of common frustrations in the genesis of social delinquent acts. This emphasis is particularly clear in the "reaction formation" theories of subcultural delinquency advanced by Cohen (1955) and by Cloward and Ohlin (1960). Cohen interprets subcultural delinquency as the eventuation of frustrated efforts to attain middle class status and prerogatives in a reactive endorsement of antisocial values. Through this reaction pattern, Cohen continues, a youngster can "retaliate against the norms at whose impact his ego has suffered, by defining merit in terms of the opposite of those norms and by sanctioning aggression against them and those who exemplify and apply them" (p. 168). Cloward and Ohlin similarly argue that "pressures toward the formation of delinquent subcultures originate in marked discrepancies between culturally induced aspirations among lower class youth and the possibilities of achieving them by legitimate means" (p. 78).

The "cultural transmission" theories of subcultural delinquency also invoke a prominent element of frustration. Shaw and McKay (1942), for example, who describe delinquency as a group tradition transmitted from older youngsters to younger ones in neighborhoods where parental authority is ineffective, traced the lack of constructive parental influence in the Chicago neighborhoods they studied in part to the frustrated efforts of native-born youngsters to identify comfortably with the standards of their immigrant parents.

These and other major contributions to the sociology of subcultural delinquency have recently been reviewed by Glaser (1965) and Short (1965) and are not elaborated here. It should be noted, however, that social-disability interpretations of delinquent behavior pertain primarily to the disadvantaged youngster and cannot account for the delinquent acts of youngsters with broad social, cultural, and economic horizons. Social-disability theories of delinquency are further compromised by clear evidence (a) that most lower class youths do not become chronically delinquent and (b) that patterns of relationship within their individual families significantly influence the likelihood of antisocial behavior in young people (see Glueck and Glueck, 1962, pp. 97–136; Nye, 1958; Peterson and Becker, 1965; Wirt and Briggs, 1959).

Yet it is just as simplistic to overlook sociological determinants of delinquency in favor of exclusively psychological hypotheses. To the extent that shared frustrations of lower social class membership can generate cooperative delinquency, psychological approaches are no more adequate than sociological formulations to explain all delinquent behavior. It has been suggested, for example, that a delinquent is a youngster "who never was properly or healthfully related to his family" (Church, 1944, p. 144) or whose "ego has failed in its fundamental role of synthesizing agent and mediator" (Bernabeu, 1958, p. 386), and that "if one is even to begin treating delinquents, it is absolutely necessary to recognize the pervasiveness of his personality distortions" (Schulman, 1955, p. 35). Such views fail to embrace the adaptive-social type of delinquency that develops primarily in deteriorated neighborhoods and is relatively independent of significant psychological disturbance or problems of early socialization.

Thus both group-sociological and individual-psychological perspectives are necessary to an adequate understanding of delinquent behavior. Despite some overlap and imprecision in the adaptive-social and maladaptive-solitary categories of delinquency, therefore, these labels refer to a meaningful distinction between the apparently primary influence of sociocultural determinants in generating some delinquency and of psychological determinants in producing other delinquent behavior.

Lower Class and Middle Class Delinquency

Delinquent behavior has been studied and interpreted primarily as a lower class phenomenon; for example, the extensive contributions of Glueck and Glueck (1950, 1956, 1960, 1962) are based largely on comparisons between 500 reform school boys, almost all of whom were drawn from underprivileged neighborhoods, and a control sample of nondelinquent boys from comparable neighborhoods. Glueck and Glueck attribute their selection of such a disadvantaged population to their particular interest in determining what factors would predict nondelinquency even in the face of adverse social conditions that are often presumed to augur against it (1950, pp. 14–15).[3]

Research with such restricted samples overlooks delinquent behavior among middle class youth and tends to yield results that say more about lower class life than about the origins of delinquency. Thus Glueck and Glueck (1950, pp. 109–110) report that delinquency is significantly asso-

---

[3] For a critical review of the Gluecks' work and other prediction studies of delinquency the reader is referred to Briggs and Wirt (1965).

ciated with lack of cultural refinement in the home and lack of family ambition, yet "cultural refinement" was absent in 82% of their nondelinquents' homes (as against 92% for delinquents) and "family ambition" was negligible for 70% of the nondelinquents (90% for delinquents).

When differences between lower class and middle class delinquency have been considered, the usual tendency has been to regard adaptive-social delinquency largely as a lower class phenomenon and maladaptive-individual delinquent behavior as the characteristic form of delinquency among middle class, socially advantaged youngsters. For example, Cohen (1955, p. 73) and Cloward and Ohlin (1960, p. 28) concur that delinquent subcultures arise primarily within the working class, and Randolph et al. (1961) present some evidence that solitary delinquents are more likely to come from the upper socioeconomic levels. As these writers acknowledge, however, such a class distinction is far from exclusive.

In the first place it is obviously as possible for a lower class as a middle class youngster to engage in individual delinquent acts motivated by underlying psychological disturbances. Second, middle class youngsters are no strangers to delinquent gangs, even though the primary locus of delinquent subcultures is in working-class neighborhoods; for example, Robins (1966, p. 189) reports that in her large clinic sample 26% of the boys from better neighborhoods had participated in "trouble-making" gangs, as compared with 53% of the boys from slum areas. According to Wattenberg and Balistrieri (1952), furthermore, at least one form of group delinquency, auto theft, occurs more commonly among advantaged than among lower class youngsters.

The task remains, then, to account for delinquency in the absence of the social and economic disadvantages to which delinquent behavior, especially when cooperative, has so frequently been attributed. Elkind (1967) suggests that middle class delinquency is essentially antifamilial rather than antisocial and represents retaliation against parents whom the youngster feels to be subverting his needs to their own. Cohen (1955) interprets male delinquency in middle class families as efforts to cope with basic sex-role anxieties by exhibiting masculine assertiveness. Other hypothesized sources of delinquent behavior in the middle class adolescent, as reviewed by Shanley (1967), include resentment of maternal dominance in the home, impatience with the protracted dependency of middle class adolescents on their parents, the upward diffusion of lower class values antithetical to achievement through deferred gratification, and ineffective early childhood training combined with inadequate parent-child relationships during adolescence.

However relevant such variables might be to delinquency, none is specific for delinquency or even unique to the middle class social context.

In fact, the more closely the distinction between middle class and lower class delinquency is examined, the more such a distinction appears to consist of little more than the difference in socioeconomic status of the delinquent. Bohlke (1961) has challenged even this distinction by suggesting that many apparently "middle class" delinquents come from families that have lower class backgrounds and values or are downwardly mobile.

Similar overlaps cloud efforts to relate lower class delinquency to deviant norms erected in reaction to frustrated aspirations or limited opportunity, and middle class delinquency to masculine-proving behavior. Elliott (1962) presents evidence that delinquent youths at every social class level perceive fewer opportunities than nondelinquents for achieving their desired adult goals. Bloch and Niederhoffer (1958) postulate that all delinquent behavior, regardless of the society in which it emerges, is a device by which a boy struggling for adult power can prove his manliness to himself and his peers. Marwell (1966) argues that adolescents independently of their social class membership experience a relative lack of social power in the larger society and utilize delinquent acts as part of an attempt "to augment their personal power by manipulation of their situation" (p. 40). Other empirical data reflect such overlaps between lower and middle class delinquency:

"Recent statistical studies of the class distribution of delinquency suggest that within any single school district there is little difference between delinquency rates of children from diverse class backgrounds, but that there is much more delinquency in predominantly lower class school districts than in more middle class districts. This can be interpreted as indicating that delinquency is acquired primarily by diffusion, as a subculture pervading a neighborhood, rather than emerging as a reaction of lower class youth to their difficulties in meeting middle class standards" (Glaser, 1965, p. 57).

It is furthermore apparent that lower class and middle class youths commit essentially the same kinds of delinquent acts. Nye, Short, and Olson (1958, p. 27) report no generally significant social class difference in the delinquent behavior admitted by several hundred high school boys and girls representing a broad socioeconomic range. Herskovitz, Levine, and Spivack (1959) reviewed the offenses of middle class delinquent adolescents at the Devereux Foundation and found the nature of the delinquent acts to be almost entirely consistent with the offenses typically observed among lower class delinquents, with the exception of auto theft (slightly more common among middle class delinquents) and burglary (committed more often by lower class offenders). Herskovitz et al. conclude that, with these two exceptions, "delinquency seems to be delinquency, irrespective of slums or suburbs, material advantages or under-privilege, gangs or no" (p. 473).

DELINQUENCY AS A NEUROTIC SYMPTOM

Psychologically determined delinquency, as distinguished from sociological delinquency developing in the relative absence of individual psychological difficulty, comprises three patterns of disturbance. In one of these patterns the delinquent behavior is primarily a neurotic symptom that expresses some underlying intrapsychic or intrafamilial conflict; in a second pattern the delinquent acts reflect a characterologically asocial personality style marked by chronically irresponsible, aggressive, and inconsiderate behavior; and in the third pattern antisocial behavior results from the generally deleterious effects of psychotic or organic disturbances on judgment, impulse control, and other ego functions.

Distinctions among sociological, symptom neurotic, characterological, and psychotic or organic delinquency are consistent with clinical observations reviewed by Finch (1960, pp. 302–309) and with available empirical data. For example, Reiss (1952), in summarizing a social-psychological study of the records of some 1100 delinquent boys, separates "relatively integrated" delinquents from those who display either markedly weak ego controls or relatively defective superego controls. Peterson, Quay, and Tiffany (1961), studying by factor analysis extensive questionnaire data from institutionalized delinquent boys and control samples of high school students, report one second-order factor of Delinquent Background, associated with environmental delinquency in the absence of any clear expression of personality disturbance, and two other relatively distinct second-order factors of Neurotic Delinquency and Psychopathic Delinquency. This and the next two sections elaborate delinquency as a neurotic symptom, the role of psychopathic personality in generating delinquent behavior, and psychotic and organic disturbances that may be implicated in delinquent behavior.

The symptomatic expression of psychological conflict through delinquent behavior usually represents (a) communication of needs that the youngster cannot otherwise impress on his environment, (b) the effects of inadvertent parental fostering of antisocial behavior, and (c) "scapegoating," the unconscious selection of a particular youngster to receive the family's implicit encouragement to delinquency. As illustrated below, these three influences often interact in motivating an individual adolescent to antisocial behavior.

Communication of Needs

A youngster who commits delinquent acts is often attempting to elicit environmental response to pressing needs that are being overlooked or ignored. The specific needs most commonly underlying such neurotic communicative efforts are needs to be punished, needs to be recognized, admired, and accorded status, and needs to receive help.

Need for Punishment. The utilization of delinquent behavior to communicate needs for punishment was first explicated in psychoanalytic studies of individuals whose motivation to illegal acts seemed rooted in guilt feelings. As suggested by Freud (1916, pp. 332–333) and later elaborated by Alexander (1930) and Friedlander (1947, pp. 149–150), the "criminal from a sense of guilt" violates the law specifically in order to be caught and punished. Such offenders usually harbor guilt over previous transgressions, real or fantasied, for which their punishment provides the needed expiation that has not previously been exacted by their environment.

Other psychoanalytic writers (e.g., Johnson and Szurek, 1952) contend that the criminal who desires to be caught is much less likely to be reacting to a sense of guilt than he is to be groping for protection against committing more or even worse crimes. William Heirens, the infamous teenage murderer of two women and a six-year-old girl whose body he dismembered, vividly demonstrated this phenomenon when he scrawled in one of his victim's apartments, "For heaven's sake catch me before I kill more; I cannot control myself" (see Kennedy, Hoffman, and Haines, 1947). Nevertheless, the demonstrable implications of masochistic needs for a variety of maladaptive behaviors (see Bergler, 1959; Reik, 1941) justify attention in the individual case to the possibility that a youngster's antisocial behavior is motivated by unfulfilled needs to be punished.

Needs for Recognition, Admiration, and Status. The needs to be recognized, admired, and accorded status are frequently communicated through delinquent acts by youngsters who feel isolated or ignored in their family and peer groups. Misbehavior generally draws attention to its perpetrator, and a youngster dismayed at the limited impact he is making on his environment may correctly anticipate that a detected delinquent act will command the attention of teachers, police, and other important adults; will forcibly engage his parents in court, school, or clinical deliberations concerning him; and will enhance his notoriety among his peers.

In this last regard Erikson (1956, p. 88) has noted in his concept of the "negative identity" that many adolescents would prefer to be "somebody bad" than "not-quite-somebody." The "masculine proving" ascribed to some male delinquency by Cohen, by Bloch and Niederhoffer, and by others illustrates such a quest for identity through deviant behavior, and Blaine and McArthur (1961) have similarly interpreted the colorful anti-establishment behavior of some college students as attempts to establish a definite public identity. Certainly the very small minority of college students who have battled police and vandalized property during the campus demonstrations of the late 1960s, whatever their professed motivations, have earned themselves a degree of public attention they would otherwise have been unlikely to command.

Among girls, needs for identity and recognition frequently contribute to sexual delinquency. "Feminine proving" girls sometimes seek through intercourse and pregnancy to bolster their sense of femininity and publicly proclaim their womanhood. For many unwed pregnant adolescents studied, for example, by Visotsky (1966) and Gottschalk et al. (1964), engaging in intercourse represented being attractive and feminine, and pregnancy was associated with peer-group respect for girls who have a lover and become pregnant by him. Conversely, Vincent (1961, pp. 253–254) concludes from an extensive research project that the development of a positive self-identity from infancy through adolescence effectively deters illegitimate pregnancy.

In many instances illegitimate pregnancy also communicates a girl's anger toward her parents, especially when she despairs of other ways of getting through to them. Fleck (1956) reports that rebelliousness and needs to punish their mothers figured prominently in the motivations of 100 unmarried pregnant girls he studied, and Barglow et al. (1967) observed a temporal association between becoming pregnant and a disruption in verbal communication with their mothers among many unwed adolescent girls they interviewed.

For any youngster who feels ignored and unrecognized, public antisocial behavior may thus serve multiply to focus attention on him, to enhance his sense of identity and his visibility among his peers, and to punish his now embarrassed or inconvenienced parents for their previous disregard. The following case illustrates such motivations in a 13-year-old girl:

> Wilma was an academically average, plain-looking eighth-grade student without previous indications of emotional disturbance who lived in the shadows of her family and peer-group life. Her father owned a small business that monopolized his time, and her mother—a youthful, attractive, and fashionable woman whose appearance contrasted markedly with Wilma's characteristic drabness—was actively engaged in a business career of her own. During their limited moments at home both parents concentrated their attention on Wilma's two younger brothers, to her great resentment. Although the parents perceived Wilma's chagrin at her brothers' favored position, they felt that she was being adequately cared for and had no grounds for her frequent griping and sullenness.
>
> Among her peers Wilma typically tagged along as a silent, unobtrusive participant rather than as a highly valued or important group

member; if she were suddenly to disappear, she presumed, her friends would probably not miss her or even notice her absence. Interestingly, many of her preferred companions were youngsters of whom her parents disapproved, primarily because of their purportedly sloppy dress, unkempt'appearance, and undisciplined behavior. Despite their constant complaints about her friends, however, Wilma's parents had never actually forbidden her to see them, nor had they criticized her for dressing as they did (her father in fact gave her his old shirts to wear), nor had they insisted that she behave differently from her friends in any way. Wilma's choice of friends thus appeared to represent in part an attempt to anger her parents and force them to pay more attention to her, whereas their failure to enforce their vocalized objections connoted both disinterest and covert approval of her behavior (see p. 306 ff.).

Wilma's antisocial efforts to communicate began when she overheard some classmates agreeing that recent bomb scares at several nearby schools had been "sharp," "cool" pranks. That same day she went to a telephone booth between classes, called the principal's office, and anonymously reported a bomb in the school. Within a few minutes an alarm was sounded, the building was evacuated, and the police arrived to search the school.

Since Wilma had boasted of her escapade to several classmates, her guilt quickly came to light. Her parents were called in to meet with school officials and the police, who referred the family to juvenile court. Subsequent legal proceedings required many hours of her parents' time, their continuing attentiveness to her activities became a judicial directive, and everybody in her school now knew precisely who she was and what she had done. For better or worse, her action had at least for the moment pulled her from the shadows into the spotlight.

Need for Help. A youngster who recognizes in himself psychological disturbances that are not sufficiently appreciated by others may utilize delinquent behavior to communicate his need for help. Such a youngster may have directly petitioned his parents for professional help with the matters troubling him. Yet some parents are unable to accept the possibility of psychological disturbance in their family and respond to such requests by depreciating the severity of the problem; others are embarrassed that their child might need psychotherapy and encourage him to work things out by himself with "common sense"; and still others resent the implication that their ministrations are inadequate and insist that, if he needs to talk to someone, "that's what parents are for." A youngster thus rebuffed often resorts to public antisocial acts to convince his parents of his needs and to elicit the insistence of teachers, police, or judges that he receive professional counsel.

In many other instances a troubled youngster feels too embarrassed or estranged from his parents to confess concern about his psychological state, even when he could anticipate a positive response to his request for professional guidance. Especially if the overt manifestations of his disturbance are subtle and fleeting or his parents are generally oblivious to matters he does not directly bring to their attention, a dramatic or illegal act may be his only way to communicate his need and receive the desired help:

> Jack was a 15-year-old high school sophomore whose mother had died several months before his first visit to the psychologist. Jack's mother had been his major source of affection and support, his older brother with whom he had a good relationship was now away at college, and his father, although devoted to him, was a busy professional man who could not fill both maternal and paternal roles for his son. Jack missed his mother acutely, and, in the absence of even any partial replacement for the nurturance she had provided him, he had slipped slowly into a mild but persistent depression. He had lost interest in school and other activities, grown listless and lethargic, and become uncharacteristically preoccupied with the bleakness of his future.
>
> Because for the most part Jack's superficial behavior remained unremarkable, no one seemed aware of his need for help with these ego-alien symptoms. He was reluctant to tell his father that he was troubled, primarily because he sensed that the father was still struggling with his own grief. In this setting Jack's behavior underwent a dramatic change. He began writing hammer-and-sickle emblems on his papers and textbooks, carrying around the *Communist Manifesto,* and monopolizing class discussions to extoll the merits of socialist states. Before long he was labeled and teased by his classmates as "the Commie," which made him a distinct object of attention but did little to meet his needs for support and nurturance.
>
> Jack then somehow acquired a master key to his school and began using it to "borrow" tape recorders and other equipment. He promptly returned these items, but always in a way that compounded his risk of being caught, which he soon was. Because of his previously exemplary conduct and strong academic record, the school deferred any disciplinary action and recommended to his father that Jack

receive professional help. Significantly, Jack's attention-seeking and delinquent behavior at school ceased abruptly after his very first interview, in which a regular schedule of return visits was agreed upon.

This instance of delinquent behavior in a previously conforming youngster after the death of a parent illustrates the already noted relationship between delinquency and depression (see p. 165). The general importance of considering depressive components in delinquent behavior has recently been supported by Chwast (1967), who rated the test protocols of 121 boys and girls referred by the police for psychological evaluation on a five-point scale for intensity of depression (none, little, somewhat, substantial, predominant). He found that 80% of these youngsters were at least somewhat depressed and almost half were substantially or predominantly depressed.

Because Chwast's sample comprised adolescent offenders referred for psychological examination, presumably because there already was some reason to suspect psychological problems in the etiology of their behavior, his data may overestimate the incidence of depression among delinquents in general. The clinical and research data in this regard are nevertheless sufficiently clear to recommend careful consideration of possible underlying depression in youngsters whose delinquent behavior arises independently of obvious sociological or characterological determinants.

Sexual promiscuity among girls in particular should be assessed for the extent that it communicates ungratified needs for affection and thus reflects underlying depression. Toolan (1962) and others have noted that a depressed youngster may seek sexual intercourse not for erotic reasons but as a means of establishing intimate contact with another human being, and persistent depression may motivate such a youngster to repetitive, indiscriminate sexual activity. Studies by Palmgren (1966) furthermore suggest that the excitement and intense personal engagement of a sexual encounter may be very appealing to a youngster who desperately needs to combat feelings of apathy and enervation.

> At 17 Patty was brought for consultation by her mother, who was concerned about her declining school performance and recent episodes of shoplifting and drinking. Patty herself, readily and with apparent relief, admitted to other, more serious concerns and behavior problems. Tearfully she complained that she felt dumb and unattractive, that her friends were snubbing her, and that life did not seem much worth living, and she reported transient thoughts of committing suicide. She then described her wish at least to find some boy who would "stick by me," and she confessed to "one-night stands"

with a large number of boys to whom she offered herself sexually in her search for someone "who would accept me and give me a reason for living."

The degree of depression or other psychological disturbance underlying premarital intercourse in adolescent girls will usually be indicated by the extent to which their sexual conduct is promiscuous. Although it may legally constitute delinquency, premarital intercourse in the context of a close, trusting, exclusive, and relatively enduring relationship has far fewer pathological implications than has promiscuity, which entails concurrent sexual liaisons with more than one partner or rapid transit from one sexual relationship to another. Walters (1965) has cogently pointed out that promiscuity implies both a lack of discrimination in the choice of sexual partner and a failure to defer sexual relations until a faithful relationship is established, neither of which is necessarily the case with premarital intercourse.

It needs also to be recognized that illegitimate pregnancy, although often rooted in neurotic determinants (see pp. 302 and 310), is not tantamount to promiscuity. A large sample of the unwed mothers studied by Pope (1967) were found for the most part to have dated their sexual partners exclusively for six months or longer and to feel committed to them in a love relationship. Seldom was this relationship outside the social circle of the girl's family and friends or unknown to them. Furthermore, whereas premarital intercourse and pregnancy may be relatively common and acceptable in some sociocultural settings, promiscuity is not. Available evidence indicates that even in neighborhoods that tolerate considerable teenage sexual activity, sexual promiscuity among girls seldom constitutes a subculturally sanctioned, sociologically determined delinquency pattern (see Rainwater, 1966; Visotsky, 1966); accordingly, its occurrence in any teenage girl should alert the clinician to significant underlying psychological disturbance.

Parental Fostering of Antisocial Behavior

Although an adolescent's conscience may at times motivate him to delinquent behavior through which he seeks punishment to assuage burdensome guilt feelings, such "punitive superego" factors play a much smaller role in generating antisocial acts than the relative lack of superego strictures and controls. In the symptomatically delinquent youngster such defects in conscience tend to be highy selective rather than pervasive, a phenomenon that was formalized by Adelaide Johnson (1949) in her concept of "superego lacunae."

The lacunar superego is neither absent nor generally weak, but rather, together with some normal and perhaps even some punitive aspects, it contains circumscribed gaps, or "lacunae." It is these gaps that allow an otherwise conforming youngster to engage in certain specific kinds of delinquent act without hesitation, guilt, or remorse (Giffin, Johnson, and Litin, 1954). Beginning with the work of Szurek (1942), clinical investigation has traced such selective superego defects to the implicit fostering of parents who covertly stimulate and inadvertently reinforce antisocial behavior in their youngsters.

Covert Stimulation. Covert stimulation to delinquent behavior commonly proceeds through two somewhat different patterns of family interaction. In one pattern the parents display superego defects in their own behavior and thereby present a lacunar model with which their child comes to identify. Generally law-abiding parents who, for example, regularly take unjustified deductions on their income tax returns or drive over the speed limit communicate to their youngster the acceptability of such illegal acts. When the parent additionally takes obvious pleasure in his law breaking ("I've figured out a nifty way to charge off our vacation as a business expense"), blandly dissembles when apprehended ("Honest, officer, I had no idea I was going over 35"), and remains unabashed if proved guilty ("It was worth a try; I'll be more careful next time"), he teaches his youngster that flaunting the law may be desirable as well as acceptable. Similarly, when a youngster has regularly been made partner to various deceptions ("Scrunch down so you won't look so tall, and maybe we can get you in at half-fare"), he is likely to conclude that lying and cheating are appropriate and expected modes of behavior.

In this pattern of parental fostering it is the modality and not necessarily the specific nature of the illegal act that is communicated as acceptable. Because of superficial differences between an adolescent's delinquent acts and the behavior of his fostering parents, the parents may frequently be amazed at their youngster's misbehavior and unaware of their role in encouraging it. The father who distorts his income tax return but is completely taken aback when his son is discovered embezzling from his class treasury fails to appreciate the similar modality in his son's behavior and his own—that is, a juggling of financial records to divert to one's own pocket money that legally belongs elsewhere. In the same vein Szurek (1949) describes the dismayed father of a 16-year-old check forger who himself at age 16 had proudly falsified his age to enlist in the Marine Corps, and Wallinga (1964) reports that one of the fathers of a group of adolescent auto thieves had previously instructed his son in the technique of jumping ignition wires.

In the other pattern of covert stimulation parents whose overt behavior is above reproach but who harbor latent antisocial impulses implicitly encourage their children to act out their impulses for them. Such parents typically incite delinquent behavior by unnecessary prohibitions that (a) identify the specific transgressions that will provide them vicarious gratification and (b) communicate an anticipation that their youngster will commit them. Parents who vigorously and repetitively caution their youngster against driving recklessly, drinking, fighting, stealing, misbehaving sexually, or hanging around with unsavory companions convey their expectation that he will do one or another of these things. Especially when he has previously given them no cause for such concern, the youngster is likely to interpret this expectation as the parents' wish that he misbehave, which it usually is. He may then decide to please them by fulfilling their expectations, and their subsequent protests or overt dismay will seldom alter his perception of their secret pleasure in his escapades.

Such parents are also quick to infer delinquent behavior from minimal evidence. Noticing a new possession, they assume that their son has stolen it, without first asking him where he got it, and if their daughter returns home late or disheveled, they suspect her of promiscuity before asking for an explanation. A youngster who is constantly accused by his parents of shoplifting, drinking, sexual misconduct, or other illicit adventures eventually realizes that they would be gratified to hear of his doing such things; typically in such instances the behavior is rationalized with "I'm getting blamed for it all the time, I might as well be doing it."

Inadvertent Reinforcement. Once a delinquent act has been committed, whether parentally abetted or otherwise stimulated, parental sanctions figure prominently in reinforcing the antisocial behavior and implicitly encouraging its repetition. The parent who sanctions superego lacunae lacks basic conviction that particular delinquent behaviors are wrong, and he accordingly disciplines his misbehaving youngster in an ambivalent, inconsistent manner that tacitly communicates approval. He varies protracted periods of permissiveness with sudden angry outbursts and punishments that are disproportionate to the offense. He deplores the delinquent behavior but collaborates to prevent its being detected; should the youngster be caught, he minimizes the significance of the offense to the authorities. He accepts flimsy excuses for misdeeds and describes them to others in a tone of bemused tolerance. He criticizes the outcome of the offense but pays scant attention to the offense itself: "If you had to speed, why did you have to do it right in the center of town where you were sure to be caught," or "Next time you want to get sloppy drunk, do it at home and don't make a public spectacle of yourself," or "If you want to fight, you could at least tangle with a kid you can handle."

These and similarly ambivalent parental responses have been consistently observed by Johnson and Szurek (1954), Johnson and Burke (1955), and Carek, Hendrickson, and Holmes (1961) in their work with adolescents manifesting parentally sanctioned delinquency. Johnson (1959, p. 846) comments specifically on the demeanor of the sanctioning parent as he learns of his youngster's antisocial tendencies:

"The entranced parental facial expression apparent to the child describing a stealing episode, a sexual misdemeanor, or a hostile attitude toward a teacher conveys to the child that the parent is achieving some pleasurable gratification. No amount of subsequent punishment will act as a deterrent against the recurrences of the acting out. A child wishes to do the thing which he senses gives the parent pleasure, even though he may be punished."

Although the evidence for parental sanctioning of delinquent behavior is largely clinical, it is of interest to note some supportive empirical data reported by Gallenkamp and Rychlak (1968). These investigators administered to the parents of delinquent boys and nondelinquent controls a "sanctioning of delinquent behavior" scale comprising items on parental expectations, parental discipline, and parental modeling of antisocial behavior. The parents of the delinquent boys demonstrated noticeably more sanctioning of delinquent behavior than the parents of the controls, and comparisons between just the fathers of the two groups yielded a highly significant difference in the expected direction.

The symptomatically delinquent youngster, particularly when his antisocial behavior is occasional or circumscribed, may initially present a puzzling clinical picture. He is likely to be one whose delinquency is not sociological in origin, who demonstrates neither sociopathic tendencies nor other marked psychopathology, who is deriving no obvious gratification from his misbehavior, such as enhanced status among his peers, and whose parents are apparently stable, conforming adults who profess complete perplexity concerning their youngster's misadventures. In such instances the clinician needs to look carefuly for subtle, covert defects in the parents' code of values and behavior, and for equally subtle ways in which they are fostering superego lacunae in their youngster. More often than not a thorough search for parental actions and attitudes that may have fostered the youngster's particular antisocial acts will reveal parental fostering that has not been so subtle after all.

Parental Fostering of Sexual Delinquency. Particularly blatant parental fostering usually emerges in clinical studies of sexually delinquent youngsters. Although not limited to symptomatically delinquent youngsters, sexual misconduct is usually associated with the same patterns of delinquent modeling, unnecessary prohibitions, unjustified accusations, and ambivalent responses to misbehavior by which parents foster and reinforce symptomatic delinquency in general. Whereas the already noted influence of depression on symptomatic sexual delinquency has implications primarily for sexual promiscuity in girls (see p. 305), delinquency-fostering patterns of family interaction participate in a broad range of sexual misconduct in both sexes.

The extent of sexual misconduct among delinquent boys and girls is probably much greater than court and clinic statistics reveal; for example, Markey (1950) provides evidence that the great majority of boys and girls referred to juvenile court for general delinquency have been sexually active in much the same manner as those charged with some form of sexual misconduct. Outpatient psychiatric clinics report a less than 1% incidence of diagnosed sexual deviation among 10- to 19-year-old patients (Rosen et al., 1965, p. 1567), but Atcheson and Williams (1954) found in a 10-year study of over 3000 juvenile delinquents referred to a court clinic that 5.8% of the boys and 34.5% of the girls had been involved in sexual misbehavior.

As these data demonstrate, sexual misconduct accounts for a considerably larger proportion of female than of male delinquency. Within the sexually delinquent population, furthermore, boys and girls differ sharply in the nature of the illegal acts they are likely to commit. Sexual delinquency among boys usually involves such specific perversions as exhibitionism, voyeurism, sodomy, and public masturbation, whereas in girls sexual delinquency consists largely of promiscuity. In the sample studied by Atcheson and Williams (1954) 68.9% of the sexually delinquent boys were charged with some specific perverse act or sexual assault, whereas 79% of the sexually delinquent girls were facing nonspecific charges related chiefly to sexual promiscuity.

The role of parental fostering in promiscuity and illegitimate pregnancy has been demonstrated in a number of studies. The data of Gottschalk et al. (1964) on illegitimately pregnant girls suggest that, aside from the already mentioned peer-group influence, becoming pregnant was heavily influenced by having (a) a mother or sister who herself had given birth as a teenager and (b) a seductive father or brother. Thus a girl's need to emulate her mother's womanhood in a setting that stimulates and implicitly sanctions her heterosexual impulses tends to encourage her becoming illegitimately pregnant. The role of incestuous attachments to the father and competitive attitudes toward the mother in stimulating illegitimate pregnancy has similarly been emphasized by Fleck (1956), who found inadequately resolved oedipal conflicts to be the most common single conflict influencing the sexual behavior of the unmarried pregnant girls he studied.

Implicit parental sanction involving an initial negative reaction that incorporates encouragement and a subsequent reinforcing expression of pleasure is vividly illustrated in Marans' (1966, p. 132) observations on the mothers of young pregnant girls:

"They would ask in frustration, 'Do you want to end up like me with 10 kids?' Yet it was not uncommon for a mother to arrange the traditional baby shower for her daughter toward the end of the pregnancy with warmth and expectant happiness."

Even in such a deviant and almost universally condemned sexual crime as father-daughter incest, blatant parental fostering and implicit sanction are usually in evidence. Case material presented by Cavallin (1966), Cormier, Kennedy, and Sangowicz (1962), Lustig et al. (1966), Machotka, Pittman, and Flomenhaft (1967), Weiner (1962), and others (see Weiner, 1964) clearly demonstrates (a) that incest seldom occurs without the collusion of all family members and (b) that the mother, far from being the injured party, has usually helped to create a sexualized relationship between her husband and daughter and then managed to deny or ignore the incestuous relationship she has fostered. For example, Kaufman, Peck, and Taguiri (1954) describe a mother who abdicated the marital bed because her husband's snoring disturbed her and then sent her teenage daughter in to sleep with him "so he wouldn't be lonely."

Similarly among sexually delinquent boys unconcern about the behavior or obvious stimulation of it by the parents often attests their fostering influence. Waggoner and Boyd (1941) found among a series of boys charged with perverse sexual behavior that two-thirds of the parents could be characterized as indifferent, disinterested, amused, unconcerned, or extremely protective and resentful of court and psychiatric interference. Shoor, Speed, and Bartelt (1966) likewise comment on the characteristic lack of remorse they noted in the parents of a group of boys who had sexually molested younger children. Litin, Giffin, and Johnson (1956) describe and illustrate the role of parental fostering in a variety of unusual sexual behaviors occurring primarily in boys, including the following response by a mother upon learning that her 14-year-old son was smelling and wearing her soiled underwear: "For heaven's sake, if you must do that, at least take some of my clean things" (p. 40). The following case illustrates the manner in which a mother's own sexual curiosity appeared to contribute to voyeurism in a boy whose father's punitive orientation blocked him from more adaptive expressions of heterosexual interest:

The parents sought consultation after 16-year-old David was caught peering over the stalls in the women's toilet of a public building. The mother expressed general concern about her physically mature son's sexual instincts, adding that she frequently noticed him to have erections in her presence and was keeping constant watch on him to determine when he was in a state of erection and when he was not. The father stated his readiness to go along with whatever was recommended to abrogate his son's peeping and frequent erections— whether drugs, hospitalization, "or an operation."

Studies by McCord, McCord, and Verden (1962) of 115 sexually deviant boys in the Cambridge-Somerville study (see Powers and Witmer, 1951) confirm that sexual deviation among adolescent boys is frequently associated with marked sexual anxiety in the mother and authoritarian punishment of heterosexual behavior by the father.

Selecting a Scapegoat

Parental fostering of delinquent behavior is usually concentrated on one or more children in the family who are selected as scapegoats. It is this youngster in particular to whom illegal acts are confided with pride, whose aid is enlisted in perpetrating various deceptions, and who bears the brunt of his parents' unnecessary prohibitions and ambivalent responses to misdeeds. As within other social or political units, the scapegoat thus selected and victimized soon becomes essential to the group's equilibrium. In emerging as the family "black sheep" and the bane of his parents' existence the youngster who is encouraged to delinquent behavior serves his family's needs in several ways: he discharges antisocial impulses that might otherwise be disconcerting to his parents; he allows his parents and siblings to enhance their self-image by contrasting their "record" with his; and through his penchant for getting into trouble he provides a ready cause to which any family difficulties or dissension can be attributed. He unites his family in common concern about his misbehavior, and they are spared from having to squabble with each other by being able to direct all squabbling at him. These dynamics of the scapegoating phenomenon have been related by Counts (1967, p. 67) to the resolution of some family crisis:

"Scapegoating an adolescent is selected as the means of solving the crisis. Pressure is brought to bear by the parents, and the youngster acts in some impulsive and self-defeating manner. The family equilibrium may or may not be reestablished by this action; but if it is restored, the new equilibrium will generally be predicated on the fiction that the family is in difficulty because of the disruptive behavior of the adolescent member, and not because of some underlying problem related to one or both parents."

The scapegoating phenomenon helps to explain the fact that often only one of the children of delinquency-fostering parents displays antisocial tendencies. Just as interfamily differences can explain why some but not all youngsters growing up in a deteriorated, high-delinquency neighborhood become delinquent, intrafamily differences account for one child of fostering parents but not his siblings becoming delinquent. The special parent-child relationship that encourages antisocial behavior is reserved for the youngster selected as scapegoat, and his siblings are spared significant exposure to the parents' superego-lacunae sanctioning attitudes.

Several considerations influence which youngster is selected by his parents for the parental fostering that renders him delinquency prone. Above all, the scapegoated youngster typically stands out from his siblings in some way that is important to the parents. He may have provoked their anger by being an unplanned or unwanted child; by being a boy when they wanted a girl, or vice versa; or by being sickly or for some other reason making unusual demands on their time, energy, and resources. As noted by Johnson (1949), the child who becomes scapegoated for having angered his parents gratifies them not only by acting out their forbidden impulses but also by being caught and punished, which satisfies their hostile, destructive feelings toward him.

In other instances the scapegoat is chosen and victimized on the basis of positive traits that distinguish him from his siblings; for example, parents with unresolved conflicts about being surpassed by their children (see p. 273) may select the brightest, ablest, or most talented of their youngsters as the object of their covert encouragement to self-defeating antisocial behavior. Still other delinquency-fostering parents appear to be threatened by the youngster who most resembles them. Whether because he challenges their own identity more than their other children or because he demonstrates more clearly their undesirable traits, the youngster most resembling his parents has been found in clinical investigations of families with scapegoated children to be the one who is frequently selected for this role (Vogel and Bell, 1960).

The scapegoating phenomenon, like the communication and parental fostering aspects of antisocial behavior, bears significantly on the clinical evaluation of symptomatically delinquent youngsters. When parental fostering appears to have elicited the misconduct and when some but not all of the children in the family have displayed antisocial behavior, the clinician can assume that one or more of the delinquent youngster's personal characteristics have made him the special target of his parents' sanctioning behavior. Since these characteristics will have participated significantly in the neurotic patterns of family interaction that gave rise to the delinquent behavior, their identification is an important aspect of the treatment.

It should finally be emphasized in this section that diagnostic attention to the role of communication needs, parental fostering, and scapegoating in the genesis of antisocial behavior contributes significantly to the differentiation of symptomatic delinquency from characterological delinquency and from delinquency deriving from psychotic or organic disturbances. Although these three phenomena can appear in any form of psychologically determined delinquency, they are essential and defining characteristics only of those antisocial tendencies that arise as symptoms of intrapsychic or intrafamilial conflict. Failure to document one or more of these phenomena in the life experience of the psychologically disturbed delinquent youngster will thus contradict a symptom neurosis interpretation of his antisocial behavior and instead point to characterological, psychotic, or organic sources of his delinquency. The clinical differentiation between delinquency as a neurotic symptom and delinquency as a characterological orientation is elaborated in the following discussion of antisocial personality style.

DELINQUENCY AS A CHARACTEROLOGICAL ORIENTATION

Psychologically determined delinquent behavior occurs in some youngsters not as a neurotic symptom but as the reflection of an asocial characterological orientation. This characterological pattern—in which acquisitive, aggressive, and pleasure-seeking impulses are translated into immediate action—is variously labeled *psychopathic personality, sociopathic personality, impulse-ridden personality,* and, in the most recent psychiatric nomenclature, *antisocial personality* (*Diagnostic and Statistical Manual,* 1968).

Psychopathic personality was first distinguished from neurosis and psychosis and elaborated clinically by Hervey Cleckley (1959, 1964), whose *The Mask of Sanity* appeared in 1941. Cleckley identified psychopathy as a condition that is marked by persistent and inadequately motivated antisocial behavior, irresponsibility, pathological lying, inability to accept blame, failure to learn by experience, incapacity for love, inappropriate or "fantastic" reactions to alcohol, lack of insight, shallow and impersonal responses to sexual life, self-defeating behavior, and unexplained life failures, all in the absence of neurotic anxiety or impaired cognitive capacities. The work of Cleckley and other early contributors is reviewed by McCord and McCord (1964, Chapter 2), who summarize the defining characteristics of psychopathy as follows:

"The psychopath is asocial. His conduct often brings him into conflict with society. The psychopath is driven by primitive desires and an exaggerated craving for excitement. In his self-centered search for pleasure, he ignores restrictions of his culture. The psychopath is highly impulsive.

He is a man for whom the moment is a segment of time detached from all others. His actions are unplanned and guided by his whims. The psychopath is aggressive. He has learned few socialized ways of coping with frustrations. The psychopath feels little, if any, guilt. He can commit the most appalling acts, yet view them without remorse. The psychopath has a warped capacity for love. His emotional relationships, when they exist, are meager, fleeting, and designed to satisfy his own desires. These last two traits, guiltlessness and lovelessness, conspiciously mark the psychopath as different from other men" (pp. 16–17).

The last part of this description is particularly important, because it is above all the psychopath's underdeveloped conscience and inability to identify with other people that distinguish him from other disturbed persons. Jenkins (1960, p. 323) likewise concludes from his studies of delinquent behavior that guiltlessness and lovelessness are the essential defining characteristics of psychopathy: "The psychopath lacks the capacity for loyalty and is distinguished from others by this lack."

These two central characteristics of psychopathic personality disorder distinguish psychopathy from antisocial behavior in general and from professional criminality. Because of his generally asocial, aggressive attitudes, limited frustration tolerance, and lack of concern for the welfare of others, the psychopathic individual is highly prone to commit antisocial acts. As the above definition indicates, however, it is his defective conscience and incapacity for loyalty that mark his personality disturbance, rather than any particular frequency of antisocial acts. Neurotically and psychotically disturbed people may be as repetitively and seriously antisocial as the psychopath, and Robins (1966, p. 159) reports that even in the most antisocial group of youngsters in her large sample a diagnosis of sociopathy was made in only about half the cases.

As for criminality, most workers in the field concur that there is little necessary relationship between the professional criminal and the psychopath. Whereas psychopaths may become inveterate criminals, most professional criminals demonstrate capacities for planning, exerting self-control, and learning from experience that are not shared by psychopaths, and many are free from the intense aggression, impulsivity, guiltlessness, and shallow emotional relationships that mark psychopathy:

"The contrast between the psychopath and the professional criminal is far greater than the contrast between the professional criminal and the law-abiding citizen. Both of the latter normally pursue occupational goals, one legal, the other illegal. Both are in part motivated by the desire for financial gain, either as a means or as an end in itself. Both learn by experience. Both plan their behavior and modify and adapt it according to the circumstances which they meet. Both understand each other far better than either can understand the psychopath" (Jenkins, 1960, p. 321).

On the other hand, the clinician should not be too restrictive in diagnosing psychopathic personality disorder. Psychopathy, like schizophrenia and depression, occurs in degrees of severity. The fact that a person has made a friend or two, or has married, or has some capacity to profit from his experience, or has some appealing personal qualities does not eliminate the diagnosis. Psychopathy implies a noticeable extent of at least some of the defining characteristics of this disorder, but it does not entail extreme, unrelieved manifestations of all the personality distortions that are associated with sociopathic personality formation.

Although psychopathy has most frequently been studied as an adult disturbance, it is not uncommon in office, clinic, and institutional work with children and adolescents. Schmideberg (1935) in her psychoanalytic experience, Jenkins from his extensive guidance-clinic and reform-school samples (see p. 293), and Serrano et al. (1962) in their already mentioned outpatient-clinic study (see p. 85) describe significant numbers of disturbed adolescents whose uncontrolled aggressive behavior, impulsiveness, low frustration tolerance, lack of guilt, incapacity for love, and failure to make affective contact with their peers point to psychopathic personality disorder. Ackerman (1958, p. 235) concludes from his broad clinical experience not only that psychopathy occurs in adolescence but that "insofar as psychopathic conduct can become entrenched as a habitual pattern of interpersonal adaptation, it is most apt to occur during adolescent maturation."

Origins of Psychopathic Personality Disturbance

There is considerable evidence that psychopathic personality disturbance most commonly arises in the setting of early and severe parental rejection that generates deep reservoirs of anger, resentment, suspicion, and distrust. The youngster who is deprived from an early age of his parents' affection and interest develops little capacity for interpersonal warmth and compassion, seldom expects consideration or nurturance from others, and feels little restraint in unleashing his bitterness and hostility against a world he experiences as hostile and uncaring.

As noted on p. 293, the essentially psychopathic "unsocialized aggressive" youngsters studied by Jenkins had consistently experienced early parental rejection, and intensive studies of aggressive antisocial adolescent boys by Bandura and Walters (1958, 1959) have further demonstrated the role of parental rejection and inadequate socialization in the genesis of this personality disorder. From their interviews with these boys and

their parents Bandura and Walters (1959, p. 32) conclude that characterologically aggressive, antisocial behavior originates primarily in the disruption of a child's dependency relationship to his parents:

"The frustration of the child's dependency needs through a lack of
affectional nurturance on the part of one or both of his parents provides
the child with continuing instigation to hostility and aggression. The disruption of the dependency relationship also has important effects on the course
of the socialization process. . . . An impaired dependency relationship
may not only be a source of aggressive feelings, but may also limit a
child's capacity to handle such feelings adequately once they are aroused."

Such early disturbed parent-child relationships, especially maternal failure to gratify an infant youngster's emotional needs, have also been observed in clinical studies of characterologically antisocial youngsters by
Bender (1961), Berman (1959), Bowlby (1944), and Friedlander (1949,
pp. 89–90). These and other studies indicate the following:

1. That the vast majority of psychopaths have been rejected in
childhood.

2. That aggression is the dominant reaction to such rejection.

3. That rejected or institutionalized children often, though not invariably, exhibit psychopathic personality disturbance (see McCord and Mc-
Cord, 1964, pp. 70–83).

Discipline. Parental rejection in the case of the budding psychopath
typically involves not only maternal deprivation in early childhood but
also the parents' subsequent failure to provide adequate discipline and
supervision. Robins (1966, pp. 167–168) reports that only 9% of the
youngsters in her sample who were disciplined adequately or strictly by both
parents were diagnosed as sociopathic as adults. In contrast, where one
or both parents were described as too lenient 29% of the youngsters were
diagnosed as sociopathic as adults, and where one or both exerted no
discipline at all 32% became sociopathic. McCord and McCord (1959,
p. 77) similarly report a positive relationship between parental disinterest,
leniency, and inconsistent discipline and subsequent convictions for illegal
acts, and the aggressive boys in the Bandura and Walters (1959) study
were found to have been subjected to many fewer restrictions, demands,
and controls than the control youngsters.

Other work has demonstrated the particular importance of the father's
failure to discipline in the genesis of characterological delinquency. Becker
et al. (1959) observed more arbitrary discipline in the families of uncon-
trollably aggressive youngsters they studied than in the parents of a control
sample of normal youngsters, with the fathers much more often failing

to enforce regulations. Anderson (1968) reports considerably more paternal deprivation in the histories of 15- to 18-year-old delinquent boys than in those of nondelinquent controls. The difference between Anderson's groups both in the actual absence of the father and "under the roof alienation" from the father had begun to appear as the boys passed age 4 and had become highly significant by age 12.

In assessing parental strictness, however, it is important to distinguish between physical abuse and harsh discipline. Random parental cruelty and physical abuse serve no disciplinary purpose and communicate to a youngster his parents' essential disinterest in him, whereas severe punishment addressed to a specific misbehavior, however much resented at the time, demonstrates parental concern and capacity to exert authority. It is similarly erroneous to mistake the cold, stern parent for a rejecting parent. The cold, stern parent, despite his undemonstrativeness, often conveys through his painstaking surveillance and legislative rulings an abiding interest in his youngsters' welfare. Thus in addition to noting an inverse relationship between adequate or strict discipline and subsequent sociopathy, Robins (1966, p. 161) found that physical abuse yielded a slightly elevated rate of sociopathy, but that the children of cold, stern parents who were not physically abusive demonstrated a particularly low incidence of subsequent sociopathy.

Parental Fostering. Beyond failing to gratify their youngster's emotional needs early in life and neglecting to discipline and supervise him adequately in childhood and adolescence, the parents of the psychopathic youngster have usually encouraged him to aggressive, delinquent, and irresponsible behavior through the same patterns of parental fostering observed in symptomatic delinquency: by setting antisocial models, by anticipating delinquent behavior before it has occurred, and by responding ambivalently to such behavior once it has begun (see pp. 306–312). The role of parental fostering in psychopathy has been documented in the clinical experience of Kaufman et al. (1963) with over 800 antisocial youngsters seen in various court and child guidance clinics. Concerning the impulse-ridden, character-disordered delinquent youngsters in their sample Kaufman et al. conclude, "The parents of this group largely tend to be impulse-ridden, character-disordered personalities themselves, and either directly by their actions or covertly condone and stimulate the delinquency in their child" (p. 316).

Robins (1966, pp. 160–161) presents corroborating evidence that perhaps the most reliable predictor of sociopathy is growing up in a home in which the parents, particularly the father, are prominently antisocial. In families where the parents had no known psychological disturbances or had demonstrated non-antisocial behavior disorders, one of every seven youngsters in her child patient sample developed subsequent psychopathy. However, when the father or mother had a history of arrest or desertion, or when the father was chronically unemployed, about one-third of these disturbed youngsters were later diagnosed as sociopathic personality, and a significantly increased risk of sociopathy also occurred when the father drank excessively or had failed to support his family. For both boys and girls, interestingly, paternal antisocial behavior was the more significant predictor of subsequent sociopathy; although having a behaviorally disturbed mother in addition to an antisocial father slightly increased the likelihood of sociopathy in the child, the risk of sociopathy when only the mother displayed behavior problems was no greater than when she did not.

Despite superficial appearances to the contrary, identification seldom plays a significant role in such familial incidence of psychopathy. Not only does the developing psychopath by definition lack capacity to identify with others, but the dominant importance of the father's pathology for nascent psychopathy in girls as well as boys transcends the sex-role influences usually associated with identification. Rather, the striking relationship between paternal psychopathy and antisocial personality formation appears to derive primarily from the pathogenic child-rearing practices of the antisocial father: the psychopathic father is a particularly likely candidate to ignore his children and to abdicate his disciplinary responsibilities for them.

The major role of pathogenic child-rearing rather than identification in producing psychopathy is also reflected in the Robins data. She reports that the relationship between paternal and child sociopathy is markedly diminished when discipline and supervision have nevertheless been adequate, whereas about as many children without antisocial fathers as with them become sociopathic in the absence of adequate discipline and supervision (p. 170). Robins furthermore suggests that the frequently reported relationship of broken and discordant homes to delinquency (see Glueck and Glueck, 1950, pp. 115 and 261; Monahan, 1957; Nye, 1958, pp. 41–52) may also constitute a derivative effect of the antisocial father's impact on his family. Specifically, the characterological aberrations of the antisocial father may simultaneously generate both antisocial behavior in his children and marital disharmony eventuating in a broken or discordant home (Robins, 1966, p. 179). The following case illustrates many of the parental patterns that contribute to sociopathic personality formation.

> Martin was 13 when his school principal recommended professional help for him. The referral was precipitated by the latest episode in Martin's long history of aggressive behavior, which had included numerous unprovoked beatings of younger children. Martin had also

been unruly and disruptive in class and he had recently begun to yell out, "I hate everyone." According to the principal, Martin was "the worst boy we've ever seen at his age."

Martin's father did most of the talking during the initial interview with the parents, both of whom were high school teachers. He deplored his son's aggressive and destructive behavior in school, and he also complained that Martin was a lazy, easily frustrated boy who wanted to achieve without working, could not tolerate losing in any endeavor, and lied constantly. The father could suggest no explanation for Martin's misbehavior, except that possibly he had just been "born bad." Yet he also made a point of emphasizing that he was a stern disciplinarian and had no difficulty with Martin at home, and that perhaps Martin's teachers, by not being sufficiently firm and by picking on him whenever there was a class disturbance, were culpable in his record of poor conduct.

This initial information gave little clue to the genesis of Martin's antisocial conduct. In a subsequent meeting with just his mother, however, she volunteered some highly significant observations she had been reluctant to divulge during the previous joint interview for fear of incurring her husband's wrath. She reported that her husband's entire description of their son was as applicable to him as to Martin. Despite considerable capacity for impressing others with his maturity, competence, and sincerity, she continued, her husband was an irresponsible, lazy, dishonest man who delegated all financial and other family responsibilities to her and frequently absented himself from the home without explanation. She labeled much of what he had said about himself, especially his stern disciplining, as a bald lie: "He likes to think of himself as a big man, but he's never done anything constructive to discipline Martin; when he is home, which isn't often, he couldn't be bothered."

This new information clarified the likely relation of Martin's behavior problems to a characterologically asocial orientation stimulated by a father who failed to discipline him and set a psychopathic example for him to imitate. In restrospect, furthermore, the father's comments implicating the school in his son's difficulties could be seen as reflecting the father's antisocial orientation and his fostering of such attitudes in his son. By blaming the school he both evaded any sense of personal responsibility and suggested to his son the appropriateness of denying guilt and externalizing blame for difficult situations.

Thus this diagnostic study suggested developing psychopathy despite the comfortable middle class circumstances, apparent stability, and superficial social conformity of Martin's parents. His father emerged as a dishonest, irresponsible, self-centered, and self-aggrandizing man and his mother as a woman who castigated her husband behind his back but tolerated his behavior, perhaps out of her own masochistic needs, and was helpless either to stand up to him on her son's behalf or to fill the gap left by his abdication of responsibility. The frequency with which such parental patterns generate psychopathy has recently been reviewed by Manne (1967, p. 802):

"The family in which the sociopath-to-be develops is often one in which both parents perceive society as hostile and aggressive. The father figure is often an exaggeration or caricature of masculine attributes. He is often a transient, hedonistic individual who functions as an absolute monarch in his home. He may be brutal towards his wife and children in maintaining his absolute authority. He satisfies his own needs at the expense of family members' needs. The father's pathology frequently complements the mother who is often a masochistic, martyr-like, chronic complainer. Both parents attempt to push the child into acting out aggressive behavior with peers in order to satisfy vicariously their own needs to rebel against what they perceive as a hostile environment."

Differentiating Characterological and Symptomatic Delinquency

Occasionally the differentiation between characterological and symptomatic delinquency is apparent in the particular nature of a youngster's delinquent behavior; for example, repetitive and poorly controlled aggressive outbursts more frequently indicate a characterologically asocial orientation than a symptomatic effort to resolve neurotic conflicts. Additionally, as discussed in Chapter 5, delinquent behavior arising specifically as a depressive equivalent can usually be distinguished from psychopathy by its precipitous onset in the wake of demonstrable object loss and in the absence of previous antisocial tendencies (see pp. 172–175; see also case of Jack, pp. 304–305). However, most types of antisocial behavior may reflect either characterological disorder or neurotic symptom formation, and symptomatic delinquency may include patterns of antisocial behavior that are as insidiously developing, chronic, and repetitive as those associated with psychopathic personality formation.

The generally most reliable basis for differentiating characterological from symptomatic delinquency consists of the youngster's basic personality style as inferred from interview and psychological test data. The more a delinquent youngster demonstrates lack of remorse, lack of personal loyalties, and a disinclination to precede action with thought, and the greater his display of shallow interpersonal relatedness, underdeveloped affectional needs, incapacity to delay impulses, limited time perspective, and intolerance for anxiety or frustration—the more likely it is that his delinquency is a concomitant of psychopathic personality formation. Conversely, the less prominently he manifests such personality characteristics, especially when neurotic concerns and parental fostering adequate to account for his antisocial behavior are in evidence, the more probably his delinquency is symptomatic in nature.

Psychodiagnostic test indices of psychopathic personality characteristics are reviewed by Pope and Scott (1967, pp. 266–271) and Schafer (1948, pp. 53–57) and will not be elaborated here. It should be emphasized, however, that the various personality characteristics mentioned above and their test manifestations pertain specifically to the distinction between characterological and symptomatic delinquency, and do not necessarily differentiate the delinquent from the nondelinquent youngster. Reviews of the Rorschach and Wechsler scales have stressed that such measures cannot meaningfully discriminate delinquent from nondelinquent youngsters, primarily because delinquency is a broad behavior category comprising divergent demographic and personality patterns (Guertin et al., 1966; Schachtel, 1951).

The heterogeneity of delinquent youngsters and the irrelevance of efforts to discriminate delinquents from nondelinquents on the basis of personality variables has similarly been noted by Tiffany, Peterson, and Quay (1961, p. 19): "Students of the problem are coming to recognize that 'juvenile delinquency' lacks any stable, unitary referent, and that knowledge gained from the study of juvenile delinquents, otherwise unspecified, is likely to be limited by the notorious heterogeneity of the group." In a subsequent review of the research on personality patterns in delinquency Quay (1965, p. 166) further shows that seeking the causes and correlates of the personality dimensions by which delinquent youngsters can be grouped is likely to be more fruitful than efforts to study *the* delinquent.

PSYCHOTIC AND ORGANIC DELINQUENCY

Although symptom neuroses and character disorders account for most psychologically determined delinquency, it is important to recognize that psychotic and organic disturbances may also be implicated in instances of antisocial behavior. London and Myers (1961, pp. 280–281) report the following outcome of diagnostic studies with 85 consecutively jailed young offenders:

"The discovery of seven schizophrenics and two mental defectives seems to justify in itself the psychiatric screening of youthful offenders. The schizophrenics, seriously ill and in need of treatment in the view of trained psychiatric observers, apparently did not appear disturbed enough by the courts to be judged psychotic. Of the two mental defectives, one was retarded enough to require commitment to a training school for defectives after he left the jail."

Psychotic delinquency emerges primarily in the schizophrenic or incipiently schizophrenic youngster whose unrealistic perception of his environment, impaired judgments concerning the impact of his actions on others, and problems with impulse control may lead him into antisocial behavior (see Chapter 4). For example, Kaufman et al. (1963) note that the schizophrenic youngster may utilize delinquent behavior as a defense against unrealistic fears of being overwhelmed by his anxiety or annihilated by his environment. Easson (1967, p. 232) similarly describes psychotic youngsters seen at the Menninger Foundation whose projective defenses precipitated apparently motiveless crimes: "Such crimes are not based on reactions to a reality based environment but are activated by totally self-centered perceptions in the patient."

Organic factors participating in delinquency proneness include mental retardation, minimal brain dysfunction, and certain patterns of epileptic disturbance. Regarding mental retardation, empirical studies by Peterson, Quay, and Cameron (1959) have demonstrated a factor of inadequate delinquency that participates with factors of neurotic delinquency and psychopathic delinquency in describing the personality patterns of delinquent boys, and this factor bears a significant negative relationship to measured intelligence (Quay, Peterson, and Consalvi, 1960). The retarded adolescent who suffers feelings of inadequacy in relation to his handicap may be drawn to delinquency primarily as a means of seeking status and acceptance among his peers. Participation with other delinquents—for whom he is an ever-willing aide, dupe, and errand boy—may be such a youngster's major source of acceptance, attention, and praise.

Minimal Brain Dysfunction

Minimal brain dysfunction has already been noted to contribute to impulsive, defiant, unmanageable behavior (see pp. 248–250), and many minimally brain-damaged youngsters first come to clinical attention for suspected behavior disorders (Grubler and Gochman, 1962; Laufer, 1962). The possible etiology of delinquent behavior in brain disturbance has been pursued in a number of electroencephalographic (EEG) studies. In one of the early such studies Jenkins and Pacella (1943) found a high incidence of EEG abnormalities among 14- to 17-year-old institutionalized delinquent boys and concluded that brain dysfunction contributes to an appreciable proportion of delinquent behavior, either as a direct cause for delinquent acts or an indirect source of improper socialization.

Significantly, however, they noted that the delinquent behaviors to which brain abnormalities contribute consist mostly of assaultive tendencies related to emotional instability, irritability, and poor self-control.

Subsequent work has suggested a specific relationship between episodic aggressive behavior in young people and an EEG abnormality defined by 6- and 14-cycle/second spiking (see Woods, 1961). Unfortunately many recent studies of this "6 and 14 syndrome" have failed to distinguish episodically aggressive from nonaggressive delinquents and, perhaps in consequence, have yielded inconsistent results. For example, Assael, Kohen-Raz, and Alpern (1967) describe a higher incidence of 6- and 14-cycle/second spiking in delinquent than in normal youngsters, whereas Loomis (1965), Loomis, Bohnert, and Huncke (1967), and Wiener, Delano, and Klass (1966) report no association between delinquency and such EEG abnormalities and criticize other writers for stressing organic factors in the etiology of delinquent behavior.[4]

Whatever its precise incidence in delinquent youngsters, minimal brain dysfunction must be considered in the clinical evaluation of antisocial behavior. Even convincing evidence that delinquents as a group are no more likely than nondelinquent youngsters to manifest indices of brain dysfunction would not eliminate the possibility of organic determinants in a given instance of delinquent behavior, especially in view of the known implications of organic impairment for impulsiveness, irritability, poor judgment, and impaired planning capacity.

Epilepsy

Some forms of epileptic disorder may also contribute to explosive outbursts of angry, assaultive, antisocial behavior that resemble manifestations of psychopathy. Most significant in this regard are psychomotor seizures, sometimes referred to as temporal lobe epilepsy because of the usual temporal focus of the brain-wave abnormalities associated with this condition (see DeJong, 1957; Stevens, 1966). As described by Sakel (1958, pp. 33–37) and Garvin (1953), psychomotor seizures occurring independently or in combination with other types of epileptic attack are characterized by a precipitous onset of apparently unmotivated action patterns that have little relevance to the matter at hand and may border on the

---

[4] Studies of psychopathic adults, on the other hand, have fairly uniformly identified an unexpected incidence of EEG abnormalities. These studies indicate that psychopaths exhibit EEG abnormalities more frequently than normal persons and furthermore that a greater proportion of psychopaths than of normal persons demonstrate abnormalities on gross neurological examination and have an early history of the types of illness that increase the risk of brain injury (see McCord and McCord, 1964, pp. 60–70).

bizarre or inappropriate. During the attack, which may last from a minute to several hours, the person persists in a stereotyped fashion to complete the actions he has begun, and the slightest effort by others to restrain him or to alter his behavior often evokes combative rage. The following case illustrates the significance of an epileptic condition in an assaultive youngster who presented numerous superficial indications of an acting-out character disorder.

Johnny was 14 when his parents sought help in connection with a four-month history of temper tantrums and violent aggressive outbursts. They associated the onset of his disturbed behavior with the birth of their youngest child, whose advent Johnny had specifically protested. According to the parents, he had complained bitterly that the family was already too large (the newcomer was the fifth child) and required more sharing of things than he could put up with. In the four months since the birth he had been unable to tolerate not having his own way and at the slightest frustration or provocation would storm around the house, yelling, throwing things, and striking out physically at his siblings.

Further inquiry revealed that Johnny's penchant for poorly controlled aggressive outbursts had existed for a number of years and had merely been intensified by the birth of the new baby. The parents reported that he had always had a quick temper and had been the most demanding of their children, with little capacity to withstand delays in the meeting of his needs. He had characteristically been cruel and mean to his siblings, he had been consistently unruly, inattentive, and combative in school, and for the most part he was inconsiderate of others and showed no remorse concerning his physical attacks on them.

Johnny came for his first interview angry, sullen, and suspicious, and he alternated throughout between smoldering resentment at having been forced to come and attempts to treat the situation as a lark. These initial data pointed to psychopathy, expressed in an unsocialized aggressive behavior pattern, and the fact that the father had impressed the interviewer as being himself a physically aggressive, short-tempered, self-centered person supported such a diagnostic inference. However, further attention to a detailed developmental history identified some birth complications and some delay in Johnny's early developmental landmarks (see pp. 250–251). Neurological consultation was accordingly utilized, and Johnny's EEG revealed paroxysmal abnormalities, consistent with convulsive disorder, with a midtemporal focus.

Subsequent clinical evaluation of Johnny's behavior disturbance did reveal some psychopathic personality features and some intrafamilial conflicts of which his misbehavior was symptomatic. The interviewer also sensed beneath his hard exterior latent capacities for warmth and loyalty that offered some promise for psychotherapeutic intervention. Nevertheless, he also suffered an epileptic disorder, and not only could some of his losses of control be understood as seizure discharges but it seemed likely that he had derived some of his abrasive personality characteristics from being reacted to by others as an aggressive, unpredictable boy. In subsequent psychotherapy, which successfully helped him work through many of his problems in relating to his parents, siblings, teachers, and peers, anticonvulsant medication prescribed and regulated by his pediatrician played a significant role in minimizing the extent and frequency of his temper tantrums and aggressive outbursts.

TREATMENT

The treatment of delinquent youngsters varies with the extent to which their antisocial tendencies are sociological in origin, symptomatic of neurotic conflicts, representative of a characterological orientation, or derived from psychotic or organic disturbance. Where schizophrenia, mental retardation, or organic brain dysfunction appears to be primarily responsible for the antisocial conduct, the therapy will follow principles specific to the treatment of these conditions, as discussed or referenced in preceding chapters (see pp. 144–149, 245, 278–279). The remainder of the present chapter discusses guidelines for the differential treatment of primarily sociological, symptomatic, and characterological delinquency.

Sociological Delinquency

Because sociological delinquency represents group endorsement of antisocial behavior in the relative absence of individual disturbance, efforts to combat it have focused more on prevention through social change than on treatment. These efforts have included such social-action programs as the organization of neighborhood citizen's committees, large-scale provision of recreational and group-work facilities, job-upgrading projects, home-study programs, youth conservation corps, and the like. The details and scope of these and similar delinquency-prevention programs are reviewed by Amos, Manella, and Southwell (1965), Rhodes (1965), and Witmer and Tufts (1954, pp. 9–23).

The socialized, psychologically stable delinquent youngster is seldom motivated to participate meaningfully in psychotherapy, nor does he suffer the kinds of neurotic conflicts or concerns that call for this treatment modality. As in the case of the sociocultural underachiever (see pp. 279–280), however, certain types of relationship, educational, and psychosocial approaches may implement changes in the value systems that guide his conduct.

The relationship approach to delinquent youngsters has been elaborated by Ernst Papanek (1958, 1964), former executive director of the Wiltwyck school described in the autobiographies of such well-known reformed delinquents as Claude Brown (1965) and Floyd Patterson (1962). Whereas sociologically delinquent youngsters are usually immune to efforts to analyze or suppress their antisocial tendencies, they can respond favorably to an opportunity for positive, nondelinquent relationships with adults, peers, and institutions:

"It was acceptance, it was friendship, it was being taken seriously, being regarded as a responsible human being, being respected as an individual in a democratic community where he, therefore, could also dare to respect each and every other member" (Papanek, 1964, p. 424).

Jenkins (1955) and Topping (1943) have similarly stressed that, because of the socialized delinquent's capacity for loyalty, the addition to his loyalty group of socialized adults may provide an effective basis for fostering behavior change.

Educational efforts with the sociological delinquent should focus on demonstrating to him (a) the self-defeating aspects of his life pattern and (b) some nondelinquent alternatives by which he can enhance his satisfactions, especially in relation to the fuller utilization of his capacities for academic and occupational advancement. To be effective, however, academic and vocationally oriented treatment programs must relate meaningfully to the youngster's environment as well as his talents. This treatment requirement has been translated into a number of promising psychosocial approaches to the sociological delinquent.

Miller (1965), for example, experimented with a halfway house in which institutionalized delinquent boys from lower class neighborhoods spent several months gradually getting accustomed to life and work outside of the institution. The recidivism rates for youngsters with this halfway-house experience were lower than those for other groups of delinquents he studied who were discharged directly to the community (pp. 196–198). Persons (1966, 1967) similarly reports from a study of institutionalized delinquent boys that, whereas psychotherapy yielded better subsequent community adjustment and lower recidivism than a no-treatment condition, best results occurred when a successful treatment experience within the institution was combined with adequate community placement and employment after discharge.

The psychosocial approach has also been demonstrated on an outpatient basis by Massimo and Shore (1963; see also Shore and Massimo, 1966a), who utilized a vocationally oriented psychotherapeutic approach with delinquent boys who had dropped out of school or been expelled. In this program the therapist first contacted each boy in terms of helping him to get a job and then provided preemployment counseling, instruction and active assistance in such tasks as opening a bank account and getting a driver's license, and psychological support as necessary, including discussions of work problems once a job was begun. Short-term and two- to three-year follow-up data have indicated positive results for this combined psychotherapy, remedial education, and job-placement approach not only in relation to overt behavior but also to academic learning, time perspective, and interpersonal attitudes (Ricks, Umbarger, and Mack, 1964; Shore and Massimo, 1966b; Shore et al., 1966; Shore, Massimo, and Mack, 1965).

Symptomatic Delinquency

The application of psychological principles in the treatment of delinquent adolescents was pioneered by August Aichhorn, who established a residential treatment center for delinquent boys and girls in post-World War I Austria. Describing his work in *Wayward Youth,* Aichhorn (1925, Chapter 1) distinguished between youngsters whose delinquency was not neurotically determined and who could respond only to educational programs and environmental manipulation, and disturbed delinquents who were amenable to psychotherapy.

Psychotherapy usually is the treatment of choice for the symptomatic delinquent. The youngster whose misbehavior communicates needs for help may rapidly curtail his antisocial tendencies as soon as he becomes involved in psychotherapy, as did Jack (see pp. 304–305). Particularly when depression related to object loss has precipitated the delinquent behavior, the additional regular relationship with an understanding and interested adult often attenuates a youngster's antisocial motivations, whatever the specific content of the treatment sessions.

Symptomatic delinquency derived from needs for attention and status is less likely to remit solely in response to a therapist's interest and respect. In such instances the therapist needs within the context of a positive treatment relationship first to aid the youngster in recognizing the attention- and status-seeking motives of his misbehavior and its inevitably self-defeating consequences and then to help him identify and carry out more constructive means of gaining the notice and respect of his parents, teachers, and peers. For example, in the case of Wilma (see pp. 302–303) treatment focus on the various punishments and embarrassing notoriety with which she paid for a brief moment of glory paved the way for exploring ways other than bomb scares of capturing attention and winning respect.

To the extent that parental fostering and scapegoating have generated the symptomatic delinquency, the therapist needs also to help the youngster recognize the relationship of his misconduct to his neurotic interactions with his parents. Without necessarily calling attention to the parents' motives or their latent antisocial impulses, the therapist can identify for the youngster the contingencies between his delinquency and their unnecessary prohibitions and ambivalent responses. If the youngster can be made aware that his delinquency relates more closely to the actions and reactions of his parents than to his own needs and goals, he may then be able to break out of the tight circle of neurotic family interaction that has fostered and reinforced his misbehavior. Thus the therapist may observe, "It sounds like you did it more because your father was making such a fuss about it than for anything it really meant to you" or "I get the impression that wanting to see the expression on your mother's face had more to do with it than anything you really got out of it."

Involving the Parents. Successful dissolution of the bonds of parental fostering and scapegoating that stimulate symptomatic delinquent behavior usually requires the involvement of the parents as well as of the youngster. Johnson (1959, p. 850) in fact considers intensive analytic therapy for both the fostering parents and their delinquent youngster to be essential to a satisfactory outcome. In practice, however, financial considerations and limited professional time often preclude intensive treatment for all family members, and many parents may furthermore be unwilling or psychologically unable to participate in a treatment approach aimed at uncovering their neurotic conflicts and their vicarious gratification in the youngster's delinquency.

On the other hand, a supportive relationship with delinquency-fostering parents may be utilized to considerable advantage in the treatment of the symptomatic delinquent. First, it may be only in the context of ongoing discussions with the parents that the therapist can identify the exact statements and actions by which they are inadvertently fostering their youngster's delinquency, and such knowledge will facilitate his helping the youngster recognize his parents' influence on him. Second, he may help the parents curtail their scapegoating by discussing with them the specific characteristics of their youngster that appear to have influenced their attitudes toward him. Third, without making interpretations to the parents the therapist can recommend changes in certain delinquency-stimulating or reinforcing aspects of their behavior. Although the parents' needs will probably prevent them from heeding such suggestions fully, even slight alterations in their approach to the youngster may help considerably in moving him toward a nondelinquent motivational system.

In discussing their success in modifying patterns of parental fostering Carek et al. (1961) additionally stress the importance of a supportive relationship with the parents at the time when the youngster begins to improve. Because of their unconscious investment in his delinquent behavior and its usual contribution to the family equilibrium, the parents may become significantly anxious when he begins to give up his role as scapegoat and troublemaker. At this crucial point in the treatment parents who have not been effectively engaged are likely to intensify their fostering behavior or in some way to sabotage the treatment, as by summarily sending the youngster off to summer camp. A continuing supportive relationship with the parents can help them deal with anxiety stirred by their youngster's behavior changes and can also anticipate and avert potentially destructive actions on their part. Such supportive work with delinquency-fostering parents—without interpreting their unconscious conflicts or in other ways making demands on them that would increase their levels of anxiety, guilt or anger—is also recommended by Gordon (1960, p. 760):

"Our purpose is to facilitate the adolescent's full use of the therapeutic experience without precipitating an even more serious crisis in the family. We know from sad experience that pathology in one child often permits a family to maintain a level of adjustment which had best not be disturbed without extreme caution."

The Treatment Relationship. As for the actual treatment relationship with the symptomatic delinquent, effective engagement of the adolescent in psychotherapy generally requires considerable therapist activity to establish a positive relationship and tune in on the central conflicts; a relatively neutral and unfocused psychotherapeutic approach is likely to produce a silent, unproductive, and prematurely terminated relationship (see Chapter 9). However, the necessity for being active poses some unique difficulties in the treatment of the symptomatic delinquent, especially when parental fostering has figured prominently in stimulating the delinquency. For the therapist to be warm, friendly, and engaging without referring to the antisocial behavior, represents permissive whitewashing and implicit sanction of the delinquency; yet to concentrate heavily on it casts the therapist as a hostile, disapproving inquisitor or as a sanctioning parent whose interest in its details suggests tacit approval and vicarious gratification.

Hence the therapist must steer a delicate middle course between skirting the delinquent behavior and meeting it head on. Without setting about actively to explore the delinquent behavior and its origins, he needs explicitly to acknowledge its relevance to his meeting with the youngster. At the same time he needs to communicate by his attitude that he has not prejudged the youngster and is open to being favorably impressed with his interests, desires, goals, talents, and virtues: "We both know you're here because you've been caught several times shoplifting; but I'd like to hear generally how things are going for you and what you enjoy doing."

This therapeutic strategy will invariably be tested by the youngster through "relapses" of misbehavior once the therapy is under way. In the middle and later stages of an extended treatment relationship with the symptomatic delinquent the therapist may be able to relate recurrent acting out to ongoing events or aspects of the treatment relationship. In the context of a briefer treatment and in the early stages of therapy, however, the therapist's most helpful response will usually be a sincere, nonpunitive effort to clarify for the youngster the ultimately self-defeating aspects of his antisocial behavior and to identify nondelinquent responses to the situations that have provoked it.

By emphasizing nondelinquent solutions to problems the therapist provides the youngster with a positive system of values and goals that can insulate him against antisocial pressures stemming from his intrapsychic or intrafamilial conflicts. The extent to which the delinquent adolescent incorporates such values and goals will depend both on the youngster's personality style and the therapist's skill in fostering identification with him.

In successful psychotherapy with the symptomatically delinquent adolescent identification with the therapist usually becomes apparent in the middle stages of the treatment, after the initial fencing and testing phase has drawn to a close. For example, the youngster reports assuming big-brother relationships with other youngsters, talks about future careers for himself in the helping professions, shows increased interest in learning about the therapist's background, attitudes, and family life, and the like. In the absence of such clear indications of positive identification the therapist needs to consider either that his patient is seriously limited in capacity for identification or that his conduct of the treatment has not been sufficiently skillful to promote this necessary identification pattern. In either case he has reason to doubt whether the treatment is leading toward enduring behavior change.

Role Modeling. Some recent studies suggest that identification with the therapist's nondelinquent personality attributes can sometimes be facilitated by planned exercises in role modeling; for example, Sarason (1968) describes a project in which delinquent boys admitted to a reception-diagnostic center were engaged in a series of 15 modeling sessions emphasizing effective, socially appropriate behavior. In these sessions each youngster role played from a prepared script such activities as applying for a job, resisting temptation by peers to engage in antisocial acts, and deferring immediate for more significant future gratifications. Each modeling session was followed by free discussion of the particular coping techniques that were demonstrated in the role-playing situation.

Sarason's initial data indicate that delinquent boys exposed to this observational modeling treatment are more likely to demonstrate positive changes in behavior and attitudes than nontreated control youngsters. Interestingly, however, this difference obtained primarily among demonstrably anxious boys, whereas the 15-session observational experience had little impact on boys with minimal anxiety. It seems reasonable to infer that Sarason's relatively nonanxious delinquent youngsters were unresponsive to the modeling procedure because of psychopathic personality features that contributed both to their freedom from anxiety and their inability to form a positive identification in the context of such a brief exposure.

Characterological Delinquency

The delinquent youngster who is characterologically asocial typically lacks the psychological stability, impulse control, judgment, and capacity for loyalty that provide remedial openings in work with the primarily sociological delinquent, and his relative incapacity for identification, distrust of others, and inability to delay gratification or to plan ahead initially obstruct the type of relationship in which the procedures helpful with the symptomatic delinquent can be implemented:

"It is to be expected that the child will treat the therapist in essentially the same way as he relates to others. Initially, he has no desire to collaborate in the treatment relationship. The defensive narcissistic quality of the child's personality and his incapacity to love or trust cause him to keep the therapist at a distance. He quickly lets the therapist know that he is not interested in changing his behavior so that it is socially acceptable, and he is determined to make a shambles out of the treatment. He feels that his behavior is of no real concern to anyone but himself" (Berman, 1964, pp. 27–28).

Aichhorn (1925) similarly identified the essentially psychopathic quality of his "aggressive group" from their inability to engage in the milieu treatment groups that yielded good results with the majority of his patients. Impressed by the aggressive group's bitter hostility and their history of early affectional deprivation, he recommended a thoroughly permissive treatment approach for them. No pressures were to be brought to bear, restrictions were to be imposed only as absolutely necessary to prevent physical injury, and the focus was to be on "a consistently friendly attitude, wholesome occupation, plenty of play to prevent aggression, and repeated talks with the individual members" (p. 172).

Subsequent clinical experience has indicated that such permissive warmth seldom achieves any genuine change in the attitudes and behavior of the psychopathic adolescent. The developing psychopath shuns personal intimacy and distrusts demonstrations of warmth and affection. Intimacy threatens him with the bitter pill of subsequent rejection, which he has been swallowing most of his life. Adults who invariably meet his hatred and misconduct with tolerance and love impress him as inadequate or insincere, either of which means that they can neither be trusted nor relied on to help him. He consequently reacts to warmth and efforts at interpersonal closeness with denial, inattention, or increasingly aggressive behavior intended to keep others at a distance. Sobel (1949), from his experience at the Hawthorne Cedar-Knowles school, similarly emphasizes that, when hostility has become an integral part of a youngster's character, the loving approach is doomed to failure: "The friendlier I am, the more the child rejects the relationship" (p. 301).

As for permissiveness, Hacker and Geleerd (1945) have concluded from their work at the Southard School that—despite the apparent logic of treating emotionally deprived youngsters with unbounded love, affection, praise, and reward—such management impedes effective treatment engagement and increases rather than alleviates the youngsters' behavior problems. They report that when acting-out adolescents were treated in an atmosphere of restrictions, the results were considerably better than those obtained under conditions of unlimited freedom. The same is reported by Craft, Stephenson, and Granger (1964), who assigned institutionalized psychopathic adolescents alternately to an authoritarian and a democratic ward on admission. The authoritarian ward stressed individual treatment and strictly enforced regulations; no noise or disarray was tolerated, and patients were required to stand when senior staff or visitors entered the room. The democratic ward had an extensive group program and enjoyed considerable self-government and a relatively equal relationship with the staff. Postdischarge studies indicated that significantly fewer subsequent delinquent acts were committed by the authoritarian-ward than by the democratic-ward youngsters.

Bromberg and Rodgers (1946) also emphasize from their treatment experience with late adolescent delinquents that the youngster with inadequate superego formation requires an authoritarian treatment approach. They point out that a passive or permissive approach is likely to be interpreted as identical with the confused or hostilely disinterested response of the parents, whereas solidly established therapist authority, including the therapist's ability to respond humanely but firmly to misbehavior meant to test his potency and concern, will provide an atmosphere in which superego development may take place.

By recognizing the drawbacks of a permissively warm treatment approach to the psychopathic delinquent, the therapist can minimize the frequency of prematurely terminated or deceptively collaborative treatment relationships that fail to penetrate the youngster's defenses against intimacy. Deceptive collaboration consists of mutually comfortable conversation between patient and therapist without any basic change in the youngster's behavior, and the therapist should be alert to this possibility whenever he experiences an early apparently positive working relationship and a smooth treatment course with the psychopathic adolescent.

Beyond avoiding a permissive approach, the therapist often must initially employ a number of unconventional treatment techniques to establish a positive working relationship with the psychopathic delinquent. These techniques include the following:

1. Forming a narcissistic collusion around the youngster's current needs.
2. Exercising power on the youngster's behalf.
3. Promulgating variegated and stimulating treatment sessions.
4. Demonstrating by deed as well as words his readiness to give of himself for his patient's benefit.

Narcissistic Collusion. Narcissistic collusion requires interested and sympathetic involvement with the delinquent youngster's antisocial activities. To be effectively collusive the therapist must not only encourage the youngster to discuss the details of his misbehavior but also find enough psychopathy within himself to share the youngster's enjoyment of having manipulated or exploited his environment and even to suggest ways in which it could have been done better.

Noshpitz (1957), Schwartz (1967), and others have elaborated a threefold rationale for this initially collusive approach. First, the psychopathic delinquent's alienation from social values is so great that any apparent opposition to his behavior, either by direct criticism or detached efforts to discuss the ethics of interpersonal relations, will be so foreign as not to capture his attention or so inimical as to harden his resistance further. Second, this initial sharing of positive interest in the youngster's antisocial behavior may provide the only topic with which the therapist can establish a pattern of mutual communication, whereas efforts to discuss almost anything else initially might fall on deaf ears. Third, the therapist's sustained interest in learning the details of the youngster's antisocial acts may have the seemingly paradoxical effect of diminishing their frequency. To the extent that a sociopathic youngster's misbehavior, especially his aggressive outbursts, are motivated by his needs to ward off intimacy and fuel his conviction that he stands alone against an unsympathetic world, the therapist's active and interested response to this behavior negates its intended effect and tends to diminish its utility.

To avoid certain dangers inherent in the collusive technique the therapist must be careful not to suggest antisocial acts beyond those the youngster has committed and not to tolerate manipulations aimed directly at him. He must also avoid expressing so much pleasure in the youngster's misconduct that a developing positive relationship serves to increase rather than diminish the antisocial behavior. On the other hand, the sanctioning of delinquent behavior by pressing for its details is much less antitherapeutic with the psychopathic than with the symptomatic delinquent. Psychopathic delinquency originates in personality distortions that are much more basic than the patterns of parental fostering usually associated with symptomatic delinquency, and some increment in sanctioning is a small price to pay for establishing a relationship in which it may ultimately be possible to ameliorate the psychopathic delinquent's long-standing hatred and distrust and insensitivity to others.

Exercising Power. The supportive exercise of power often proves to be effective in convincing the psychopathic delinquent that his advantage lies on the therapist's good side, and his self-interest can then be relied on to foster a positive treatment relationship. Typically the therapist's allegiance and power will be tested early in the treatment by requests that he intercede with parents, teachers, or other authorities about some issue. At this point the youngster is all too ready to perceive the therapist as having little influence or, when the chips are down, siding with the establishment against him. Either way he can feel reinforced in his belief that he can rely only on himself, and he can then justify to himself no further engagement in the treatment. Thus it may initially be very important for the therapist to be able and willing to influence the youngster's environment on his behalf—for example, in prevailing on the parents to rescind a previous veto on his attendance at some social function or in persuading a teacher to allow him to make up an examination from which he was inexcusably absent.

In exercising such power to build the relationship the therapist must guard against being manipulated rather than tested. For the youngster to ask the therapist himself to engage in antisocial behavior (e.g., participating in or helping to plan a criminal act), to use his resources to get the youngster into trouble rather than out of it (e.g., providing him with amphetamines or other nonindicated prescription drugs), or to do the patently impossible (e.g., getting him a high school diploma without his completing the minimum requirements) represents provocation rather than a meaningful test of the therapist's power and interest, and must be responded to as such. Repetitive demands for the exercise of the therapist's power, without any significant progress in the relationship, similarly indicate manipulation. Each demonstration by the therapist of power and willingness to intercede should be followed by noticeably more positive participation by the youngster in the relationship. Furthermore, after a few such demonstrations testing should give way altogether to infrequent, modest appeals for help that can appropriately be given.

Stimulating and Variegated Sessions. The need for a stimulating and variegated treatment approach derives from the psychopathic youngster's characteristically nonverbal orientation, short time perspective, and boredom with the familiar. Attempts to treat the adolescent psychopath through regular, orderly conversations within the office hold little promise of success, no matter what the content of the conversations. Eissler (1950) and Gladstone (1962) among others have observed that many of these youngsters utilize antisocial acts to overcome boredom and make their lives more interesting and that their treatment accordingly requires a sufficient element of surprise to keep them stimulated and interested: "The earlier the delinquent is given an opportunity of experiencing the analyst's presence as something new, unforeseen, and surprising, the greater is the hope that the delinquent's treatment will take an effective course" (Eissler, 1950, p. 108).

To some extent such surprise is accomplished by the therapist's initially collusive approach; for example, Eisner (1945), in a session with a sexually delinquent girl at Cedar-Knowles who was caught running off with a boy just one day after promising she would never do it again, criticized her not for the broken promise but for her poor handling of the affair, including her selecting such an obvious place to run to that she was quickly discovered. In addition to saying the unexpected, the therapist must be ready to stop talking and leave the friendly confines of his office on the spur of the moment. A spontaneous visit to the coffee shop or the ping-pong table, a sudden shift of focus in the middle of a session ("It's too nice a day to stay inside—why don't you take me outside and show me the car you've been working on"), and similar variations from standard procedure are vital to gaining and sustaining the attention and interest of the psychopathic delinquent, aside from their obvious implications for building a positive treatment relationship.

Demonstrating Readiness to Give. The therapist must be able and willing to display deep and sustained interest in the mundane as well as in the abnormal aspects of the psychopathic delinquent's life, and he must also be prepared to back up his interest with concrete gifts of advice and sometimes money. If a boy wants to talk for hours about his search for a certain-size double-barrel carburetor, then the therapist must become an avid fan of double-barrel carburetors and perhaps educate himself on the subject with supplementary reading, even if he has never previously been motivated to raise the hood of his own car.

In line with the collusive approach, advice in this relationship-building phase refers not to advice on ethical conduct but rather specific help in coping with various life situations, as in the psychosocial approaches mentioned on page 328. As for gifts of money, Eissler (1950) comments that he has never treated a male delinquent without the necessity arising of giving him money, although such gifts are therapeutic only when they are expected and given without conditions attached. Routine gifts, gifts granted on demand or in response to promises of good behavior, and predictable gifts will do no more for building a relationship than the lavish favors of insensitive parents who attempt to purchase their youngster's affection with material gifts rather than by giving of themselves.

If these initial, relationship-building techniques successfully engage the psychopathic delinquent in treatment, he will gradually begin to identify with the therapist's nondelinquent behavior and attempt to suppress or control some of his own antisocial tendencies. Although it is occasionally suggested that the psychopathic youngster's incapacity for identification prevents any meaningful psychotherapy with him, it must be kept in mind that the pure psychopath, totally lacking in identificatory capacity, is as hypothetical as the individual who is thoroughly and unremittingly schizophrenic (see p. 316). Thus, although to the extent that his identificatory capacity is impaired the sociopathic delinquent will present special difficulties in the early stages of treatment, these difficulties are not necessarily insurmountable for the skilled and determined therapist who is able to implement the above-mentioned techniques.

Once the psychopathic youngster begins to incorporate some of his therapist's standards and behavior patterns, he will also begin to experience intrapsychic conflict. Since these therapeutically stimulated intrapsychic conflicts typically generate anxiety and neurotic symptoms similar to those experienced by the symptomatically delinquent youngster, the treatment can at some point be adjusted to emphasize these conflicts and the self-defeating consequences of delinquent behavior. In other words, the initial phase of treatment for the psychopathic delinquent can be construed in part as an effort to generate sufficient anxiety to develop him into a neurotically disturbed delinquent, at which point treatment for symptomatic delinquency can be instituted. Blos (1961) and Unwin (1968) have similarly stressed the technical necessity with such youngsters of turning their delinquency into a neurotic symptom: "The usual aim with these patients is to bring about the conversion of alloplastic behaviour into autoplastic symptoms" (Unwin, 1968, p. 115).

It must be recognized, however, that a considerable expenditure of time and energy may be necessary to generate neurotic symptoms in the psychopathic youngster. The therapist experienced mainly with symptomatic delinquents, whose antisocial behavior often diminishes soon after treatment is begun, may become too quickly discouraged in his efforts to help the psychopathic youngster; for example, Edwalds and Dimitri (1959, p. 615) report, "The adolescents with sociopathic personality disorders had to be discharged after one or two months in the hospital, since this type of adolescent exhibited little or no capacity for internalized anxiety, or for close relationships with others." Yet in Noshpitz' (1957) successful experience with such youngsters at the Topeka State Hospital, *two to four months* of the initial "psychopathic" treatment approach to such youngsters was necessary before shifts to neurotic symptom formation and improved behavior were noted. It is finally of interest to note Szurek's (1949, p. 123) comments that the appropriate treatment for such youngsters

". . . may offer a chance that such a child will become attached to the adult, and *if the relationship is continued long enough,* begin to identify with the adult's ideals, the adult's wishes for his own welfare, and to acquire a new sense of his own worth as a person. In short, he may be able to integrate the beginnings of a new self-respect, of a conscience or more conscience, and of more self-restraint."

REFERENCES

Ackerman, N. W. *The Psychodynamics of Family Life.* New York: Basic Books, 1958.

Aichhorn, A. (1925) *Wayward Youth.* New York: Viking, 1935.

Alexander, F. The neurotic character. *International Journal of Psychoanalysis,* 11:292–311, 1930.

Amos, W. E., Manella, R. L., and Southwell, M. A. *Action Programs for Delinquency Prevention.* Springfield, Ill.: Thomas, 1965.

Anderson, R. E. Where's Dad? Parental deprivation and delinquency. *Archives of General Psychiatry,* 18:641–649, 1968.

Assael, M., Kohen-Raz, R., and Alpern, S. Developmental analysis of EEG abnormalities in juvenile delinquents. *Diseases of the Nervous System,* 28:49–54, 1967.

Atcheson, J. D., and Williams, D. C. A study of juvenile sex offenders. *American Journal of Psychiatry,* 111:366–370, 1954.

Bandura, A., and Walters, R. H. Dependency conflicts in aggressive adolescents. *Journal of Social Issues,* **14**:52–65, 1958.

Bandura, A., and Walters, R. H. *Adolescent Aggression: A Study of the Influence of Child-Training Practices and Family Interrelationships.* New York: Ronald, 1959.

Barglow, P., Bornstein, M. B., Exum, D. B., Wright, M. K., and Visotsky, H. M. Some psychiatric aspects of illegitimate pregnancy during early adolescence. *American Journal of Orthopsychiatry,* **37**:266–267, 1967.

Becker, W. C., Peterson, D. R., Hellner, L. A., Shoemaker, D. J., and Quay, H. C. Factors in parental behavior and personality as related to problem behavior in children. *Journal of Consulting Psychology,* **23**:107–118, 1959.

Bender, L. Psychopathic personality disorders in childhood and adolescence. *Archives of Criminal Psychodynamics,* **4**:412–415, 1961.

Bergler, E. *Principles of Self-Damage.* New York: Philosophical Library, 1959.

Berman, S. Antisocial character disorder: Its etiology and relationship to delinquency. *American Journal of Orthopsychiatry,* **29**:612–621, 1959.

Berman, S. Techniques of treatment of a form of juvenile delinquency, the antisocial character disorder. *Journal of the American Academy of Child Psychiatry,* **3**:24–52, 1964.

Bernabeu, E. P. Underlying ego mechanisms in delinquency. *Psychoanalytic Quarterly,* **27**:383–396, 1958.

Blaine, G. R., and McArthur, C. C. Basic character disorders and homosexuality. In G. R. Blaine and C. C. McArthur, eds., *Emotional Problems of the Student.* New York: Appleton-Century-Crofts, 1961, pp. 100–115.

Bloch, H. A., and Niederhoffer, A. *The Gang: A Study in Adolescent Behavior.* New York: Philosophical Library, 1958.

Blos, P. Delinquency. In S. Lorand and H. I. Schneer, eds., *Adolescents: Psychoanalytic Approach to Problems and Therapy.* New York: Hoeber, 1961, pp. 132–151.

Bohlke, R. H. Social mobility, stratification inconsistency, and middle-class delinquency. *Social Problems,* **8**:351–363, 1961.

Bowlby, J. Forty-four juvenile thieves: Their characters and homelife. *International Journal of Psychoanalysis,* **25**:19–53, 107–128, 1944.

Briggs, P. F., and Wirt, R. D. Prediction. In H. C. Quay, ed., *Juvenile Delinquency: Research and Theory.* Princeton, N.J.: Van Nostrand, 1965, pp. 170–208.

Brigham, J. C., Ricketts, J. L., and Johnson, R. C. Reported maternal and paternal behaviors of solitary and social delinquents. *Journal of Consulting Psychology,* **31**:420–422, 1967.

Bromberg, W., and Rodgers, T. C. Authority in the treatment of delinquents. *American Journal of Orthopsychiatry,* **16**:672–685, 1946.

Brown, C. *Manchild in the Promised Land.* New York: Macmillan, 1965.

Carek, D. J., Hendrickson, W., and Holmes, D. J. Delinquency addiction in parents. *Archives of General Psychiatry,* **4**:357–362, 1961.

Carr, L. J. *Delinquency Control,* revised edition. New York: Harper, 1950.

Cavallin, H. Incestuous fathers: A clinical report. *American Journal of Psychiatry,* **122**:1132–1138, 1966.

Church, A. S. Adolescence and juvenile delinquency. *Nervous Child,* **4**:142–146, 1944.

Chwast, J. Depressive reactions as manifested among adolescent delinquents. *American Journal of Psychotherapy,* **21**:575–584, 1967.

Cleckley, H. M. Psychopathic states. In S. Arieti, ed., *American Handbook of Psychiatry,* Vol. I. New York: Basic Books, 1959, pp. 567–588.

Cleckley, H. *The Mask of Sanity,* 4th edition. St. Louis: Mosby, 1964.

Cloward, R., and Ohlin, L. E. *Delinquency and Opportunity: A Theory of Delinquent Gangs.* New York: Free Press of Glencoe, 1960.

Cohen, A. K. *Delinquent Boys: The Culture of the Gang.* Glencoe, Ill.: The Free Press, 1955.

Cormier, B. M., Kennedy, M., and Sangowicz, J. Psychodynamics of father-daughter incest. *Canadian Psychiatric Association Journal,* **7**:203–217, 1962.

Counts, R. M. Family crises and the impulsive adolescent. *Archives of General Psychiatry,* **17**:64–71, 1967.

Cowden, J. E. Differential test responses of two types of delinquent girls under authoritarian and permissive conditions. *Journal of Clinical Psychology,* **21**:397–399, 1965.

Craft, M., Stephenson, G., and Granger, C. A controlled trial of authoritarian and self-governing regimes with adolescent psychopaths. *American Journal of Orthopsychiatry,* **34**:543–554, 1964.

DeJong, R. N. "Psychomotor" and "temporal lobe" epilepsy: A review of the development of our present concepts. *Neurology,* **7**:1–14, 1957.

Diagnostic and Statistical Manual of Mental Disorders, 2nd edition. Washington, D.C.: American Psychiatric Association, 1968.

Easson, W. M. Projection as an etiological factor in "motiveless" delinquency. *Psychiatric Quarterly,* **41**:228–237, 1967.

Edwalds, R., and Dimitri, K. Treatment of the adolescent patient in a state hospital. *Psychiatric Quarterly,* **33**:615–622, 1959.

Eisner, E. A. Relationships formed by a sexually delinquent adolescent girl. *American Journal of Orthopsychiatry,* **15**:301–308, 1945.

Eissler, K. R. Ego-psychological implications of the psychoanalytic treatment of delinquents. *Psychoanalytic Study of the Child,* **5**:97–121, 1950.

Elkind, D. Middle-class delinquency. *Mental Hygiene,* **51**:80–84, 1967.

Elliott, D. S. Delinquency and perceived opportunity. *Sociological Inquiry,* **32**:216–227, 1962.

Erikson, E. H. The problem of ego identity. *Journal of the American Psychoanalytic Association,* **4**:56–121, 1956.

Ferdinand, T. N. *Typologies of Delinquency: A Critical Analysis.* New York: Random House, 1966.

Finch, S. M. *Fundamentals of Child Psychiatry.* New York: Norton, 1960.

Fleck, S. Pregnancy as a symptom of adolescent maladjustment. *International Journal of Social Psychiatry,* **2**:118–131, 1956.

Freud, S. (1916). Some character-types met with in psychoanalytic work. *Standard Edition,* Vol. XIV. London: Hogarth, 1957, pp. 311–333.

Friedlander, K. *The Psycho-Analytic Approach to Juvenile Delinquency.* New York: International Universities Press, 1947.

Friedlander, K. Latent deliquency and ego development. In K. R. Eissler, ed., *Searchlights on Delinquency.* New York: International Universities Press, 1949.

Gallenkamp, C. R., and Rychlak, J. F. Parental attitudes of sanction in middle-class adolescent male delinquents. *Journal of Social Psychology,* **75**:255–260, 1968.

Garvin, J. S. Psychomotor epilepsy: A clinicoencephalographic syndrome. *Journal of Nervous and Mental Disease,* **117**:1–8, 1953.

Giffin, M. E., Johnson, A. M., and Litin, E. M. Specific factors determining anti-social acting out. *American Journal of Orthopsychiatry,* **24**:668–684, 1954.

Gladstone, H. P. A study of techniques of psychotherapy with youthful offenders. *Psychiatry,* **25**:147–159, 1962.

Glaser, D. Social disorganization and delinquent subcultures. In H. C. Quay, ed., *Juvenile Delinquency: Research and Theory.* Princeton, N.J.: Van Nostrand, 1965, pp. 27–62.

Glueck, S., and Glueck, E. T. *Unraveling Juvenile Delinquency.* New York: Commonwealth Fund, 1950.

Glueck, S., and Glueck, E. *Physique and Delinquency.* New York: Harper and Bros., 1956.

Glueck, S., and Glueck, E. *Predicting Delinquency and Crime.* Cambridge, Mass.: Harvard University Press, 1960.

Glueck, S., and Glueck, E. *Family Environment and Delinquency.* Boston: Houghton-Mifflin, 1962.

Gordon, S. A psychotherapeutic approach to adolescents with character disorders. *American Journal of Orthopsychiatry,* **30**:757–766, 1960.

Gottschalk, L. A., Titchener, J. L., Piker, H. N., and Stewart, S. S. Psychosocial factors associated with pregnancy in adolescent girls: A preliminary report. *Journal of Nervous and Mental Disease,* **138**:524–534, 1964.

Grubler, E. R., and Gochman, S. I. Statistical observations regarding the clinical diagnosis of brain damage. *Psychological Reports,* **11**:221–222, 1962.

Guertin, W. H., Ladd, C. E., Frank, G. H., Rabin, A. I., and Hiester, D. S. Research with the Wechsler intelligence scales for adults: 1960–1965. *Psychological Bulletin,* **66**:385–409, 1966.

Hacker, F. J., and Geleerd, E. R. Freedom and authority in adolescence. *American Journal of Orthopsychiatry,* **15**:621–630, 1945.

Halleck, S. L. *Psychiatry and the Dilemmas of Crime.* New York: Harper and Row, 1967.

Herskovitz, H. H., Levine, M., and Spivack, G. Anti-social behavior of adolescents from higher socio-economic groups. *Journal of Nervous and Mental Disease*, **125**:1–9, 1959.

Jenkins, R. L. Adaptive and maladaptive delinquency. *Nervous Child*, **11**:9–11, 1955.

Jenkins, R. L. Motivation and frustration in delinquency. *American Journal of Orthopsychiatry*, **27**:528–537, 1957.

Jenkins, R. L. The psychopathic or antisocial personality. *Journal of Nervous and Mental Disease*, **131**:318–334, 1960.

Jenkins, R. L. Diagnoses, dynamics, and treatment in child psychiatry. *Psychiatric Research Report, American Psychiatric Association*, **18**:91–120, 1964.

Jenkins, R. L. Psychiatric syndromes in children and their relation to family background. *American Journal of Orthopsychiatry*, **36**:450–457, 1966.

Jenkins, R. L., and Boyer, A. Types of delinquent behavior and background factors. *International Journal of Social Psychiatry*, **14**:65–76, 1968.

Jenkins, R. L., and Glickman, S. Patterns of personality organization among delinquents. *Nervous Child*, **6**:329–339, 1947.

Jenkins, R. L., NurEddin, E., and Shapiro, I. Children's behavior syndromes and parental responses. *Genetic Psychology Monographs*, **74**:261–329, 1966.

Jenkins, R. L., and Pacella, B. L. Electroencephalographic studies of delinquent boys. *American Journal of Orthopsychiatry*, **13**:107–120, 1943.

Johnson, A. M. Sanctions for superego lacunae of adolescents. In K. R. Eissler, ed., *Searchlights on Delinquency*. New York: International Universities Press, 1949, pp. 225–245.

Johnson, A. M. Juvenile delinquency. In S. Arieti, ed., *American Handbook of Psychiatry*, Vol. I. New York: Basic Books, 1959, pp. 840–856.

Johnson, A. M., and Burke, E. C. Parental permissiveness and fostering in child rearing and their relationship to juvenile delinquency. *Proceedings of Staff Meetings, Mayo Clinic*, **30**:557–565, 1955.

Johnson, A. M., and Szurek, S. A. The genesis of antisocial acting out in children and adults. *Psychoanalytic Quarterly*, **21**:323–343, 1952.

Johnson, A. M., and Szurek, S. A. Etiology of antisocial behavior in delinquents and psychopaths. *Journal of the American Medical Association*, **154**:814–817, 1954.

Juvenile Court Statistics, 1966. Washington, D.C.: U.S. Children's Bureau Statistical Series, No. 90, 1967.

Kaufman, I., Durkin, H., Frank, T., Heims, L. W., Jones, D. B., Ryter, Z., Stone, E., and Zilbach, J. Delineation of two diagnostic groups among juvenile delinquents: The schizophrenic and the impulse-ridden character disorder. *Journal of the American Academy of Child Psychiatry*, **2**:292–318, 1963.

Kaufman, I., Peck, A. L., and Taguiri, C. K. The family constellation and overt incestuous relations between father and daughter. *American Journal of Orthopsychiatry*, **24**:266–279, 1954.

Kennedy, F., Hoffman, H. R., and Haines, W. H. A study of William Heirens. *American Journal of Psychiatry,* **104**:113–121, 1947.

Kvaraceus, W. C., and Miller, W. B. *Delinquent Behavior, Culture, and the Individual.* Washington, D.C.: National Educational Association, 1959.

Laufer, M. W. Cerebral dysfunction and behavior disorders in adolescents. *American Journal of Orthopsychiatry,* **32**:501–506, 1962.

Leventhal, T. Control problems in runaway children. *Archives of General Psychiatry,* **9**:122–128, 1963.

Lindesmith, A. R., and Dunham, H. W. Some principles of criminal typology. *Social Forces,* **19**:307–314, 1941.

Litin, E. M., Giffin, M. E., and Johnson, A. M. Parental influence in unusual sexual behavior in children. *Psychoanalytic Quarterly,* **25**:37–55, 1956.

London, N. J., and Myers, J. K. Young offenders: Psychopathology and social factors. *Archives of General Psychiatry,* **4**:274–282, 1961.

Loomis, S. D. EEG abnormalities as a correlate of behavior in adolescent male delinquents. *American Journal of Psychiatry,* **121**:1003–1006, 1965.

Loomis, S. D., Bohnert, P. J., and Huncke, S. Prediction of EEG abnormalities in adolescent delinquents. *Archives of General Psychiatry,* **17**:494–497, 1967.

Lustig, N., Dresser, J. W., Spellman, S. W., and Murray, T. B. Incest: A family group survival pattern. *Archives of General Psychiatry,* **14**:31–40, 1966.

McCord, W., and McCord, J. *Origins of Crime.* New York: Columbia University Press, 1959.

McCord, W., and McCord, J. *The Psychopath: An Essay on the Criminal Mind.* Princeton, N.J.: Van Nostrand, 1964.

McCord, W., McCord, J., and Verden, P. Family relationships and sexual deviance in lower-class adolescents. *International Journal of Social Psychiatry,* **8**:165–179, 1962.

Machotka, P., Pittman, F. S., and Flomenhaft, K. Incest as a family affair. *Family Process,* **6**:98–116, 1967.

Manne, S. H. A communication theory of sociopathic personality. *American Journal of Psychotherapy,* **21**:797–807, 1967.

Marans, A. E. The psychological impact of pregnancy on the adolescent girl. In F. P. Heald, Ed., *Adolescent Gynecology.* Baltimore: Williams and Wilkins, 1966, pp. 130–147.

Markey, O. B. A study of aggressive sex misbehavior in adolescents brought to juvenile court. *American Journal of Orthopsychiatry,* **20**:719–731, 1950.

Marwell, G. Adolescent powerlessness and delinquent behavior. *Social Problems,* **14**:35–47, 1966.

Massimo, J. L., and Shore, M. F. The effectiveness of a comprehensive, vocationally-oriented psychotherapeutic program for adolescent delinquent boys. *American Journal of Orthopsychiatry,* **33**:634–642, 1963.

Miller, D. *Growth to Freedom: The Psychosocial Treatment of Delinquent Youth.* Bloomington, Ind.: Indiana University Press, 1965.

Miller, W. B. Lower-class culture as a generating milieu of gang delinquency. *Journal of Social Issues,* **14**:5–19, 1958.

Monahan, T. P. Family status and the delinquent child: A reappraisal and some new findings. *Social Forces,* **35**:250–258, 1957.

Murphy, F. J., Shirley, M. M., and Witmer, H. L. The incidence of hidden delinquency. *American Journal of Orthopsychiatry,* **16**:686–696, 1946.

Noshpitz, J. D. Opening phase in the psychotherapy of adolescents with character disorders. *Bulletin of the Menninger Clinic,* **21**:153–164, 1957.

Nye, F. I. *Family Relationships and Delinquent Behavior.* New York: Wiley, 1958.

Nye, F. I., Short, J. F., and Olson, V. J. Socio-economic status and delinquent behavior. In F. I. Nye, ed., *Family Relationships and Delinquent Behavior.* New York: Wiley, 1958, pp. 23–33.

Offer, D., Sabshin, M., and Marcus, D. Clinical evaluation of normal adolescents. *American Journal of Psychiatry,* **121**:864–872, 1965.

Palmgren, L. Sociopsychiatric investigation of teenage girls with gonorrhea. *Acta Psychiatrica Scandinavica,* **42**:295–314, 1966.

Papanek, E. Re-education and treatment of juvenile delinquents. *American Journal of Psychotherapy,* **12**:269–296, 1958.

Papanek, E. Management of the acting-out adolescent. *American Journal of Psychotherapy,* **18**:418–434, 1964.

Patterson, F. *Victory Over Myself.* New York: Bernard Geis Associates, 1963.

Persons, R. W. Psychological and behavioral change in delinquents following psychotherapy. *Journal of Clinical Psychology,* **22**:337–340, 1966.

Persons, R. W. Relationship between psychotherapy with institutionalized boys and subsequent community adjustment. *Journal of Consulting Psychology,* **31**:137–141, 1967.

Peterson, D. R., and Becker, W. C. Family interaction and delinquency. In H. C. Quay, ed., *Juvenile Delinquency: Research and Theory.* Princeton, N.J.: Van Nostrand, 1965, pp. 63–99.

Peterson, D. R., Quay, H. C., and Cameron, G. R. Personality and background factors in juvenile delinquency as inferred from questionnaire responses. *Journal of Consulting Psychology,* **23**:395–399, 1959.

Peterson, D. R., Quay, H. C., and Tiffany, T. L. Personality factors related to juvenile delinquency. *Child Development,* **32**:355–372, 1961.

Pope, B., and Scott, W. H. *Psychological Diagnosis in Clinical Practice.* New York: Oxford University Press, 1967.

Pope, H. Unwed mothers and their sex partners. *Journal of Marriage and the Family,* **29**:555–567, 1967.

Porterfield, A. L. Delinquency and its outcome in court and college. *American Journal of Sociology,* **49**:199–208, 1943.

Powers, E., and Witmer, H. *An Experiment in the Prevention of Delinquency: The Cambridge-Sommerville Youth Study.* New York: Columbia University Press, 1951.

Quay, H. C. Personality and delinquency. In H. C. Quay, ed., *Juvenile Delinquency: Research and Theory.* Princeton, N.J.: Van Nostrand, 1965, pp. 139–169.

Quay, H. C., Peterson, D. R., and Consalvi, C. The interpretation of three personality factors in juvenile delinquency. *Journal of Consulting Psychology,* **24**:555, 1960.

Rainwater, L. Some aspects of lower class sexual behavior. *Journal of Social Issues,* **22**:96–108, 1966.

Randolph, M. H., Richardson, H., and Johnson, R. C. A comparison of social and solitary delinquents. *Journal of Consulting Psychology,* **25**:293–295, 1961.

Reik, T. *Masochism in Modern Man.* New York: Farrar Strauss, 1941.

Reiss, A. J. Social correlates of psychological types of delinquency. *American Sociological Review,* **17**:710–718, 1952.

Rhodes, W. C. Delinquency and community action. In H. C. Quay, ed., *Juvenile Delinquency: Research and Theory.* Princeton, N.J.: Van Nostrand, 1965, pp. 209–262.

Ricks, D., Umbarger, C., and Mack, R. A measure of increased temporal perspective in successfully treated adolescent delinquent boys. *Journal of Abnormal and Social Psychology,* **69**:685–689, 1964.

Robey, A., Rosenwald, R. J., Snell, J. E., and Lee, R. E. The runaway girl: A reaction to family stress. *American Journal of Orthopsychiatry,* **34**:762–767, 1964.

Robins, L. N. *Deviant Children Grown Up: A Sociological and Psychiatric Study of Sociopathic Personality.* Baltimore: Williams and Wilkins, 1966.

Rosen, B. M., Bahn, A. K., Shellow, R., and Bower, E. M. Adolescent patients served in outpatient psychiatric clinics. *American Journal of Public Health,* **55**:1563–1577, 1965.

Sakel, M. *Epilepsy.* New York: Philosophical Library, 1958.

Sarason, I. G. Verbal learning, modeling, and juvenile delinquency. *American Psychologist,* **23**:254–266, 1968.

Schachtel, E. G. Notes on Rorschach tests of 500 juvenile delinquents and a control group of 500 non-delinquent adolescents. *Journal of Projective Techniques,* **15**:144–172, 1951.

Schafer, R. *Clinical Application of Psychological Tests.* New York: International Universities Press, 1948.

Schmideberg, M. The psycho-analysis of asocial children and adolescents. *International Journal of Psycho-Analysis,* **16**:22–48, 1935.

Schulman, I. Dynamics and treatment of antisocial psychopathology in adolescents. *Nervous Child,* **11**:35–41, 1955.

Schwartz, L. J. Treatment of the adolescent psychopath: Theory and case report. *Psychotherapy: Theory, Research, and Practice,* **4**:133–137, 1967.

Sellin, T., and Wolfgang, M. E. *The Measurement of Delinquency.* New York: Wiley, 1964.

Serrano, A. C., McDonald, E. C., Goolishian, H. A., MacGregor, R., and Ritchie, A. M. Adolescent maladjustment and family dynamics. *American Journal of Psychiatry,* **118**:897–901, 1962.

Shanley, F. J. Middle-class delinquency as a social problem. *Sociology and Social Research,* **51**:185–198, 1967.

Shaw, C. R., and McKay, H. D. *Juvenile Delinquency and Urban Areas.* Chicago: University of Chicago Press, 1942.

Shellow, R., Schamp, J. R., Liebow, E., and Unger, E. Suburban runaways of the 1960's. *Monographs of the Society for Research in Child Development,* **32**:1–51, 1967.

Shinohara, M., and Jenkins, R. L. MMPI study of three types of delinquents. *Journal of Clinical Psychology,* **23**:156–163, 1967.

Shoor, M., Speed, M. H., and Bartelt, C. Syndrome of the adolescent child molester. *American Journal of Psychiatry,* **122**:783–789, 1966.

Shore, M. F., and Massimo, J. L. Mobilization of community resources in the outpatient treatment of adolescent delinquent boys: A case report. *Community Mental Health Journal,* **2**:329–332, 1966a.

Shore, M. F., and Massimo, J. L. Comprehensive vocationally oriented psychotherapy for adolescent delinquent boys: A follow-up study. *American Journal of Orthopsychiatry,* **36**:609–615, 1966b.

Shore, M. F., Massimo, J. L., Kisielewski, J., and Moran, J. K. Object relations changes resulting from successful psychotherapy with adolescent delinquents and their relationship to academic performance. *Journal of the American Academy of Child Psychiatry,* **5**:93–104, 1966.

Shore, M. F., Massimo, J. L., and Mack, R. Changes in the perception of interpersonal relationships in successfully treated adolescent delinquent boys. *Journal of Consulting Psychology,* **29**:213–217, 1965.

Short, J. F. Social structure and group processes in explorations of gang delinquency. In M. Sherif and C. W. Sherif, eds., *Problems of Youth: Transition to Adulthood in a Changing World.* Chicago: Aldine, 1965, pp. 155–188.

Sobel, R. Treatment of character-conditioned hostility in adolescents. *Nervous Child,* **8**:301–310, 1949.

Stevens, J. R. Psychiatric implications of psychomotor epilepsy. *Archives of General Psychiatry,* **14**:461–471, 1966.

Szurek, S. Notes on the genesis of psychopathic personality trends. *Psychiatry,* **5**:1–6, 1942.

Szurek, S. A. Some impressions from clinical experience with delinquents. In K. R. Eissler, ed., *Searchlights on Delinquency.* New York: International Universities Press, 1949, pp. 115–127.

Tiffany, T. L., Peterson, D. R., and Quay, H. C. Types and traits in the study of juvenile delinquency. *Journal of Clinical Psychology,* **17**:19–24, 1961.

Toolan, J. M. Depression in children and adolescents. *American Journal of Orthopsychiatry,* **32**:404–415, 1962.

Topping, R. Treatment of the pseudo-social boy. *American Journal of Orthopsychiatry,* **13**:353–360, 1943.

Unwin, J. R. Stages in the therapy of hospitalized acting-out adolescents. *Canadian Psychiatric Association Journal,* **13**:115–119, 1968.

Vedder, C. B. *Juvenile Offenders.* Springfield, Ill.: Thomas, 1963.

Vincent, C. E. *Unmarried Mothers.* New York: Free Press of Glencoe, 1961.

Visotsky, H. M. A project for unwed pregnant adolescents in Chicago. *Clinical Pediatrics,* **5**:322–324, 1966.

Vogel, E. F., and Bell, N. F. The emotionally disturbed child as a family scapegoat. *Psychoanalysis and the Psychoanalytic Review,* **47**:21–42, 1960.

Waggoner, R. W., and Boyd, D. A. Juvenile aberrant sexual behavior. *American Journal of Orthopsychiatry,* **11**:275–291, 1941.

Wallinga, J. V. A study of adolescent auto theft. *Journal of the American Academy of Child Psychiatry,* **3**:126–139, 1964.

Walters, P. A. Promiscuity in adolescence. *American Journal of Orthopsychiatry,* **35**:670–675, 1965.

Wattenberg, W., and Balistrieri, J. Automobile theft: A favored group delinquency. *American Journal of Sociology,* **57**:575–579, 1952.

Weiner, I. B. Father-daughter incest: A clinical report. *Psychiatric Quarterly,* **36**:607–632, 1962.

Weiner, I. B. On incest: A survey. *Excerpta Criminologica,* **4**:137–155, 1964.

Wiener, J. M., Delano, J. G, and Klass, D. W. An EEG study of delinquent and nondelinquent adolescents. *Archives of General Psychiatry,* **15**:144–150, 1966.

Wirt, R. D., and Briggs, P. F. Personality and environmental factors in the development of delinquency. *Psychological Monographs,* No. 73 (Whole No. 485), 1959.

Wirt, R. D., and Briggs, P. F. The meaning of delinquency. In H. C. Quay, ed., *Juvenile Delinquency: Research and Theory.* Princeton, N.J.: Van Nostrand, 1965, pp. 1–26.

Witmer, H. L., and Tufts, E. *The Effectiveness of Delinquency Prevention Programs.* Washington, D.C.: U.S. Children's Bureau Publication No. 350, 1954.

Woods, S. M. Adolescent violence and homicide: Ego disruption and the 6 and 14 dysrhythmia. *Archives of General Psychiatry,* **5**:528–534, 1961.

CHAPTER 9

Psychotherapy

Psychotherapy with disturbed adolescents is a demanding task that is sought by some clinicians, approached with trepidation by many, and eschewed by most. The reluctance of otherwise skilled clinicians to grapple with adolescent problems and the very small cadre of therapists who are competent in work with his age group are well known to practitioners in the field. Empirical data indicate that adolescents are the largest users of psychiatric clinics in the United States but that only one-third receive treatment in these clinics, with the remainder receiving only intake or other diagnostic services (Rosen et al., 1965, p. 1565). In contrast, 55.7% of the 18- to 64-year-old patients terminated from psychiatric clinics in 1966 had received treatment (*Outpatient Psychiatric Clinics,* 1966, p. 14). Although these findings could reflect greater need for treatment among adult than among adolescent patients, they also suggest the hypothesis of many lost opportunities to help young people avert subsequent, more serious psychological breakdown.

The difficulties of psychotherapeutic work with adolescents have been stressed even by clinicians who are distinguished for their contributions in this area. Anna Freud (1958, p. 261) describes the analytic treatment of adolescents as "a hazardous venture from beginning to end"; Josselyn (1957, p. 13) considers treatment of the young adolescent "perhaps the most challenging, the most frustrating, the most baffling, the most anxiety-arousing . . . experience a psychiatrist can have"; and Lorand (1961, pp. 239–240) comments that the adolescent's characteristic impatience, uncommunicativeness, lack of insight, and refusal to cooperate can often discourage a therapist from even trying to create a therapeutic atmosphere.

Such cautions notwithstanding, most disturbed adolescents are remarkably accessible to psychotherapeutic intervention. The major personality developments that occur during the teenage years and the adolescent's usual freedom from crystallized patterns of psychological disturbance frequently provide therapists a unique opportunity to facilitate positive behavior change (see Harris and Heald, 1957; Martin, 1963; Nichols and Rutledge, 1965). Gallagher and Harris (1964, p. 64) conclude from their experience at the Boston Children's Hospital that adolescents "because of their flexibility and resilience . . . usually respond with gratifying ease and speed to proper treatment." Balser (1966) reports that approximately 80% of the psychological disturbances that develop during adolescence respond well to short-term therapy, with only a minority requiring long-term treatment or hospitalization.

Although adolescents are accessible to psychotherapy and able to derive considerable benefit from it, their treatment usually requires frames of reference that differ from those that guide work with child or adult patients. Most children are brought by their parents for help, are engaged primarily through play techniques, and relate to the therapist as to a benign, understanding parent. The typical adult patient voluntarily seeks help for matters of concern to him, participates in psychotherapy primarily through spontaneously reported thoughts and feelings, and construes the situation as a cooperative endeavor to comprehend and resolve his difficulties. The adolescent, because of his transitional point in the life cycle, is often too old to accept the adult therapist as a substitute parent and too mature to utilize play techniques, yet still too young to recognize and seek help for his psychological difficulties and too immature to communicate his underlying concerns and fantasies through free-associative techniques (see Axelrod, Cameron, and Solomon, 1944; Hellman, 1964; Schaeffer, 1962).

In practice the appropriate psychotherapeutic approach to the adolescent youngster will vary considerably with his particular level of development. The younger and less mature he is, the more properly his treatment will incorporate aspects of child therapy, especially games; the older and more mature he is, the more likely he will be to desire treatment for himself and to understand its necessity, and the more closely his therapy will resemble that of an adult with similar problems (Fraiberg, 1955; Geleerd, 1957). The following examples indicate the importance of a youngster's maturity rather than his chronological age in determining the style in which his therapy can best be approached.

> Joseph at 15 was an undersized, childish-looking, only child who spent most of his time with his parents at the expense of meaningful peer-group engagements. He was a well-dressed, polite, composed boy who made a good impression on adults and responded intelligently to their questions. Conversational therapy could easily have been initiated with him but probably would have continued indefinitely in an unspontaneous, affectively bland, and unproductive fashion.

However, recognizing the pseudomaturity of his overt behavior and his underlying emotional immaturity, the therapist utilized competitive games as the main currency of the treatment. As in child therapy, the give-and-take around these games resulted in considerable affective interchange and the generation of thoughts and feelings that might otherwise have remained inaccessible.

Alan J———, on the other hand, who at 16 was only one year older than Joseph, was a tall, grown-up looking, deep-voiced boy who arrived for his first interview in suit and vest and introduced himself as "Mr. J———." Although Alan was underachieving in school, primarly in relation to conflicts involving his father, and was viewed by his peers as somewhat pompous and stuffy, the clinical data suggested that his rush to maturity was in the main adaptive and consistent with his basically pedantic, intellectual personality style. Without overtly admitting to personality problems Alan professed from the beginning of his therapy a sincere interest in being helped to improve his grades. Throughout the treatment the therapist addressed him as "Mr. J———," as he would an adult patient, and conducted the interviews in the relatively unstructured fashion appropriate to intensive psychotherapy with adults.

The following sections elaborate several key aspects of psychotherapy with the adolescent: depth and goals, initiating the treatment, building the relationship, termination, and work with parents. Although the discussion is directed primarily toward individual, dynamically oriented, outpatient treatment, many of the principles outlined have relevance for other modalities of treating disturbed youngsters.[1] It should also be noted that these general principles do not transcend the specific guidelines for treating schizophrenic, depressed, suicidal, school-phobic, underachieving, and delinquent youngsters, which are reviewed in Chapters 4 through 8.

DEPTH AND GOALS

Psychotherapy must always be planned in terms of the treatment depth and goals that are most appropriate to the needs, motives, and personality

---

[1] Other modalities that are commonly applied to the treatment of adolescents include group psychotherapy (see Clements, 1966; Godenne, 1964; MacLennan and Felsenfeld, 1968; Slavson, 1965), family psychotherapy (see Ackerman, 1966, Chapter 8; Kimbro et al., 1967; McGregor et al., 1964), behavior modification (see Kolvin, 1967; Schwitzgebel, 1967; Weiner, 1967), and residential treatment (see Beckett, 1965; Beskind, 1962; Greaves and Regan, 1957; Holmes, 1964, Chapters 12–15).

resources of the individual patient. As traditionally defined, depth of treatment pertains to the extent to which a patient's defenses are to be probed for whatever unconscious conflicts and previous painful experiences have generated them or are instead to be supported and strengthened in reference to conscious concerns and current problem solving. The goals of the treatment correspondingly involve the degree to which therapist and patient aim at significant increments in self-understanding and personality reorganization—or rather at stabilization and improved functioning without major personality change.

For most adolescents psychotherapy cannot be usefully directed toward stripping away the defensive structure, reworking previous experience, achieving deep insights, or reorganizing the personality. Teenage youngsters are integrating hosts of new biological, social, heterosexual, and academic experiences, and adolescent personality development is largely defined by a major thrust toward the establishment and consolidation of a consistent style of coping with life events. In moving toward identity consolidation most youngsters are experimenting with a variety of coping styles to which they have no deep or lasting commitment. Hence, since much of the adolescent's behavior does not reflect stable or well-defined defenses that systematically cover underlying conflicts, psychotherapeutic efforts to weaken and penetrate his defensive style tend to be unproductive.

Efforts to strip away defenses are furthermore likely to mobilize considerable anxiety in the adolescent youngster, to the detriment of his engagement in the treatment. Repetitive interpretations of his coping behavior not only constrain a youngster from the normal adolescent business of experimenting but also convince him that the therapist is picky, hostile, disapproving, or pessimistic about his future. For the therapist to focus extensively on irrational and unconscious motives for his behavior tends to communicate to the youngster, "I don't think much of you" or "I don't see much hope for you," both of which darken his perceptions of the treatment relationship.

As for achieving deep insights and reworking previous experience, the adolescent typically has little patience with rehashing the vicissitudes of his earlier years. The present, with its manifold complexities and uncertainties, is too much with him for him to spare energy or concern on matters he considers over and done with. Furthermore his needs to view himself as a maturing, almost adult, almost self-sufficient individual make it embarrassing and distasteful for him to review his childish foibles of only a few years earlier. Laufer (1964a) similarly notes that the recovery of past events and affects may threaten an adolescent's efforts to free himself from the past, and Miller (1959, p. 774) observes that youngsters are usually correct in their conviction that current rather than past experiences are more relevant to resolving their psychological difficulties: "For an adolescent in search of an identity, overcoming the fears and failures of the moment is much more important than knowing the events which led up to them."

These reservations concerning a depth approach apply even to many late adolescents. Blaine (1961) and Braiman (1967) endorse nonanalytic psychotherapeutic intervention as the treatment of choice in the college setting, and Farnsworth (1966, p. 34) draws the same conclusion from his experience with college students:

"The problems of adolescence usually cannot be treated by the development of deep insights. Sometimes the youngsters are angered by attempts to get at the deeper reasons for their behavior. There is little to be gained by such attempts. Instead, work should be done on the present situation, on the ego strength."

The concept of personality reorganization is similarly inappropriate to the goals of adolescent psychotherapy. Personality structure is usually still in a formative stage during the adolescent years, and most troubled teenagers have no firm personality organization that needs undoing before more adaptive developments can be fostered:

"Treatment which is directed toward the dissolution of past difficulties will not assist him sufficiently in his search for ways to invest his new drives and interests. The treatment of the adolescent must accordingly be an active process directed toward what he is able to become" (Robinson, 1957, p. 77).

This emphasis on personality development and consolidation in adolescent psychotherapy has been formulated by Berman (1957), Gitelson (1948), Josselyn (1952, Chapter IX), Wittenberg (1955), and others in terms of promoting ego adequacy and synthesis. From this point of view the goal of psychotherapeutic work with adolescent youngsters is to provide them a new emotional experience that will strengthen the functions of their ego and permit adaptive character synthesis. Adaptive character synthesis is achieved when a youngster can manage his biological tensions and other impulses comfortably, can relate realistically to his parents and other adults, and can channel his creative and productive energies into rewarding social and educational accomplishments.

Despite its emphasis on immediacy, the ego-synthesis approach to psychotherapy of the adolescent does not preclude efforts to enhance the youngster's self-understanding. To consolidate rewarding patterns of managing needs and impulses, relating to others, and channeling creative and productive energies the disturbed adolescent needs to understand to the limit of his capacity the manner in which his current attitudes, feelings, and behavior may be impeding such consolidation. Masterson (1958, p. 513) summarizes this treatment focus in the following way:

"The therapist does not expect the patient to locate and identify emotions but rather attempts to anticipate and clarify the patient's emotional reactions for him, pointing out the distortions. He minimizes the historical aspect of the relationship by focusing treatment on the contemporary level, clarifying present reactions, pointing out distortions, and responding in such a way as to give the patient a corrective emotional experience."

Specifically, then, psychotherapy of the adolescent will typically not involve an ontogenetic reconstruction of his personality style, but it will encourage him to look critically at his current behavior patterns and recognize their unrealistic, self-defeating characteristics. Interpretations of present rather than past experiences will be the most common aspect of this limited-insight approach, as illustrated in the following types of therapist observation: "It sounds like you're afraid to speak up to your father but get back at him by managing to get poor grades"; "I don't think it's just starting in at the high school building that's bothering you, I think you're generally not too happy with the whole idea of growing up"; "It seems to me that you're turning people off by acting more grouchy than you really feel—maybe you don't like the prospect of having people get too close to you, even though you feel you'd like to have more friends." Given adequate personality resources and the building of a positive treatment relationship, the adolescent will usually be abe to utilize such interpretations as a first step in learning new and more adequate ways of coping with his experience.

INITIATING THE TREATMENT

A swift, incisive launching of the treatment relationship is vital to successful psychotherapeutic work with the adolescent, often more so than with other age groups. Most children are oblivious to the significance of therapy and come prepared to play some games in the office or "the school part of the hospital"; adults, whatever their knowledge or estimation of psychotherapy, typically come prepared to see what talking with a professional person will be like and to make a judgment of whether psychotherapy might benefit them. The adolescent has neither the naivete of the child nor the options of the adult. He knows full well that he is being brought to the "shrink" by others who are empowered to legislate his continued attendance at sessions. Even if he has realized some of his personal problems, he is likely to be acutely embarrassed at having actually been brought for help and to welcome any excuse for summarily deciding that therapy is irrelevant to his needs or that the particular therapist is insensitive to his problem.

In view of the adolescent's customary apprehension and aversion, the therapist should consider that his most important task in the first session will usually be to conduct it in such a way that the youngster returns willingly for a second. In other words, "The first order of business in the treatment of the adolescent is to get him into treatment, and the next is to keep him there" (Holmes, 1964, p. 123). In the absence of emergency situations requiring immediate diagnostic judgments, such as the need for hospitalization or precautions against suicide, the therapist should therefore concentrate initially on fostering the youngster's willingness to participate in a treatment relationship. To generate such willingness the therapist must strive in the initial interviews (a) to allow the youngster to be comfortable, (b) to engage him beyond the level of the superficial and obvious, and (c) to get him to acknowledge and respect his own role in determining the course of the treatment.

Allowing Comfort

The adolescent usually begins the first interview uncertain of what to expect and hard put to suppress his apprehension. Children can turn to play and adults can occupy themselves with presenting their complaints, symptoms, and social history while they are appraising the situation. But the adolescent cannot be directed toward the toy chest, and for the most part he has no verbal content with which to begin. The complaints and symptoms that have brought him are largely the concern of his parents, school, or pediatrician, and he sees little reason to review his background with a total stranger whose role is unclear to him.

Hence, if initially undirected, tested with unstructured questions, requested to expose deep personal feelings, or challenged to account for problem situations, most youngsters will become extremely uncomfortable. Some will angrily refuse to respond, some will squirm in painful silence, some may even burst into tears and dash out of the office. To avoid such an impasse the therapist needs to minimize the youngster's initial discomfort by actively directing the interview toward benign factual information and by not asking him to explain his behavior or elaborate on his feelings.

The therapist's opening remarks should be carefully weighed in terms of these guidelines for promoting comfort. Even an apparently innocuous invitation to discuss the problem ("What brings you here?") may unnecessarily increase the adolescent's initial anxiety level. He may be unsure why he has been brought, in which case he is embarrassed at having no answer to the question; or he knows the reason—which is almost always some inadequacy, failure, or misbehavior on his part—and is now in the position of having been asked to put his worst foot forward. Furthermore an initial question like "What brings you here?" is likely to suggest to the youngster that the therapist has not bothered to acquaint himself in advance with the situation that precipitated the referral, in which case he appears to be disinterested and inert; or that he is asking a question to which he already knows the answer, which will stamp him as devious and untrustworthy in the youngster's eyes.

In contrast, a beginning like "I understand you've been having some problems in school—what's it like?" is straightforward without restricting the youngster's alternatives in responding. He can plunge right in with talk about his poor grades or unruly behavior, if these are the problem, or he can temporize with superficial, "safe" comments about what the school is objectively like—its building, classes, students, teachers, and so forth. Mention of any such subjects provides an opening for further specific inquiries ("How many are there in your class?" "Do you have men or women teachers, or both?") that yield potentially useful information and at the same time facilitate an active, relatively comfortable verbal interchange.

With regard to explaining behavior and elaborating feelings, such questions as "Why do you think you've been taking things from stores?" or "How do you feel about your father?" will seldom stimulate a productive exchange early in the treatment relationship. Because of embarrassment, concern about being criticized, or uncertainty about how far the therapist can be trusted, the youngster will be reluctant to dredge up and share intense feelings with him. On the other hand, a differently phrased question such as "What's your father like?" allows the youngster the option of venting feelings, if he is ready to do so, or of maintaining comfortable communication with a simple description of the father's objective physical characteristics.

Although comfortable, mutual communication is necessary in initiating the treatment of adolescents, the therapist can and should modify his primary focus on comfort as soon as the youngster is ready. A consistently comfortable treatment relationship is as detrimental to effective psychotherapy as an initial failure to make the youngster comfortable. Continuing smooth, pleasant conversations with the adolescent patient, unmarred by rapid shifts in his willingness to talk, repetitive questions about the purpose of his coming, and expressions of dissatisfaction with the therapist's efforts constitute deceptive collaboration (see p. 334) and indicate failure to achieve the second crucial element in initiating psychotherapy—namely, engagement.

Achieving Engagement

To engage his adolescent patient the therapist must impress him that this relationship will differ significantly from most relationships he has experienced with parents, peers, teachers, and other well-meaning people who have attempted to help him with his difficulties. Specifically, the therapist needs to demonstrate that his special knowledge and training allow him to perceive thoughts and feelings that are not put into words, and that he furthermore intends to use this sensitivity to help the youngster understand himself better and develop more rewarding ways of coping with his experience.

The therapist displays his ability and willingness to go beyond the face value of things by beginning as soon as he feels the youngster can tolerate it to challenge or interpret superficial aspects of his behavior in the interview situation: "I find it hard to believe that *all* of your teachers have it in for you" or "You say you couldn't care less, but from the look on your face I'd say you were pretty burned up about it." Without such therapist efforts at engagement the adolescent is unlikely to regard treatment as anything more than a pleasant interlude in which he can discuss mundane topics of his choice with an accepting, unthreatening adult. He will not come to perceive the relationship or the therapist as being able to offer anything special or different from what other kindly, attentive adults provide him. For some emotionally deprived youngsters pleasant interpersonal interludes may in themselves be significantly therapeutic. Most adolescents, however, will soon tire or despair of a comfortable but nonengaging treatment relationship, because it presents them no evidence that the therapist has any particular capacity to understand or help them modify their behavior.

Whereas efforts to achieve engagement typically follow the establishment of comfort in the youngster who comes to his first session overtly apprehensive, different priorities obtain for the teenager who has steeled himself before hand to remain uninvolved in the proceedings. Without appearing anxious or blocked, this type of youngster sits steadfastly in his chair, steeped in petulance and scorn, and refuses to respond beyond an occasional grunt or uninformative monosyllable; or he fixes the therapist with a hostile stare and tells him in no uncertain terms that he was forced to come, that there is nothing the matter with him, and that he is not about to have anything to do with any psychology business; or he maintains a derisive, patronizing smirk, answering questions politely but all the while conveying the impression of laughing up his sleeve; or he uses a buddy-buddy, it's-all-a-big-mistake approach, in which he affects a friendly nonchalance, points out at length how well he is getting along, and emphasizes,

"It's got nothing at all to do with you, Doc, you seem like a nice guy, but you should work on all those kids that really have troubles and need you—I just don't."

Although such initial behaviors derive from underlying discomfort, they insulate the youngster from situational anxiety so well that efforts to promote his comfort make little headway. With such a youngster the therapist must immediately search for some means of engaging him; of penetrating his facade of anger, scorn, or bravado; and of shaking him free from his disengaged stance long enough to allow some real relationship to be engendered. The following exchanges illustrate initial attempts to engage youngsters who presented in this way:

PATIENT: I don't mind being here, but I want you to know there's no reason for it.
THERAPIST: So why did you come?
PATIENT: My mother told me I had to.
THERAPIST: Do you always do what your mother tells you to?

[This question obliges the youngster to admit either (a) that he is totally dependent on, and subservient to, his mother, (b) that some type of bribe or condition was attached to his coming, or (c) that, if he denies total subservience to his mother, there must be something more than her request involved in his actually keeping the appointment. Each of these alternatives has some potential for injecting engagement into the patient-therapist communication.]

THERAPIST: You seem awfully mad that I'm asking a few questions. What's bothering you?
PATIENT: I've already made up my mind I'm not going to talk to you.
THERAPIST: Why not?
PATIENT: There's nothing wrong with me, I don't have any problems, and it's none of your business anyway.
THERAPIST: Maybe there is nothing wrong with you and maybe it is none of my business. But don't tell me you don't have any problems. Your folks are fed up with you and your principal's getting ready to bounce you out of school; that adds up to trouble no matter how you slice it. Maybe it's not your fault, but I'd at least like to hear your side of the story.

[The opportunity to defend himself is hard to resist for the youngster who feels put upon, and his self-justifications usually provide openings for engaged communication; similarly, for the therapist thus to identify trouble and offer to help with it, without assuming or implying that the youngster is responsible for the trouble, often softens an initial refusal to talk.]

The therapist should balance these comfort and engagement techniques in his initial approach to an adolescent patient according to the youngster's needs. From observing his new patient in the waiting room, exchanging greetings with him, and getting him seated in the office, the therapist should already have a fairly good idea of whether the youngster is anxious and frightened and needs first to be made comfortable or is hostile and resistive and requires above all to be engaged. As the initial treatment phase proceeds it will be important for the therapist to shift his emphasis as the occasion demands, pressing engagement when the youngster appears comfortable enough to tolerate it and providing comfort in response to exacerbations of anxiety.

Establishing Motivation

The initial contact with the adolescent patient must begin to establish his motivation for psychotherapy or at least for indicated return visits. The motivation necessary for the adolescent patient to participate profitably in psychotherapy differs from what is usually requisite for adults. Whereas the adult patient needs at least consciously to endorse a course of psychotherapy addressed to his difficulties, such expressed motivation rarely occurs in adolescents and is largely unnecessary to their successful treatment. Just as the adolescent seldom seeks treatment voluntarily, he cannot be expected to embrace it warmly when it is offered to him. He is either unaware of his psychological difficulties or too embarrassed, frightened, or counterdependent to ask directly for help with them.

Thus the adolescent will not initially be saying that he has enjoyed this chance to discuss his problems with someone and thinks that further talks would prove helpful, nor is he likely to report that he has been considering the idea of psychotherapy and would definitely like to arrange for regular visits. At best, given a reasonably well-handled first interview in which the therapist has been able to achieve a good blend of patient comfort and engagement, the adolescent patient will respond to the idea of returning with such comments as "I don't mind," "Today wasn't so bad—I suppose I could come another time," "Sure, if you think it will do any good," or "I don't see much purpose in it, but if you can put up with me, I guess I can take you."

Each of these apparently noncommittal, lukewarm comments represents for the adolescent a very significant endorsement of the therapist as a potentially helping person and of talking as a potentially helpful means of resolving difficulty. To expect any more than this from most adolescent patients is unrealistic, and to view such remarks as reflecting insufficient motivation for psychotherapy is to misunderstand the adolescent's style of approaching treatment, even when he feels strong need for it. By and large the only expression of motivation necessary to initiating the treatment is the adolescent's stated willingness to return for further talk with the therapist.

Comments expressing willingness to return should be elicited from the adolescent patient during the first interview. Sometime near the end of the session, preferably after some channels of communication have been established, the therapist needs to ask the youngster something like "What thoughts did you have about coming in to talk with me today?" Such a question gives the patient a chance to air his preconceptions, apprehensions, or hopes in coming for the session, if these have not already come up for discussion, and to contrast what the experience has been like with what he thought, feared, or wished it would be. From this material the therapist can identify and correct as necessary any misconceptions the youngster may have had (e.g., "You thought I was going to lay you out on a couch and let you do all the talking, but as you see we've just been sitting here by the desk and talking back and forth"; "You expected me to lecture you about doing what your parents and teachers tell you to do, but I think you realize now that I'm interested in hearing your side of the story and seeing what could help to make things better for you").

The therapist can then proceed with a question like "How would you feel about coming in again and talking further as we have today?" This inquiry into the youngster's feelings about returning is essential for establishing the necessary spirit of mutual participation in the therapeutic venture. To tell the youngster, "I'm going to give you an appointment to come in again next week" or, worse yet, merely to instruct his waiting parent to bring him for a return visit, seriously frays his dignity and integrity as a blossoming adult. Even for the 12- or 13-year-old, to be treated with such disregard for the self-sufficiency and independence he is proudly nourishing often convinces him that neither therapy nor therapist has much potential for meeting his needs.

While recognizing the crucial importance of the adolescent's participant responsibility for planning and implementing his treatment, the therapist must allow for the teenager's usual difficulty in acknowledging responsibility for his problems or admitting any need for help. Should he defer to the therapist's judgment about a return visit ("If you think I should"), the therapist will often do well to spare him from having to present a specific request for therapy: "Yes, I think we should talk again; we've already seen today that there are some things going on that you haven't quite understood, and I think it would be helpful to look at the situation some more"; or "I realize you haven't felt anything was wrong with you, but things certainly haven't been going as well for you as you like; maybe by talking further we could get some ideas about how to improve the situation"; or "You don't have to think it's a great idea or that you really need it; if you're willing to go along with the idea of coming in again I think we could talk about some things that might be helpful to you."

Even while he is directly and emphatically encouraging a return visit, however, the therapist must be sure to involve the youngster in the eventual decision to do so. To become an engaged participant who will eventually assume his full responsibility in the treatment the youngster needs to be able to say words to the effect of "I guess you've got a point, so *I* wouldn't mind coming back" or "If you think there's some reason for it, *I'm* willing to come again." The therapist should not be satisfied with responses that refer the decision entirely to someone else. To the youngster who says, "I'll come back if *you* say so," the therapist's reply must communicate, "Not because I say so; I'm saying that it would be a good idea and that I want to see you again, but whether you do or not is up to *you.*"

The therapist should likewise challenge any decision about return visits that is referred to the parents. Near the end of a comfortable but not yet engaged first interview with a 14-year-old boy the following interchange took place when he was asked his feelings about a return visit:

PATIENT: It's up to you and my folks.
THERAPIST: You've left yourself out.
PATIENT: That's the way it is. If you think I should come, my folks will send me.
THERAPIST: What if you don't want to come but I think you should?
PATIENT: I'll come; my folks would make me. (They'd make you?) Yes. (You wouldn't have any choice?) No. (You wouldn't have any control over the situation?) No.
THERAPIST: I wonder if there aren't times you get angry when you don't have any control or say in things?

[This question was followed by the patient's first significant affective engagement in the interview and his subsequent participation in deciding to return.]

BUILDING THE RELATIONSHIP

If the therapist has initiated the treatment with adequate attention to matters of comfort, engagement, and motivation, he will already have laid the foundations for an effective treatment relationship. From this point the further building of the relationship seldom proceeds in terms of well-defined, sequential therapeutic tasks. Josselyn (1957, p. 17) comments in this regard that, "the versatility required in the therapist . . . makes it extremely difficult to define in any orthodox way the therapeutic procedure," and Hendrickson, Holmes, and Waggoner (1959, p. 528) observe that "the best way to 'build a relationship' with an adolescent is to avoid scrupulously any self-conscious effort to do so." Yet the therapist can keep in mind that the therapeutic impact of the treatment relationship he builds with his teenage patient will usually depend on how well he is able (a) to maintain the flow of communication with him, (b) to foster the patient's positive identification with him, and (c) to regulate his inevitable concern about the implications of the treatment relationship for his independence.

Maintaining the Flow of Communication

With few exceptions the therapist must take major responsibility for maintaining the flow of communication with his adolescent patients throughout the course of their treatment. His main technique for maintaining a productive level of interchange with teenage youngsters will be an active and direct approach to talking with them. Although the importance of therapist flexibility limits the generalities that can be made about effective communication with the adolescent patient, some guidelines for actively and directly maintaining the flow of communication with adolescents can be specified.

Activity. The therapist needs to utilize a rapid cadence in his conversation with the adolescent, avoiding long latencies and studied musings as he formulates his responses, and to keep on talking until the youngster is ready and able to respond. The purposeful silences, pregnant pauses, and noncommittal responses that are often productive in the psychotherapy of adults serve little purpose with the adolescent, to whom they often connote a therapist's disinterest, inattention, or inability to find something relevant to say.

Although most adolescents require a considerable level of therapist activity, the therapist needs also to recognize those who find it oppressive or disconcerting and respond better to a slower pace. The low-keyed youngster or one who feels particularly subjugated and put upon by adults may communicate more easily if the therapist gives him some breathing space:

> Sally, a 16-year-old ideationally oriented youngster, appeared anxious, blocked, and disorganized during an initial interview in which the therapist utilized a rapid-cadence approach. Concerned about possible incipient schizophrenia, he decided to conduct the second interview in a relatively unstructured fashion to determine what extent of

disordered thinking or bizarre fantasy might emerge if he did not act to suppress it. Unexpectedly, in the unstructured setting Sally was relaxed, reflective, and able with little encouragement to present an orderly review of her major needs and concerns. The therapist's earlier activity had apparently been too dissonant with her personality style for her to respond comfortably.

At other times it may be necessary for the therapist to inject some nonverbal activity into the treatment session in order to repair a break in communication. Some otherwise responsive youngsters periodically become reluctant to go further into matters they have been discussing. Faced with silences that appear to reflect such resistances to content the therapist may at times do well not to interpret or probe the resistance, but rather to comment, "You don't seem to feel much like talking today, so what would you like to do?" If the youngster makes a response like "I've been learning to play chess—you wouldn't happen to have a chess set here would you?" or "My favorite hobby is drawing, that's what I really like to do most," then the therapist may be able to utilize the interaction around a chess board or his patient's art work to reopen channels of communication. Although such activity therapy has something in common with play therapy, its effectiveness is not limited to early adolescents. Schaeffer (1962) describes successful utilization of selected activities with 14- to 16-year-old school-phobic, underachieving, and delinquent youngsters who had verbalized a desire for help but had reached a conversational plateau attributable to resistance to the material.

Directness. To be direct as well as active the therapist needs to state his thoughts explicitly, phrase his questions concretely, and respond fully to requests that he explain the basis of his impressions and inquiries. Such directness and willingness to explain himself are essential to maintaining communication with the adolescent patient. The partial interpretations, veiled allusions, and nondirective probes ("What ideas do you have about why I asked you that?") that are useful with adult patients are frequently perceived by the adolescent as subterfuge or mystification.

Yet therapist directness should not be allowed to spare the youngster his share of responsibility in the treatment work. Particularly at points of obvious superficial resistance the types of partial interpretation and nondirection that the therapist would otherwise avoid will usually prove more incisive than complete and unambiguous statements. For example, in working with a youngster whose infantile attachments to his mother have stunted his emotional growth the therapist may several times have said, "It sounds to me like your mother's views about things are always more important to you than your own." Should the youngster then revert to discussing a situation from his mother's point of view, after this directly made interpretation has been worked through and integrated, the therapist may ellipticallly comment, "You're talking mother-talk again," and leave it to the patient to reconstruct the complete interpretation.

Similarly, the therapist will usually respond to "Why did you ask me that?" by indicating the considerations that led to his question (e.g., "As I recall, each time you've gone to a school dance before, you've just sort of hung around without talking to anyone, and I wondered if this last time had been any different"). But if he senses that the youngster is merely stalling or "playing dumb," then the question, "Why did you ask me that?" may call not for explication but for "You know as well as I do." In the same vein, when a youngster responds to an interpretation with "What do you mean?" it usually behooves the therapist to go over the ground again and spell out the elements of his inference. Yet there are times when the therapist has little doubt that his interpretation has incisively struck home and that superficial resistances are in play, and then his response to "What do you mean?" may well be, "Just what I said."

The therapist must also be able to recognize when it is important not to break up a flow of conversation by identifying its elements of resistance or transference:

> Andy, a surly, guarded youngster, was describing with enthusiasm and in some detail his plans to organize a rock band with Rick, a friend he had mentioned some weeks earlier. He suddenly broke off this therapeutically important and for him rare sharing of personal experience to ask, somewhat querulously, "Do you know who Rick is?" His question seemed a transparent test of whether the therapist had been sufficiently attentive and interested to remember Rick. The therapist elected not to interpret the challenge implicit in his question or to point out the underlying need for reassurance it suggested. Rather, he directly and in as much detail as had been reported to him reviewed who Rick was. Andy nodded with satisfaction and returned to his story. The therapist had prevented any intrusion on the relationship-building import of Andy's continuing with his story, and at the same time he had concretely demonstrated his interest and attention.

Fostering Positive Identification

Effective psychotherapy of the adolescent requires that the youngster identify positively with his therapist. This positive identification motivates him toward becoming a mature, successful, and sensitive adult, which he will perceive the therapist to be, and it also generates the trust and respect necessary for him to tolerate and accept the therapist's efforts to modify his attitudes and behavior. To foster such identification the therapist must be able to demonstrate his genuineness as a person, his understanding of his adolescent patient, and his liking for and interest in helping him. These parameters of therapist behavior correspond to the variables of empathic understanding, nonpossessive warmth, and therapist authenticity outlined by Truax and Carkhuff (1967, Chapters 2 and 3) as essential ingredients of effective psychotherapy.

Genuineness. The therapist presents himself to his adolescent patient as a genuine person by addressing him with the same candor, conversational tone, and affective spontaneity that he would use in talking with a casual friend, particularly with respect to his personal life and attitudes. Without going into the initimate details that he would share with his family and close friends, the therapist needs to avoid the evasive, uninformative, or interpretive style with which he might respond to an adult patient's questions about his private life; for example, if asked about a vacation trip, his best course will usually be matter-of-factly to tell the youngster where he went, what the weather was like, whether he enjoyed himself, and the like, just as he would with a casual acquaintance.

In addition to giving such facts about himself the therapist should also let his attitudes enter freely into discussions of events not directly related to the treatment. If his adolescent patient wants to know whether he is a Democrat or Republican, whether he prefers popular or classical music, or whether he likes summer sports or winter sports best, he should tell him. If there are underlying motives for such questions that need to be explored, they should be explored after the therapist has demonstrated his genuineness with a forthright response.

Even if uninvited to expess himself, the therapist should at times inject his attitudes into the discussion in order to define himself more clearly and to facilitate the youngster's identifying with him. When a youngster describes his enjoyment of a recent concert, the therapist, if he can honestly do so, should not hesitate to say "I was there too, and I agree with you that they played a nice program." Argumentative attitudes can also serve to promote the therapist's identifiability. Thus a youngster's tirade against restrictive drinking laws may give the therapist an opportunity to present his defense of the current legal drinking age. The usefulness of arguing over points of view as a means of exposing the therapist's attitudes and opening up lines of communication has been elaborated by Silber (1962) and by Holmes (1964, pp. 109–117), who also observes that the adolescent works best in therapy in response to a conversational style that would appear to an adult to be one of "abnormal candor":

"The therapist reveals much of his personality for two general reasons: (1) he can't hide it from the adolescent anyway and (2) there is no good reason to try to hide it even if it were possible. The adolescent is able to tell too much about us even when it is our intention to tell him nothing at all. Our efforts to operate as emotional technicians of some sort are transparent to him; they only increase his embarrassment and uneasiness in a situation that is already strained at best" (p. 103).

Thus the therapist's conversational tone needs to be as free of artificiality and restraint as he can make it. Most youngsters will not develop a strong positive identification with a therapist whose general way of thinking and feeling about things is unclear to them, and they will quickly spot as artificial a reserved therapist's efforts to be more open and spontaneous than is comfortable for him. For the therapist who tends to be open and spontaneous in his interpersonal relationships, therefore, fostering positive identification means just being himself. For the therapist who is by nature reticent or circumspect and does not readily convey to other people a clear idea of what he is like as a person, work with adolescents may not be the area of greatest competence or comfort:

"The easy display of feelings, the ingenuity often needed to make therapy interesting enough to be continued. the shift from dramatization to interpretation, from support to demand, from humor to surprise, these shifting attitudes, always scrutinized by their therapeutic intent, are not qualities which every therapist possesses nor can acquire" (Blos, 1953, pp. 238–239).

Concerning his display of feelings, the therapist must be able to let his affects come spontaneously into play. If something the youngster says strikes him as funny, he should laugh. If it was meant to be funny, he and his patient will have shared a genuine personal interaction. If the youngster does not see the humor in his remark, the therapist's spontaneous reaction can be used to expand his awareness of how he is perceived by others: "I can see that you meant what you said to be serious, but something about the way you said it made me laugh; the same thing must happen to you with other people, and maybe we can learn something from this about how you affect them that way without meaning to."

Similarly, if the adolescent is trying to make a joke of a serious situation, the therapist's spontaneous impatience or disapproval can be the first step in helping him to consider the extent to which his behavior in the situation was inappropriate or self-defeating. To a youngster who laughingly describes how disruptive behavior got him ejected from a classroom the therapist might respond, "I don't see anything funny in that, and I don't think you really do either; all you got from it is your teacher mad at you, and if any of the kids were laughing, they were laughing at you and not with you, and that's not what you're after."

Obviously the therapist has to exercise judgment concerning the extent of his spontaneity. When he senses a degree of distress that calls more for comfort than for challenge, he should refrain from laughing at a seriously made remark or from scowling at a jocular one. He must furthermore be sufficiently in tune with his patient to recognize occasions when motives underlying a remark call for interpretation rather than affect; for example, the boy who tells a scatological joke has something on his mind other than being amusing, and the therapist needs to respond not with laughter but perplexity at why the youngster has brought him a dirty story. Is he testing the therapist's knowledge of pornographic vernacular, is he looking for shock value or trying to assess the extent of the therapist's willingness to like him and to work with him, or does he perhaps have some disturbing sexual thoughts on his mind that he would like to approach?

Similarly, in listening to a girl tearfully describe reversals in her peer-group and family relationships that gravely concern him about the extent of her disturbance and capacity to be helped, the therapist needs to conceal his affective response. He will not help his patient by expressing his concern about her and his real sadness at sensing his inability to help her realize a comfortable and rewarding adult life. Rather, he needs to acknowledge her distress and to attempt as best he can to support her: "I know things are difficult for you, but let's see what we can do to help."

Understanding. The therapist demonstrates his understanding of his adolescent patient by his capacity to appreciate the youngster's feelings and to recognize his underlying thoughts and attitudes. To empathize with his adolescent patients the therapist must first of all be thoroughly familiar with the psychology of adolescence. He must be sensitive to teen-age vicissitudes of physical growth, making and losing friends, reaching out for the opposite sex, wresting self-determination from parents, and struggling for academic, athletic, social, and other successes, and he must quickly recognize the possible role of such concerns in the life events his adolescent patient describes to him. For example, when a 15-year-old boy complains of fatigue and says that it takes him hours to fall asleep at night, the therapist needs to appreciate and explore the significant likelihood that masturbatory impulses or sexual fantasies are contributing to the problem.

The therapist also needs to be conversant with whatever transient values, heroes, fads, and figures of speech are currently dominanting the adolescent scene. To draw a blank when his patient refers to a popular rock group or to being "up tight" stamps the therapist as out of tune with what's happening. The therapist cannot be expected to know everything and may in fact achieve therapeutic gain by expressing interest in learning from his adolescent patient: "That expression is a new one on me" or

"I really don't know much about how the dances are run at your school—can you fill me in?" On the other hand, constant unfamiliarity with what the youngster is talking about and repeated requests that he translate his parlance into the King's English will raise major doubts in the patient's mind about whether his therapist is capable of understanding and helping him.

In addition to his knowledge of adolescent psychology and teenage life the therapist's ability to communicate understanding to his adolescent patient will finally depend on the extent of his basic intuitive capacity. Intuitive capacity, the sensitivity of one person to the inner life of another, cannot be learned from didactic instruction or supervised experience as can personality dynamics and therapeutic techniques. Intuition is something the therapist will bring to his professional work to the extent that his personality style and developmental experiences have made him an intuitive person.

Personal psychotherapy and an openness to reviewing his own adolescence in the light of his classroom and clinical learning may enhance a therapist's sensitivity to his adolescent patient's experiences. Yet as a function of their own basic personality, most therapists remain intuitive to differing degrees with different kinds of patients. Some find themselves more fully intuitive with children and others with adults, some more with women and others with men, and some more with intellectually oriented patients than those with repressive defensive styles, and the effectiveness of their therapeutic work will reflect these differences. Thus some therapists will be more therapeutically empathic with teenage youngsters than others, perhaps, as Schonfeld (1967) suggests, in relation to how well they have resolved their own adolescent conflicts, and some who do well with certain kinds of youngsters will have limited success with others; for example, Gitelson (1948) reports that he has successfully treated intellectualizing and inhibited youngsters but failed with rebellious and delinquent types, whereas some of his colleagues have had the reverse experience.

Liking and Interest. The therapist proves his liking for his adolescent patients primarily through his sincere and unflagging dedication to helping them overcome their difficulties and feel better. It is essential that the adolescent perceive his therapist as respecting and valuing him as a person, especially at times when the therapist overtly disapproves of his behavior. Such positive regard cannot be communicated directly; it is no more natural for the therapist to say, "I like you" to his adolescent patient than to a casual friend, and the youngster will quickly recognize the artificiality of such comments. Even specific questions concerning the therapist's attitudes ("Do you really like me?") cannot be taken at face value without risking ungenuineness. The youngster who asks such a question has some purpose other than eliciting protestations of undying affection, and the therapist needs to respond either by exploration ("Why do you ask me that?") or, if he already has some understanding of the youngster's behavior, by affirming the indirect evidence of his positive regard: "If I didn't want to talk to you, I'd say so; you've had these problems that are giving you a hard time, and I want to help you get a better handle on them, and I'm ready to keep working at it as long as you are."

Holmes (1964, p. 16) has similarly stressed that the therapist who feels compelled to say, "I like you" to his adolescent patient "will have to work a long time to get the hook out of his mouth." Holmes points out that the teenage patient is fully aware that it would be much easier for the therapist not to have to bother with him at all and that the troubled adolescent will accordingly infer affectionate concern primarily from the therapist's determined efforts to persist in trying to help him (pp. 21, 207).

At times very simple actions above and beyond the call of duty add immeasurably to a youngster's feelings of being liked by his therapist. The therapist may suggest some reference sources to a youngster who is having difficulty in collecting material for a composition, or he may call a youngster who has missed a session because of illness to ask how he is feeling and whether there are any matters he would like to discuss over the telephone. Such concrete expressions of therapist interest, beyond what the youngster may have expected, will usually help to cement the treatment relationship. These and similar direct interventions, which are also discussed by Berryman (1960) and Gitelson (1942), demonstrate the therapist's interest in his patient far more emphatically than any explicit declaration.

Regulating Independence

Finally the therapist needs carefully to regulate the adolescent's concerns about his independence. Most teenage youngsters are simultaneously pressing for independence and yearning for the dependent gratifications of childhood. In their relationships with adults they seek to be treated as self-sufficient equals, but also to be advised, guided, and protected when they are confronting difficulties that are beyond their capacity to understand and resolve. To meet both needs in his adolescent patients the therapist must avoid as much as possible making them feel either that they are being babied or that they are being left entirely to their own devices.

Beckett (1965, p. 105) observes in this regard that the adolescent's wish for maturity and adult privileges motivates him to deny any dependence on adults whom he does not fully trust to respect him; hence a treatment relationship cannot really develop until the therapist has amply proved his regard for the youngsters dignity, integrity, and worth. Easson (1967) notes that the adolescent who cannot surrender any of his independence to the therapist may remain in therapy without ever formally beginning it, thus becoming a "continued nonpatient." And Josselyn (1952, pp. 76–77) has pointed out that, because of the importance of both freedom and guidance in work with adolescents, the therapist needs to strike a treatment relationship balance that allows the needed freedom while assuring that the youngster will accept guidance and restrictions.

Such a balance of dependence-independence must govern all phases of the adolescent's treatment. In the beginning the therapist acknowledges the adolescent's dignity and capacity for self-sufficiency by including him in the decision to embark on psychotherapy (see p. 360). At the same time he presents himself as someone who can be depended on to be available at regularly scheduled times or as otherwise necessary to listen and comment with interest and understanding. From this balanced beginning the therapist must continue to display respect for the patient's point of view and to carefully refrain from patronizing him or belittling his attitudes and pursuits. He needs also to be initially cautious about the extent to which he gives advice or offers definitive pronouncements, either of which can imply that the youngster is unable to think for himself.

In time, as the youngster comes to appreciate the therapist's regard for his prerogatives and independent capacities, advice and guidance may constructively meet his unspoken needs to rely on an interested, understanding adult who is more experienced than he in the ways of the world. To the extent that the therapist has given the impression of being a knowledgeable, clear-thinking, successful person, the youngster will be able to accept his guidance without necessarily having to think of himself as being inadequate for doing so.

In this vein Easson (1966) has observed that adolescents can often work through dependency conflicts with their parents by making an ego-ideal figure of the therapist; that is, the therapist's personification of personal adequacy makes it possible for the youngster to incorporate ideas and values from him without feeling that he is being infantilized in the process. Leventhal and Sills (1963), while focusing on the importance of patient autonomy and responsibility in the psychotherapy of adolescents, similarly encourage therapists to create an image of themselves as strong, experienced, unwavering, nonavoidant, and wise: "The more impressive the therapist is, the more likely it is that his statements will have effect and tend to be assimilated by the patient" (p. 157).

TERMINATION

The termination of psychotherapy with the adolescent patient becomes appropriate when he has achieved the limited insights and adaptive character synthesis that define the goals of psychotherapeutic work with teenage youngsters (see pp. 353–354). Because of the disturbed adolescent's relative freedom from crystallized psychopathology and his usual capacity for rapid behavior change, this termination point can often be reached in the course of brief or short-term psychotherapy. Adatto (1958), Goolishian (1962), and others have demonstrated that effective psychotherapy of the adolescent does not necessarily require intensive working through of insights or a thorough exploration of transference feelings but is likely to have occurred when the youngster has achieved sufficient relief from his anxieties and symptoms to settle down comfortably in his daily routine. Laufer (1964b) in fact suggests that to recommend extensive treatment beyond such a point may unnecessarily frighten a youngster with the specter of serious mental derangement.

The precise length of "brief" or "short-term" psychotherapy cannot be readily specified. Perez-Reyes and Lansing (1967) comment on the psychotherapeutic effectiveness of the diagnostic process alone with some young people, Bieliauskas (1968) notes largely successful outcomes in the treatment of college students seen eight times or less, and Miller (1959) describes the adequate short-term treatment of disturbed adolescents in 3 to 30 sessions. The concept of brief psychotherapy needs to be defined not so much in terms of a specific treatment length, but rather according to whatever period of time is necessary to achieve the circumscribed goals of the therapy.

However, in applying the goals of limited insight and character synthesis to decisions about terminating the psychotherapy of the adolescent, the therapist should not be too quick to capitalize on improvement. The price of prematurely terminated treatment is frequently a rapid recrudescence of the difficulties that prompted it. The therapist should thus take care to avoid treatment that is too brief or superficial to buffer the youngster against recurrent psychological disturbance. Masterson (1958, 1967), endorsing the notion that the adolescent patient will become ready for termination of treatment as his anxiety diminishes and he feels more control, similarly warns therapists not to be satisfied with symptomatic improvement in their adolescent patients when they can still identify distinct possibilities of subsequently impaired adjustment (1967, p. 162).

In deciding when an adolescent's psychotherapy is approaching termination the therapist must evaluate not only the extent of enduring behavior change but also the nature of the treatment relationship. Most important in this respect is the state of the youngster's dependence on the therapist. The more he appears no longer to need the therapist's regular presence in his life and the more he appears to resent continued treatment as an affront to his capacity for independence, the closer he is to a point at which termination is indicated. Conversely, the greater the youngster's apparent need to continue the relationship, the more cautiously the therapist should weigh broaching the idea of termination, no matter how great the youngster's symptomatic improvement and seeming resilience to subsequent emotional crises.

The adolescent patient whose increased self-awareness and enhanced coping capacity might justify termination will usually reveal in numerous ways his covert feelings about continuing the relationship. The therapist needs only to listen carefully and utilize appropriate opportunities to test the status of the relationship. The youngster who says, "I feel like I've been doing pretty well, and I wonder if I couldn't stop coming in or at least have these appointments less often," displays considerable readiness to begin the terminal phase of his treatment. The therapist's failure to consider reducing the intensity of treatment at such points may inappropriately imply the youngster's dependence on the therapist and undermine his confidence in the improvements he has made; conversely, there is often considerable therapeutic benefit in interpreting a youngster's display of self-sufficiency and social comfort as evidence of his decreased need for therapeutic contact (see Zwick, 1960).

On the other hand, the behaviorally improved youngster who still makes full and unquestioning use of the opportunity to review his activities with the therapist has probably not yet adequately replaced the treatment relationship with other interpersonal investments. Likewise the patient who asks during the session, "How much longer do I have to come here?" but at the end of the interview comments eagerly, "See you next week, right?" is probably not yet prepared to consider termination. Decreased therapeutic contact for a youngster in these circumstances is highly likely to be perceived by him as abandonment or rejection and to be followed by a depressive reaction or an exacerbation of previously remitted behavior difficulties.

Opportunities for testing the status of the relationship often arise from circumstances that interfere with the regular schedule of appointments. The therapist who must miss a session for a business trip may say to his adolescent patient, "I have to be away next Wednesday, so I won't be able to meet with you." The youngster who casually responds to this announcement with, "We'll meet again in two weeks then, huh?" is much closer to termination than the one who states, "Could I come on Tuesday or Thursday then?" If a flat statement of the therapist's impending absence does not elicit a definite response, he should pursue his patient's feelings by asking him directly, "What would you like to do?," and if this question is still too unstructured for the youngster to answer, he should specify alternative possibilities for the next visit and insist that the youngster express a preference.

While waiting for the behaviorally improved youngster himself to indicate his readiness for termination, the therapist should not overlook opportunities to suggest readiness beyond what the patient would otherwise recognize. When a youngster's treatment has been interrupted by illness, travel, or other circumstances, the therapist may be in a position to remark, "You seem to have gotten along pretty well since we met last—maybe we don't have to have our sessions as frequently as we have been." At other times he may be able directly to stimulate the youngster's thinking about such spacing of visits: "Your summer vacation is coming up in a few weeks; have you thought at all about how you'd like to work out our meetings during the summer?"

Should a youngster respond to such overtures with obvious concern or disappointment, it is usually important for the therapist promptly to reendorse the current treatment arrangement. Above all, it is necessary for him to prevent feelings of being abandoned or rejected from confounding the patient's perception of his suggesting less frequent meetings. The message implicit in the therapist's approach to termination needs to be, "I'm willing to stick with you as long as it's necessary and helpful, but it's starting to appear that you can just about handle things for yourself." Termination, in other words, must connote praise and reward, not criticism and rejection.

As indicated in the above examples, in the adolescent patient termination can usually be approached best through a plan of decreasing the frequency of interviews. Often a process of gradually halving the frequency of sessions works well in allowing the patient to test his capacity for independent functioning without feelings that all bridges to the therapist have been burned behind him. The therapist can make clear his readiness to revert to the original frequency of visits if it should become necessary, and at the same time he can utilize continued good functioning at one interval to suggest still longer ones and eventually no further appointments at all. Even at the point of arranging not to schedule a return visit the therapist should indicate that he is no further than a phone call away if the youngster should need him or even just want to let him know how things are going.

WORK WITH PARENTS

It is finally important to consider the integral role of work with the parents in the evaluation and treatment of adolescent youngsters. The particular goals and methods of approaching the adolescent's parents can be discussed in relation to the diagnostic process, treatment planning, and conduct of the psychotherapy.

The Diagnostic Process

The diagnostic evaluation of disturbed adolescents almost always requires one or more interviews with the parents. In the case of a youngster who is initially unable or unwilling to recount the difficulties that have brought him for help information obtained from the parents is essential to an adequate assessment. To begin psychotherapy without sufficient data for some tentative diagnostic formulations leaves the therapist vulnerable to numerous errors of procedure, some of which may have grave consequences. He may overlook important aspects of the patient's disturbance, such as not learning of previous suicidal threats or gestures, and fail to include appropriate precautionary measures in his therapeutic approach. Moreover his unfamiliarity with the youngster's problems, history of difficulty, family setting, and circumstances of referral may seriously compromise his efforts to allow comfort and achieve engagement.

Even when the youngster can present a detailed picture of himself and his problems, diagnostic contact with the parents is often indispensable. The therapist can usually improve his grasp of the patient's difficulties by learning the parents' view of the problem and of their youngster's impact on his environment. From talking with the parents he can also assess more fully the role of their attitudes, feelings, and personality styles in the problem. Furthermore, the parents can often help resolve important issues of differential diagnosis by providing background information that is unknown to the youngster, including the nature of his early development and any family history of disturbance.

Generally the initial diagnostic session with the parents should include *both* mother and father and should precede the first meeting with the youngster. Too often therapists underestimate the contribution of fathers to the psychological disturbances of their teenage children and are dissuaded from requiring their participation. The mother reports over the telephone that the father is only peripherally engaged with the family, the father protests the inconvenience of having to come for an appointment, and/or both parents concur that the mother by herself can provide all the necessary information. In fact; however, the mother by herself usually cannot provide all the necessary information, let alone a sample of the father's personality style. By excusing the father from the evaluation, furthermore, the therapist may be sanctioning his alienation from family affairs and from the youngster who is having psychological difficulty.

Many fathers who reluctantly agree to come for an initial interview interpret the therapist's insistence on their participation as an endorsement of their importance in the family's affairs. They are often flattered to have had their views so strongly solicited and cooperate much more fully with the diagnostic process than their original recalcitrance or their wives' statements ("Don't bother to call him—I'm sure he wouldn't be interested in talking with you") would have led the therapist to expect.

Seeing the parents first, as also recommended by Berman (1954), Fraiberg (1955), and Gallagher (1958), will give the therapist some idea of the problems that precipitated the referral before he meets with the youngster. This advance information can then guide him in probing for crucial diagnostic data and attempting to generate communication and engagement in his first meeting with the patient.

Perhaps even more importantly, the therapist can utilize an initial interview with the parents to discuss with them how to present to their youngster the idea of seeing the therapist. Even parents consciously committed to seeking professional help are often too anxious, embarrassed, or uninformed about psychotherapy to discuss arrangements for it in a direct, positive fashion. Left to their own devices, some will pick up their youngster after school and, without previous explanation, suggest "stopping by to talk with someone" on the way home. Others will tell their youngster that they have scheduled "a doctor's appointment" for him, without indicating the nature of the "doctor" or the reason for the appointment. Others will begin weeks in advance to "prepare" their teenager to see the psychotherapist, repetitively emphasizing the painlessness of the process to the point where they fill him with apprehensions and misgivings. Prepared with such deception and obfuscation, adolescents frequently bring to the first visit preconceived notions, resentments, or anxieties that hinder the therapist's efforts to communicate with and engage them.

The therapist can minimize the likelihood of such destructive preparation by suggesting to the parents some simple and straightforward methods of discussing an appointment with their youngster. Often it will suffice for them merely to mention some of their concerns about him and to suggest that it might be helpful for him to talk with a trained person who is familiar with the problems of young people. Although parents who need to sabotage treatment before it even begins will probably do so despite the therapist's efforts, preparatory guidance will help many anxious, psychologically unsophisticated parents to smooth their youngster's path to the therapist's door.

Like other aspects of therapeutic work with adolescents, however, parental participation in the diagnostic process must be handled flexibly. Generally, the younger or the less mature the adolescent and the more serious his disturbance, the more extensive will be his parents' diagnostic role.

Conversely, the parents' necessary engagement will diminish in relation to the youngster's maturity and/or psychological intactness. Such variability is reflected in the already mentioned data of Rosen et al. (1965). In their sample of youngsters seen for intake or diagnostic studies in outpatient clinics the percentage seen alone, without interviews for the parents, increased from 9.9% in the 10- to 11-year-old group to 28.7% in 16- to 17-year-olds and to 61.2% in the 18- to 19-year-olds (p. 1573).

In fact, it may be important to respect and reward the independent behavior of the late adolescent who calls for his own appointment by seeing him first. Then, to the extent the therapist feels the parents need to be involved in planning or conducting the treatment, he can discuss with the youngster his feelings about the manner in which they should be contacted. Godenne (1965) in particular has emphasized the value of allowing youngsters to express their feelings about the therapist's contact with the parents and of giving them the option of sitting in on the parents' meeting with the therapist.

Treatment Planning

In planning treatment for an adolescent patient it is essential that the therapist obtain the cooperation and support of his parents. Peltz (1957) and others have pointed out the difficulties of many parents in accepting a recommendation that their youngster receive psychotherapy, even when they have been sufficiently concerned and psychologically oriented to bring him for a diagnostic evaluation. For many parents a treatment recommendation connotes failure on their part to rear their child properly; for others it generates grave anxiety about their youngster's future; and for some it represents embarrassment, humiliation, and inconvenience imposed on them by the therapist. The anxiety, guilt, humiliation, and anger that are often evoked by a recommendation for treatment can motivate parents to deny or resist needed treatment unless the therapist can discuss their feelings with them and help them to understand and endorse the treatment that is to follow.

Two primary patterns of parental resistance, each of which can vitiate his efforts to help his adolescent patient, demand the therapist's careful attention. The first is a readily observable, overt refractoriness in which the parents express skepticism about psychological methods or their youngster's needs for professional help, or, having acceded to a treatment agreement, manage in numerous ways to prevent their child from fulfilling it. They repeatedly find themselves unable to bring him for appointments, eagerly reinforce his slightest expression of reluctance to come, and regularly report how beautifully he is behaving. Such parental ploys are usually attempts to deny the youngster's difficulties by proving that he can get along without professional assistance. The therapist must be able to help the parents resolve the anger, anxiety, or guilt that motivates these obvious resistances if he is to have much hope of initiating psychotherapy with their youngster.

The second and more subtle pattern of parental resistance is the so-called dumping syndrome. The "dumping" parents defend themselves against the implications of a recommendation for treatment by surrendering their youngster to the ministrations of the therapist, to whom they give *carte blanche,* and retreating in graceless haste to the bleachers. As far as they are concerned they have been good and dutiful parents, their youngster's problems are of his own making, and they will support his treatment responsibly without becoming involved in it. Such parents pose few overt problems for the therapist. They endorse his treatment recommendation, guarantee the youngster's regular and prompt attendance at sessions, and seldom intrude on the therapy with questions about method or progress.

Although the dumping syndrome may seem to give the therapist a free hand, it usually subverts his treatment efforts in several insidious ways. First, if the therapist allows his adolescent patient to be dumped, he permits a situation that will confirm the youngster's impressions of his parents' disinterest in him and will probably increase his alienation from his family. Second, parents who wash their hands of their youngster's treatment may nevertheless remain furious with him for the inconvenience and embarrassment his psychotherapy causes them, and they are as likely as openly resistive parents to seek subtle means of forcing its premature end. Although the dumping syndrome is most likely to be pronounced when the parents physically deposit their youngster for treatment in an inpatient setting, as observed at the Menninger Foundation by Miller (1958), it can also occur in outpatient psychotherapy unless the therapist's treatment planning prevents the parents from closeting themselves at a distance.

Conducting the Psychotherapy

Clinicians who urge ongoing psychotherapy with the parents of children in treatment generally agree that adolescents, particularly those who are not seriously disturbed, can be effectively treated without concomitant psychotherapy for the parents (e.g., Szurek, Johnson, and Falstein, 1942; Johnson and Fishback, 1944). Nevertheless ongoing psychotherapy of adolescent youngsters usually requires some continued contact with the parents to allow the therapist to keep informed about daily events in the family's life, to monitor the parents' perception of, and allegiance to, the treatment goals, and to anticipate and counter parental actions that might undermine the therapy. Particularly at points where changes in the youngster's behavior alter the family equilibrium or tax the parents' understanding of how to cope with him, preparation and guidance from the therapist can minimize their anxiety and their likelihood of reacting to it by sabotaging the treatment. Green (1964), Josselyn (1957), and others have elaborated on these benefits of continued contact with the parents.

There are several alternative modes of engaging parents in the conduct of their adolescent youngster's treatment. In deciding which to pursue the therapist needs first to evaluate the parents' needs and interest in receiving psychological help for themselves. Some parents utilize the occasion of their youngster's referral to report concerns of their own for which they would like to receive professional assistance. For such parents a course of psychotherapy independent of their youngster's treatment, provided by a different therapist, is often indicated. Hellman (1964) suggests from experiences at the Hempstead Clinic that ongoing treatment for the parents should be conducted not only by a different therapist but at a different place from where the youngster is being seen. If the therapist should recommend independent therapy for the parents of his adolescent patient, he will then have to arrange sufficient channels of communication with the other therapist to achieve the information, monitoring, and anticipatory goals of parental contact noted above.

At other times the therapist may sense that parents who would otherwise not require psychological help are so confused and distressed by their youngster's difficulties that they could benefit from continued discussion of their relationship to him and his problems. Here too a recommendation for independent treatment may be in order. Helfat (1967) points out that parents who have unwittingly complicated their youngster's development by their unfamiliarity with the needs and concerns of adolescents often lack opportunities to air their apprehensions and uncertainties and receive helpful counsel in return. She describes a discussion group for parents of adolescents in psychotherapy in which the parents reported noticeable lessening of tension and greater tolerance of adolescent behavior in themselves over the course of a dozen or fewer sessions.

Some parents express little interest in treatment for themselves and give no indication that they might profit from an opportunity to explore their feelings about themselves or their youngster. In such instances the therapist should usually refrain from suggesting independent psychotherapy for them. Not only is the suggestion likely to be rejected but it may also harden the parents' resistances to the point where treatment for the youngster becomes impracticable. Parents who present no psychological concerns of their own and hold their youngster to be primarily responsible for his difficulties are often unresponsive to a recommendation that they receive psychotherapy. The implications of parental blame and the burdens of time and expense that attend such a recommendation may raise their level of anxiety or anger to a point where they question the therapist's competence or reject the whole idea of treatment for their youngster.

With parents of this type the therapist should usually arrange a supportive relationship in which he focuses on the problems of the patient and on information, monitoring, and anticipatory functions without probing the parents' personal difficulties. This supportive role can usually be managed best by the youngster's therapist himself. Although concerns are sometimes raised about the deleterious effects on the treatment of the therapist's conferring with the patient's parents, the advantages of this procedure usually outweigh any problems it may create.

Parents who do not consider themselves as being in psychotherapy, and indeed are not, find it very awkward and artificial to be told that they must speak with someone other than their youngster's therapist to discuss his progress. The wastefulness of this procedure is highlighted when they ask questions about their youngster that their interviewer cannot answer because his communication with the therapist is imperfect, or when for the same reasons the therapist does not receive information he seeks because the parents' interviewer failed to obtain it from them.

Furthermore, as already noted, there is no reason why a meeting with the parents need exclude the adolescent patient. Kaplan (1967) suggests that the therapist periodically ask the parents to join their youngster for a family session. This procedure allows the necessary parent-therapist interaction without implying to the youngster that he is not mature enough to sit with the grown-ups, that things need to be said about him that he would not like to hear, or that the therapist's allegiance to him is secondary to his responsibility to the parents. It can also allow the therapist to assess patterns of family interaction at regular intervals and to utilize techniques of family treatment that appear indicated.

As in the diagnostic and planning phases of psychotherapy, the extent of parental involvement in the ongoing psychotherapy will vary with the extent of disturbance and maturity of the youngster. The less serious his difficulties and the more closely the adolescent is approaching adulthood, the less frequently his parents will be seen and the more his treatment will be his responsibility. The data of Rosen et al. (1965, p. 1573) indicate that well over 90% of the parents of 10- to 13-year-old youngsters treated in outpatient clinics are also seen for interviews, whereas almost 30 and 62% of 16- to 17- and 18- to 19-year-old patients, respectively, are treated without collateral interviews for the parents. During the course of psychotherapy, furthermore, behavioral improvement will indicate reduced contact with the parents just as it suggests decreasing the frequency of the youngster's sessions. In all of these judgments the therapist must be guided by whatever means he feels will stimulate, nourish, reward, and maximize the adolescent youngster's progress toward maturity.

REFERENCES

Ackerman, N. W. *Treating the Troubled Family.* New York: Basic Books, 1966.

Adatto, C. P. Ego reintegration observed in analysis of late adolescents. *International Journal of Psychoanalysis,* **39**:172–177, 1958.

Axelrod, P. L., Cameron, M. S., and Solomon, J. C. An experiment in group therapy with shy adolescent girls. *American Journal of Orthopsychiatry,* **14**:616–627, 1944.

Balser, B. H. A new recognition of adolescents. *American Journal of Psychiatry,* **122**:1281–1282, 1966.

Beckett, P. G. S. *Adolescents out of Step: Their Treatment in a Psychiatric Hospital.* Detroit: Wayne State University Press, 1965.

Berman, S. Psychotherapeutic techniques with adolescents. *American Journal of Orthopsychiatry,* **24**:238–245, 1954.

Berman, S. Psychotherapy of adolescents at clinic level. In B. H. Balser, ed., *Psychotherapy of the Adolescent.* New York: International Universities Press, 1957, pp. 86–112.

Berryman, E. The treatment of adolescents: Effecting the transference. *American Journal of Psychotherapy,* **14**:338–345, 1960.

Beskind, H. Psychiatric inpatient treatment of adolescents: A review of clinical experience. *Comprehensive Psychiatry,* **3**:354–369, 1962.

Bieliauskas, V. J. Short-term psychotherapy with college students: Prevention and cure. *Confinia Psychiatrica,* **11**:18–33, 1968.

Blaine, G. R. Therapy. In G. R. Blaine and C. C. McArthur, eds., *Emotional Problems of the Student.* New York: Appleton-Century-Crofts, 1961, pp. 232–248.

Blos, P. The contribution of psychoanalysis to the treatment of adolescents. In M. Heiman, ed., *Psychoanalysis and Social Work.* New York: International Universities Press, 1953, pp. 210–241.

Braiman, A. Therapeutic uses of the university. *Journal of the American College Health Association,* **16**:60–68, 1967.

Clements, B. E. Transitional adolescents, anxiety, and group counseling. *Personnel and Guidance Journal,* **45**:67–71, 1966.

Easson, W. M. The ego-ideal in the treatment of children and adolescents. *Archives of General Psychiatry,* **15**:288–292, 1966.

Easson, W. M. The continued nonpatient. *Archives of General Psychiatry,* **16**:359–363, 1967.

Farnsworth, D. L. *Psychiatry, Education, and the Young Adult.* Springfield, Ill.: Thomas, 1966.

Fraiberg, S. H. Some considerations in the introduction to therapy in puberty. *Psychoanalytic Study of the Child,* **10**:264–286, 1955.

Freud, A. Adolescence. *Psychoanalytic Study of the Child,* **13**:255–278, 1958.

Gallagher, J. R. Problems of the adolescent. *Pediatric Clinics of North America,* **5**:775–787, 1958.

Gallagher, J. R., and Harris, H. I. *Emotional Problems of Adolescents,* revised edition. New York: Oxford University Press, 1964.

Geleerd, E. R. Some aspects of psychoanalytic technique in adolescence. *Psychoanalytic Study of the Child,* **12**:263–283, 1957.

Gitelson, M. Direct psychotherapy in adolescence. *American Journal of Orthopsychiatry,* **12**:1–25, 1942.

Gitelson, M. Character synthesis: The psychotherapeutic problem of adolescence. *American Journal of Orthopsychiatry,* **18**:422–431, 1948.

Godenne, G. D. Outpatient adolescent group therapy. *American Journal of Psychotherapy,* **18**:584–593, 1964.

Godenne, G. D. A psychiatrist's techniques in treating adolescents. *Children,* **12**:136–139, 1965.

Goolishian, H. A. Family treatment approaches: II. A brief psychotherapy program for disturbed adolescents. *American Journal of Orthopsychiatry,* **32**:142–148, 1962.

Greaves, D. C., and Regan, P. F. Psychotherapy of adolescents at intensive hospital treatment level. In B. H. Balser, ed., *Psychotherapy of the Adolescent.* New York: International Universities Press, 1957, pp. 130–143.

Green, S. L. Psychotherapy with adolescent girls. *American Journal of Psychotherapy,* **18**:393–404, 1964.

Harris, H. I., and Heald, F. P. Psychotherapy of adolescents by pediatrician and psychiatrist at combined clinic and inpatient hospital level. In B. H. Balser, ed., *Psychotherapy of the Adolescent.* New York: International Universities Press, 1957, pp. 113–129.

Helfat, L. Parents of adolescents need help too. *New York State Journal of Medicine,* **67**:2764–2768, 1967.

Hellman. I. Observations on adolescents in psycho-analytic treatment. *British Journal of Psychiatry,* **110**:406–410, 1964.

Hendrickson, W. J., Holmes, D. J., and Waggoner, R. W. Psychotherapy of the hospitalized adolescent. *American Journal of Psychiatry,* **116**:527–532, 1959.

Holmes, D. J. *The Adolescent in Psychotherapy.* Boston: Little, Brown, 1964.

Johnson, A. M., and Fishback, D. Analysis of a disturbed adolescent girl and collaborative psychiatric treatment of the mother. *American Journal of Orthopsychiatry,* **14**:195–203, 1944.

Josselyn, I. M. *The Adolescent and His World.* New York: Family Service Association of America, 1952.

Josselyn, I. M. Psychotherapy of adolescents at the level of private practice. In B. H. Balser, ed., *Psychotherapy of the Adolescent.* New York: International Universities Press, 1957, pp. 13–38.

Kaplan, A. H. Problems of psychotherapy with the adolescent. In M. Hammer and A. M. Kaplan, eds., *The Practice of Psychotherapy with Children.* Homewood, Ill.: Dorsey, 1967, pp. 255–289.

Kimbro, E. L., Taschman, H. A., Wylie, H. W., and MacLennan, B. W. A multiple family group approach to some problems of adolescence. *International Journal of Group Psychotherapy,* **17**:18–24, 1967.

Kolvin, I. "Aversive imagery" treatment in adolescents. *Behaviour Research and Therapy,* **5**:245–248, 1967.

Laufer, M. Ego ideal and pseudo ego ideal in adolescence. *Psychoanalytic Study of the Child,* **19**:196–221, 1964a.

Laufer, M. A psycho-analytic approach to work with adolescents. *Journal of Child Psychology and Psychiatry,* **5**:217–230, 1964b.

Leventhal, T., and Sills, M. R. The issue of control in therapy with character problem adolescents. *Psychiatry,* **26**:149–167, 1963.

Lorand, S. Treatment of adolescents. In S. Lorand and H. I. Schneer, eds., *Adolescents: Psychoanalytic Approach to Problems and Therapy.* New York: Hoeber, 1961, pp. 238–250.

McGregor, R., Ritchie, A. M., Serrano, A. C., and Schuster, F. P. *Multiple Impact Therapy with Families.* New York: McGraw-Hill, 1964.

MacLennan, B. W., and Felsenfeld, N. *Group Counseling and Psychotherapy with Adolescents.* New York: Columbia University Press, 1968.

Martin, F. Technical problems in the treatment of adolescents: Beginning psychotherapy. *Journal of Child Psychology and Psychiatry,* **4**:109–124, 1963.

Masterson, J. F. Psychotherapy of the adolescent: A comparison with psychotherapy of the adult. *Journal of Nervous and Mental Disease,* **127**:511–517, 1958.

Masterson, J. F. *The Psychiatric Dilemma of Adolescence.* Boston: Little, Brown, 1967.

Miller, D. H. Family interaction in the therapy of adolescent patients. *Psychiatry,* **21**:277–284, 1958.

Miller, L. C. Short-term therapy with adolescents. *American Journal of Orthopsychiatry,* **29**:772–779, 1959.

Nichols, W. C., and Rutledge, A. L. Psychotherapy with teen-agers. *Journal of Marriage and the Family,* **27**:166–170, 1965.

Outpatient Psychiatric Clinics: Annual Statistical Report. Washington, D.C.: U.S. Department of Health, Education, and Welfare, Public Health Service Publication No. 1854, 1966.

Peltz, W. W. Psychotherapy of adolescents at private practice plus school practice level. In B. H. Balser, ed., *Psychotherapy of the Adolescent.* New York: International Universities Press, 1957, pp. 39–66.

Perez-Reyes, M., and Lansing, C. The diagnostic evaluation process: A follow-up of 49 children studied in an outpatient clinic. *Archives of General Psychialtry,* **16**:609–620, 1967.

Robinson, J. F. Psychotherapy of adolescents at school plus inpatient treatment level. In B. H. Balser, ed., *Psychotherapy of the Adolescent.* New York: International Universities Press, 1957, pp. 67–85.

Rosen, B. M., Bahn, A. K., Shellow, R., and Bower, E. M. Adolescent patients served in outpatient psychiatric clinics. *American Journal of Public Health,* **55:**1563–1577, 1965.

Schaeffer, R. L. Treatment of the adolescent. 3. An approach to therapy with the adolescent through selected activities. *American Journal of Orthopsychiatry,* **32:**390–394, 1962.

Schonfeld, W. A. Adolescent psychiatry. *Archives of General Psychiatry,* **16:**713–719, 1967.

Schwitzgebel, R. L. Short-term operant conditioning of adolescent offenders on socially relevant variables. *Journal of Abnormal Psychology,* **72:**134–142, 1967.

Silber, E. The analyst's participation in the treatment of an adolescent. *Psychiatry,* **25:**160–169, 1962.

Slavson, S. R. Para-analytic group psychotherapy. A treatment of choice for adolescents. *Psychotherapy and Psychosomatics,* **13:**321–331, 1965.

Szurek, S. A., Johnson, A. M., and Falstein, E. I. Collaborative psychiatric treatment of parent-child problems. *American Journal of Orthopsychiatry,* **12:**511–516, 1942.

Truax, C. B., and Carkhuff, R. R. *Toward Effective Counseling and Psychotherapy: Training and Practice.* Chicago: Aldine, 1967.

Weiner, I. B. Behavior therapy in obsessive-compulsive neurosis: Treatment of an adolescent boy. *Psychotherapy: Theory, Research, and Practice,* **4:**27–29, 1967.

Wittenberg, R. On the superego in adolescence. *Psychoanalytic Review,* **42:**271–279, 1955.

Zwick, P. A. Gauging dosage and distance in psychotherapy with adolescents. *American Journal of Orthopsychiatry,* **30:**645–647, 1960.

Author Index

Subject Index

Academic underachievement, and fear of failure, 269-272
and fear of success, 272-274
and sexual identity, 258
as specific aversions to learning, 263-264
definition of, 245-246
organic determinants of, 247-255; case illustration of, 253-255; treatment of, 278-279
psychological determinants of, 260-277; case illustration of, 276-277; treatment of, 280-283
role of hostility in, 265-269; case illustrations of, 267-268
role of immaturity in, 260-262
role of motivation in, 255-259
role of opportunity in, 259-260
role of other psychopathology in, 262-263
role of passive-aggressive personality in, 90, 264-277
role of rivalry in, 269-274; case illustrations of, 271-272
sex differences in, 249, 275
sociocultural determinants of, 255-260; case illustrations of, 279-280
Acting out, 88, 114-116, 164-165
see also Delinquent behavior; Psychopathic personality; Sociopathic personality
Acute schizophrenia, 105-107, 109-110, 126
Acute school phobia, 208-211
case illustrations of, 219-225
Adaptive decompensation syndrome, 189
Adaptive delinquency, 292-294
Adjustment reaction of adolescence, 87
see also Adolescent turmoil; Transient situational personality disorder
Adolescent turmoil, and diagnostic classification, 77-78, 80-81
as a myth, 24-25, 30-33, 50-54, 66-68
as deviant adjustment, 55-62

as normal development, 22, 41-42
psychoanalytic views of, 21-23, 41-42
Affective integration, 99
Alienation, 184
Antisocial personality, 314
see also Delinquent behavior; Psychopathic personality; Sociopathic personality
Anxiety reaction, 91, 203
and academic underachievement, 262
incidence of, 82
Apathy, 99, 162, 166-167

Behavior modification, 236-237, 351
Bellevue Hospital, 83, 104, 107, 147, 181
Bender-Gestalt, 253
Bethlem Royal Hospital, 139
Boston Children's Hospital, 350

California Growth Studies, 3, 14
California Personality Inventory, 58, 62
Cambridge-Somerville Youth Study, 290
Case illustrations, of acute school phobia, 219-225
of characterological delinquency, 319-320
of chronic school phobia, 225-232
of delinquency as a neurotic symptom, 302-305
of depression, 171-176
of epilepsy and delinquent behavior, 325-326
of organically-determined underachievement, 253-255
of passive-aggressive underachievement, 276-277
of psychologically-determined underachievement, 267-268, 271-272
of schizophrenia, 132-138
of sexual delinquency, 305-306, 311-312
of suicidal behavior, 185-186, 192-195